MOTIVATIONAL PRACTICE
PROMOTING HEALTHY HABITS AND
SELF-CARE OF CHRONIC DISEASES

Richard J. Botelho, B.Med.Sci., B.M., B.S., M.R.C.G.P. (UK)
Professor of Family Medicine and Nursing,
University of Rochester School of Medicine and Dentistry
Rochester, New York

Contributing Author (Chapters 1, 6 and 7)
Harvey Skinner, Ph.D.
Chair and Professor of Public Health Sciences
Department of Public Health Sciences
Toronto, Ontario

MHH Publications

Richard J. Botelho
University of Rochester School of Medicine and Dentistry
Rochester, New York 14620 USA

© 2002, 2004 by Richard J. Botelho

First edition published 2002
(Beyond Advice: 1.Becoming a Motivational Practitioner and 2.Developing Motivational Skills.)
Second edition 2004.
(This edition appears as a new title and is based on the above book series.)
Printed in the United States of America

Visit www.MotivateHealthyHabits.com to obtain contact information and
- *Learn more and get more support from a newsletter*
- *Listen to audio or watch videos*
- *Inquire about training programs, online courses and consultations*
- *Learn about the books for practitioners and lay health coaches*

Permission to Reproduce

Table 7.3
Guilford Press has given permission to adapt a table from W. R. Miller and S. Rollnick (1991), *Motivational Interviewing: Preparing People to Change Addictive Behavior.* New York: Guilford Press.

Table 7.4
Cambridge University Press has given permission to adapt a table from the chapter "Types of Self-Efficacy in Addictive Behavior" from G. A. Marlatt, J. S. Baer and L. A. Quigley, *Self-efficacy and Addictive Behavior.* In A. Bandura (ed.), *Self-efficacy in a Changing Society* (1995): Cambridge University Press.

Table 16.5
Carfax Publishing Company has given permission to adapt the Fagerström Test from T. F. Heatherton, L. T. Kozlowski, R. D. Frecker, et al. "The Fagerström Test for Nicotine Dependence: A Revision of the Fagerström Tolerance Questionnaire." *British Journal of Addiction* (1991); 86(9): 1119-1127.

To Eve, Anna and Sara with love

CONTENTS

List of Tables..xi
List of Figures xii
List of Learning Exercises...xii
Preface... 1
Acknowledgments... 1
Foreword 1: How to Motivate Healthy Behaviors 2
Foreword 2: How to Motivate Healthy Learning... 5
Introduction 9
What Is Motivational Practice? 10
An Overview of What You Could Learn 12
How to Use this Book 13
An Ecological Perspective 14

Section I. Consider Changing Yourself before Helping Others................... 17

1   When Giving Health Information and Advice Doesn't Work 18
Limitations of Giving Information and Advice.. 19
Limitations of the Best Evidence 21
Adopting New Metaphors 22
The Need for a Complementary Approach 23
Limitations of the Fix-it Role... 24
Motivating Change... 25
Consider Changing Yourself 27
Continuing Professional Development.. 34
Your Summary 35

2   Contrasting the Fix-it and Motivational Roles................................... 41
Clinical Example.. 42
Your Summary 48

3   Adapting Your Role to Patients' Needs 50
Role Characteristics... 52
Role Functions... 56
Role Boundaries 58
Role Outcomes 59
Your Choice about Roles 60
Your Summary 61

4   Becoming Aware of Assumptions 64
Range of Assumptions 65
Your Summary 70

Section II. Understanding Individual Change 73

5   **Forces of Change** 74
     The Forces of Change Model 75
     Leverage Points and Effort.. 76
     Supports and Barriers to Change (System Vectors)....................... 78
     Your Summary 82

6   **Understanding Resistance** 86
     Understanding Patient Resistance 88
     Evoking Patient Resistance 93
     How Do Patients Resist Change? 93
     Go with Resistance 94
     Your Summary 95

7   **Understanding Motivation** 97
     Concepts, Models, Theories and Clinical Approaches 98
     Likelihood-of-Action Index 105
     Your Summary 106

8   **Overview of the Six-step Approach** 109
     Six Steps 110
     The Ladder of Change 111
     A Practical Application 113
     Your Summary 116

Section III. Helping Patients Change: A Six-step Approach 119

9   **Step 1: Building Partnerships** 120
     Part A. Developing Empathy... .. 121
         Empathic Skills 122
         Your Summary 126
     Part B. Using Relational Strategies... .. 127
         Relationship Map 128
         Relational Strategies... .. 133
         Using Relational Strategies Creatively 135
         Using Role Choices Creatively 136
         Your Summary 136
     Part C. Clarifying Roles and Responsibilities............................. .. 139
         Your Patients' Confidence and Ability (Self-Efficacy) 141
         Your Patients' Motives.. .. 141
         Your Patients' Autonomy.. .. 142
         Your Use of Authority, Influence and Control 142
         Balance of Responsibilities Between You and Your Patients 146
         Your Summary 148

10   Step 2: Negotiating an Agenda **150**
    Clarifying Agendas 151
    Two Agendas 152
    Toward a Shared Agenda 154
    Your Summary 160

11   Step 3: Assessing Resistance and Motivation **162**
    Disease-centered Assessment... ..163
    Motivational Assessment 164
    Your Summary 181

12   Step 4: Enhancing Mutual Understanding **183**
    Working with Your Differences.. ..184
    Four Essential Skills 187
    Your Summary 198

13   Step 5: Implementing a Plan for Change **200**
    Evaluate Commitment Toward a Plan for Change.................. ..201
    Decide about Goals for Change 202
    Work toward Solutions 205
    Your Summary 207

14   Step 6: Following Through **209**
    Rationale, Purpose and Reasons for Follow-up 210
    Timing, Duration and Frequency of Follow-up Appointments..... ..210
    Methods to Ensure Change and Prevent Relapse................... ..211
    Your Summary 212

Section IV. Specific Behaviors **215**

15   Excessive Alcohol Use **216**
    Part A. Key Facts about Excessive Alcohol Use 217
        Specific Issues 218
        Your Summary 224

    Part B.   Reducing Alcohol Risk and Harm 229
        Step 1: Building Partnerships.. ..230
        Step 2: Negotiating an Agenda.. ..231
        Step 3: Assessing Resistance and Motivation 236
        Step 4: Enhancing Mutual Understanding 242
        Step 5: Implementing a Plan for Change 251
        Step 6: Following Through 257
        Your Summary 260

16   Tobacco Use 263

    Part A. Key Facts about Tobacco Use 264

        Specific Issues 267

        Your Summary 273

    Part B. Helping Resistant Smokers Quit 279

        Step 1: Building Partnerships 280

        Step 2: Negotiating an Agenda 281

        Step 3: Assessing Resistance and Motivation 282

        Step 4: Enhancing Mutual Understanding 287

        Step 5: Implementing a Plan for Change 292

        Step 6: Following Through 295

        Your Summary 297

17   Facilitating Self-care of Diabetes 300

        Step 1: Building Partnerships 302

        Step 2: Negotiating an Agenda 303

        Step 3: Assessing Resistance and Motivation 305

        Step 4: Enhancing Mutual Understanding 307

        Step 5: Implementing a Plan for Change 311

        Step 6: Following Through 313

        Your Summary 314

Afterword 316

        Bail-out Strategies 316

Appendices

    Worksheets for Skills Development

        Partnership-Building 318

        Agenda-Setting 319

        Assessment 320

        Developing Mutual Understanding 321

        Implementing a Plan 322

        Following Through 323

Tables

1.1. Comparing Medical and Behavioral Worldviews and Value Systems 22
1.2. Contrasting Assumptions about Patients 25
1.3. Motivational Principles 26
1.4. Six-step Approach for Negotiating Change 32
3.1. Spectrum of Role Characteristics 56
3.2. Contrasting Role Functions, Boundaries and Outcomes 59
3.3. Comparing the Fix-it and Motivational Roles 60
4.1. Reflecting about Your Assumptions 68
4.2. Patient's Perspective: Stumbling-block v. Facilitating Assumptions 69
4.3. Family's Perspectives 70
5.1. Factors Affecting the Forces of Change 77
6.1. Triggers for Patient Resistance 93
6.2. Signs of Patient Resistance 93
7.1. Stages of Change Model 101
7.2. The Pros and Cons of Change 102
7.3. Strategies for Motivation Enhancement 103
7.4. Determinants of Relapse 104
7.5. Likelihood-of-action Index 105
9.1. Separate and Shared Responsibilities for Addressing Behavior Change 147
9.2. Separate and Shared Responsibilities for Addressing Medical Complications 147
11.1. Motivational Assessment 166
11.2. Lifestyle Benefits 168
11.3. Emotional Benefits 168
11.4. Interpersonal Benefits 169
11.5. Coping Benefits 169
11.6. Social Benefits 170
11.7. Spiritual Benefits 170
11.8. Decision Balance 175
12.1. Approaches to Providing Education and Advice 188
12.2. Nondirect Interventions 190
12.3. Direct Interventions 192
12.4. Perceptions about Self-efficacy 196
15.1. Low-risk Drinking Recommendations 220
15.2. *DSM-IV* and *ICD-10* Definitions of Abuse (Harmful Use) 220
15.3. Definitions of Abuse and Dependence 221
15.4. Differences in Perspective about At-risk and Problem Drinking 222
15.5 Using the Likelihood Scale to Educate Patients about Their Alcohol Use 223
15.6. Enhancing Mutual Understanding about At-risk and Problem Drinking 224
15.7. CAGE Questionnaire 232
15.8. AUDIT Questionnaire 233
15.9. Five-shot Questionnaire 234
15.10. Performance of Screening Tests in General Practice 234
15.11. Comparing Specialist and Generalist Assessments 236
15.12. Self-evaluation for Alcohol Problems 241
15.13. Self-evaluation for Alcohol Dependence 241

15.14. Goals for Change: Hazardous and Harmful Use of Alcohol 252
16.1. Impact of Screening System for Tobacco Users in Health Care Settings 266
16.2. Impact of Clinical Interventions on Tobacco Abstinence Rates 266
16.3. Impact of Different Methods on Tobacco Abstinence Rates 267
16.4. Impact of Behavioral Methods on Tobacco Abstinence Rates 267
16.5. Fagerström Test 268
16.6. Impact of Pharmacotherapy on Tobacco Abstinence Rates 269

Figures

3.1. Factors Affecting Our Roles and Assumptions 54
3.2. Coalition against the Patient 56
3.3. Alliance with the Patient 57
5.1. Forces of Change Model 75
6.1. Benefits Continuum 91
6.2. Behavioral Risk Continuum 92
6.3. Readiness for Change Continuum 92
7.1. Self-determination Theory 101
8.1. The Ladder of Change 112
9.1. Relationship Map for Developing Effective Partnerships 129
11.1. Contrasting Disease-centered and Motivational Assessments 165
11.2. An Inverted Hierarchy of Benefits 167
12.1. Enhancing Mutual Understanding 184

Learning Exercises

1.1. Assess your overall health behaviors and life issues 29
1.2. Reflect about Mrs. S.'s decision balance 32
3.1. Anchor your learning 51
4.1. Think about a challenging patient 65
4.2. Reflect about your assumptions 67
6.1. Think of a resistant patient 88
9.1. Role clarification 140
9.2: Addressing hopelessness/helplessness 146
9.3: Unclear responsibilities 147
10.1: Review a videotape 151
10.2: Unaware patient 156
10.3: Minimizing patient 157
10.4: Nonadherent patient 158
11.1: Imagine you are a patient with a risk behavior 170
11.2: Compare concerns about staying the same 172
11.3: Compare concerns about changing 173
11.4: Compare benefits of changing 173
15.1: Drug substitute request 173
15.1: Responding to the patient's request for sleeping tablets 254

PREFACE

I am a British-trained general practitioner who has been teaching academic family medicine in the United States for over 20 years. During the past 10 years, I have done research and development in process improvement work on health behavior change. This work is part of my never-ending journey of learning how to change practitioner and patient behavior, with the goal of promoting healthy habits and self-care of chronic diseases. I hope that this book will expand my network of colleagues who share a passion for advancing and integrating this marginalized field into mainstream health care.

Students and practitioners can use this book to learn when and how to change from the advice-giving (fix-it) role to a motivational role. To assist them with this process, I have synthesized evidence, experience and wisdom from multiple sources—patients, students, colleagues, health care practitioners and expert educators, as well as integrated pragmatic approaches from selected theories, models and concepts together with research evidence from different disciplines. These eclectic resources are organized within a six-step, problem-solving approach to provide some coherence to a complex field. This clinical framework can assist practitioners with initiating the lifelong learning process of enhancing their ability to engage patients in change dialogues.

However, the magnitude of unhealthy behaviors in the general population is far too big for the health care system alone to treat everyone. Mutual aid and self-help (MASH) approaches are needed. I have also written a MASH guidebook, *Motivate Healthy Habits: Stepping Stones to Lasting Change,* to assist your patients with self-directed change (with or) without your professional assistance. This book taps into the most important yet underutilized resources: families and friends working on health behavior change in a grassroots manner.

In Foreword 1 of this book, Dr. Ian McWhinney describes the importance of learning about the therapeutic value of dialogue in helping patients change. In Foreword 2, Dr. Kirsti Lonka describes the introspective process of "higher learning" with respect to the personal and professional context of motivating behavior change.

ACKNOWLEDGMENTS
I would like to thank Ceil Goldman and Barbara Coster for their editorial support, Steve Marcus for his secretarial support, Hilliard Jason and Jane Westberg for their educational expertise, and my patients, students and professional colleagues, who contributed in countless different ways over many years.

FOREWORD 1
How to Motivate Healthy Behaviors

The information and advice we convey to our patients is often ineffective. A knowledge of risk factors alone seldom dissuades people from smoking, excessive alcohol consumption, overeating, high-risk sexual behavior or substance abuse. Knowledge itself does not change behavior. Type 2 diabetes, for example, is increasing in many Western countries, driven by epidemic obesity and physical inactivity. Yet in clinical trials, lifestyle changes (exercise, diet and weight reduction) in people with impaired glucose tolerance can reduce the incidence of type 2 diabetes by 50-66%.[1]

Why is it so difficult to apply our knowledge? The guidelines are available and quite straightforward. If results can be obtained in the tightly controlled world of the randomized trial, why can they not also be obtained in the world outside? It is tempting to blame primary care physicians, their patients or both. But let us at least consider that the way medicine is being practiced and taught is part of the problem. We practice a medicine based on the metaphor of the body as machine. Our logic is of linear, unidirectional causal chains, and our notion of therapy is a technology of control. The mechanistic approach to medicine extends not only to treatment but also to behavior modification based on control, reinforcement, conditioning and social engineering—an approach that overlooks human decision-making and autonomy. Not surprisingly, this approach has significant limitations when it comes to promoting healthy behavior and the self-care of chronic disease.

Most guidelines are the product of linear logic. Problems arise when linear logic meets complexity in the form of patients with their thoughts, beliefs, assumptions, expectations, emotions and relationships. This complexity is the reality of medical practice, and Rick Botelho's motivational approach is designed to deal with this reality. His groundbreaking book springs from advances in psychology and moves beyond the linear logic of control and behavior modification.

The sciences of complexity and organization provide a context for understanding the nonlinear process of change for both practitioners and patients. The work also challenges the simplistic notion of a unidirectional translation of research into practice, thus transcending the research-practice divide. This book liberates practitioners from the constraints of evidence-based guidelines without ignoring the guidelines' significant contributions.

We cannot continue to think only in terms of single causes, single-point interventions and predictable outcomes. When linear logic meets the nonlinear logic of complexity, meanings must also be considered. As Dr. Botelho says, giving advice (the "fix-it" role) is not enough. Patients have to be engaged where they live. It is not easy to change oneself: there have to be good reasons, and the motivation to change has to come from the heart as well as the head. We are all—practitioners and patients—very good at self-deception, at finding reasons (rationalizations) for avoiding change.

For practitioners educated in the fix-it role, adopting a motivational role requires a major shift from "doing" to "being" with patients. As Dr. Botelho so rightly says, going through behavior change ourselves can help us to empathize with patients facing similar changes. The self-knowledge that comes from reflection on experience can help us to sense the appropriate role for us to adopt for a particular patient at a particular time. In adopting the motivational role, we acknowledge that, for all of us, change has to come from within. We cannot enforce change in our patients, but we can, with their agreement, help them to work through the process, clarifying their thoughts and expectations, identifying sources of resistance, pointing out inconsistencies and correcting misconceptions.

We are fortunate in having a body of knowledge on motivation and behavioral change from other disciplines, and Dr. Botelho makes very good use of this knowledge. There are skills here that can be learned, and the format of the book helps by being that of a workbook. A step-by-step approach takes the reader through the process of motivational practice, using many case examples, strategies and exercises. This book lends itself to being studied alongside clinical practice. I visualize the reflective practitioner changing gradually as he or she goes from patient to book and back to patient, until mastery is achieved, the knowledge and skills internalized and a lasting transformation accomplished.

The book has great relevance for the patient-centered clinical method, recently conceived and developed as a successor to the method that has dominated modern medicine.[2] The previous method laid its greatest emphasis on diagnosis, as exemplified by the clinical-pathological conference. A clinician is presented with a case report and develops a differential diagnosis, which is then confirmed or otherwise by the pathologist. The injunction given to clinicians is "Either make a physical diagnosis or exclude organic pathology." With its predictive and inferential power based on organic pathology, the method has great strength. On the other hand, it makes the tacit assumption that therapy follows naturally from diagnosis. Although such is often the case, the method has little to say about the complexities of management or about the many situations in which no conventional diagnosis is appropriate. For many people, their health status is the outcome of many interrelated, complex factors, including economic, social, cultural, educational and attitudinal issues that intersect with their biological condition.

The patient-centered clinical method is designed to deal with complexity. Like the previous method, it gives clinicians a number of injunctions.[3] "Ascertain the patient's expectations" recognizes the importance of knowing why the patient has come.

"Understand and respond to the patient's feelings" acknowledges the crucial importance of the emotions. "Make or exclude a clinical diagnosis" recognizes the continuing power of correct classification. "Listen to the patient's story" recognizes the importance of narrative and context. "Seek common ground" enjoins the physician to mobilize the patient's own powers of healing. Seeking common ground is the key to therapeutic success: the method requires it but does not indicate the skills required to achieve it. With this book, Rick Botelho has fulfilled this purpose.

Pedro Lain Entralgo,[4] one of the foremost scholars of the history of clinical method, has reminded us that a part of the Hippocratic tradition was a "therapy of the word," whereby the physician tried to influence the patient to take the measures necessary to recover from his or her illness. The therapy called for all the physician's skill in rhetoric. Far from being an exercise in coercion, this was based on the skill of helping the patient to see what was in his or her own interest. Rhetoric at one time was regarded as one of the foremost and most difficult arts, worthy of its place in a classical education and in the curriculum of the medieval university, before the term and its meaning became debased in our own time. Dr. Botelho is teaching us a new therapy of the word.

I. R. McWhinney, O.C., M.D., F.R.C.G.P, F.C.F.P, F.R.C.P
Professor Emeritus
Department of Family Medicine
The University of Western Ontario
London, Ontario, Canada

REFERENCES

1. Pinkney J. Prevention and cure of type 2 diabetes. British Medical Journal 2002;325: 232-233
2. Stewart M, Brown JB, Weston WW, et al. Patient-centered medicine: Transforming the clinical method. Thousand Oaks, CA: Sage Publications; 1995
3. McWhinney IR. Textbook of family medicine, 2nd ed. New York: Oxford University Press; 1997
4. Entralgo P. The therapy of the word in classical antiquity. New Haven, CT: Yale University Press. 1961

FOREWORD 2
How to Motivate Healthy Learning

Knowledge about the best evidence does not necessarily change our professional behavior.[1;2] Even when we use evidence-based interventions (such as providing information and advice), our patients do not necessarily change their behaviors. Most of us are not well educated in how to motivate patients who resist these interventions.

The process of developing motivational skills involves higher learning about ourselves and our patients. It involves reflecting about assumptions, perceptions, mental maps (ways of thinking), and exploring our feelings and differences in values. To initiate this process of continuing professional development (CPD), you can use this book and the accompanying guidebook (described below) to address personal and professional changes that underpin the lifelong learning process of enhancing motivational skills.

- *Personal change.* Learn how to change yourself before helping others. The mutual aid and self-help guidebook *Motivate Healthy Habits: Stepping Stones to Lasting Change* invites you to change one of your own health behaviors. This book guides you through an experiential process of learning about change concepts that you can then use to help others.

- *Professional change.* Learn how to change your professional role from being a fix-it health adviser to being a motivational practitioner. This book describes a six-step approach that can help you to transform your professional role and to develop the art of dialogue with patients.

This process of higher learning prepares you to address the challenges and complexities of change when collaborating with your patients to create shared learning opportunities. Let me clarify how these books use two strategies synergistically in groundbreaking ways that epitomize what higher learning is all about.

Strategy 1. Use introspective journaling as part of your learning portfolio

In this information overload age, continuing professional education predominantly focuses on keeping up-to-date with the latest scientific discoveries. The major focus is on providing content. The self or the inner experience of the individual learner is at risk of drowning in a sea of overwhelming content. The neglect of self dehumanizes learners and places them at high risk of professional burnout, thereby losing the heart and soul of caring. Increasing considerations are given to our professional and personal growth.[3;4] We also need to develop process skills to help patients learn how to improve their health.[5]

This book integrates improvement cycles as part of the journaling process for creating your learning portfolio (a compilation of personal evidence about your ongoing professional development).[6-8] Each chapter offers you the opportunity to write a brief summary about what learning was new for you and how this new learning will change what you do. These assignments encourage you to find your personal voice by writing in the first person (I) rather than in the third person (he, she or it).

Research shows that writing is a powerful tool for this kind of higher learning.[9] However, introspective journaling goes against traditional education in health care, and students and practitioners are reluctant to engage in such a learning opportunity. And yet, it is one of the most potent ways of enhancing their continuing professional development.

Strategy 2. This book inverts the traditional hierarchy of learning
European researchers have developed a hierarchy of learning categories, ranging from superficial to deep.[10-12] A reformulation of these categories, as they relate to behavior change, is as follows:

- *Passive.* Learners remember new facts and information from external sources
- *Active.* Learners acquire knowledge from external sources and reformulate the information in a personalized way
- *Applied.* Learners acquire knowledge, principles and ideas for a practical purpose, such as solving problems
- *Meaningful.* Learners discover new perspectives and ideas to understand the complexity underlying the change process
- *Interpretative.* Learners reflect about and change their attitudes and views through the process of reconstructing their mental maps

As lifelong learners, we can continually refine our mental maps to deepen our understanding about the complexities of our clinical work, including the change process. The transformation from a novice to an expert on behavior change involves a continuous improvement process[13-15] as well as the development of emotional awareness when working with patients.[3;5] Such a learning process can enhance our capacities to help our patients find their own motives to sustain constructive behavior change.

A deeper level of learning has been added to the categories described above: *personal and professional change.*[16] Ideally, we should undergo deep change as the consequence of engaging in any significant learning process. The self-awareness process that is encouraged in this book series involves reflecting about ourselves and our patients in ways that can enable us to work with them most effectively.[4;5]

This orientation and approach are what I find particularly appealing about Dr. Botelho's work. These books incorporate the principles of modern learning theories. The CPD process used in these books begins with self-focused change, both in your personal and your professional life. Then you learn a method to expand your range of skills as a motivational coach. To work in patient-centered ways, you can use your expanded range of skills to understand better your patients' thoughts, feelings, perceptions and values and to develop an individualized process of engaging patients in the change process over time.

This "process" textbook is an invaluable resource. After reading this book, you can refer back to appropriate sections when you get stuck while working with a patient. Section IV provides key content and specific suggestions for initiating dialogues with patients about tobacco cessation, alcohol risk and harm reduction and self-care of chronic diseases, as illustrative examples, but this process can be expanded to any unhealthy behavior. You will probably find that it works best to use this book as part of an ongoing learning process, using improvement cycles (see Introduction) repeatedly over time by incorporating specific suggestions into your practice. The book can also help you initiate a learning portfolio, so that you can gather evidence about the impact of this learning process on your CPD and your work with patients.

I had the pleasure of participating in one of Dr. Botelho's workshops. I have seldom observed how the application of educational principles and methods fits so well with modern learning theories. (View the videotape used in this workshop at www.MotivateHealthyHabits.com.) He is also developing online courses based on his books, so that professional bodies and educational institutions can develop formal curricula to address this major deficiency in professional education. Ideally, students and practitioners need longitudinal curricula and continuing professional development opportunities to become better motivational coaches. This increases the chances for us to develop a learning organization, where professionals create a shared vision about patient care.[17]

This book on motivational practice captures what higher learning is all about: the cognitive, emotional, perceptual and ethical aspects of personal change. Health care professionals of the 21st century can use this book and the guidebook to assist themselves and their patients in the change process. Dr. Botelho's work gives us all hope that it is truly possible to make modern learning theories work in action, for both practitioners and patients.

Kirsti Lonka, Ph.D.,
Professor of Medical Education
Karolinska Institute, Stockholm, Sweden

REFERENCES

1. Davis DA, Thomson MA, Oxman AD, et al. Changing physician performance. A systematic review of the effect of continuing medical education strategies. Journal of the American Medical Association 1995;274: 700-705

2. Davis D, Evans M, Jadad A, et al. The case for knowledge translation: Shortening the journey from evidence to effect. British Medical Journal 2003;327: 33-35

3. Hager P, Gonczi A. What is competence? Medical Teacher 1996;18: 15-18

4. Schon DA. Educating the reflective practitioner. Toward a new design for teaching and learning in the professions. San Francisco: Jossey-Bass Publishers; 1987

5. Makoul G. The interplay between education and research about patient-provider communication. Patient Education and Counseling 2003;50: 79-84

6. Lonka K, Slotte V, Halttunen M, et al. Portfolios as a learning tool in obstetrics and gynaecology undergraduate training. Medical Education 2001;35: 1125-1130

7. Parbooshingh J. Learning portfolios: Potential to assist health professionals with self-directed learning. The Journal of Continuing Education 1996;16: 75-81

8. Snadden D, Thomas M. The use of portfolio learning in medical education. Medical Teacher 1998;20: 192-199

9. Tynjala P, Mason L, Lonka K. Writing as a learning tool: Integrating theory and practice. Studies in Writing, Vol. 7. Dordreth, The Netherlands: Kluwer Academic Publishers; 2001

10. Entwistle N, Ramsey P. Understanding student learning. London: Croom Helm; 1983

11. Lonka K, Joram E, Bryson M. Conceptions of learning and knowledge: Does training make a difference? Contemporary Educational Psychology 1996;21: 240-260

12. Lonka K, Ahola K. Activating instructions. How to foster study and thinking skills in higher education. European Journal of Psychology of Education 1995;10: 351-368

13. Chi MTH, Glaser R, Farr MJ. The nature of expertise. Hillsdale, NJ: Erlbaum; 1988

14. Glaser R, Bassok M. Learning-theory and the study of instruction. Annual Review of Psychology 1989;40: 631-666

15. Schmidt HG, Boshuizen HPA. On acquiring expertise in medicine. Educational Psychology Review 1995;5: 205-221

16. Marton F, Dall'Alba G, Beaty E. Conceptions of learning. International Journal of Educational Research 1993;19: 277-300

17. Senge PM. The fifth discipline: The art and practice of the learning organization. New York: Doubleday; 1990

INTRODUCTION

Let's use the tobacco pandemic as the leading example of how health care systems and the scientific community underestimate the complexity of changing behavior. The tobacco pandemic will reach its peak in 20 to 30 years and kill one in eight persons worldwide (20 million to 30 million deaths per year), with 70% of these deaths occurring in the developing countries. This global threat far exceeds the negative impact of all acts of wars and terrorism, alcoholism, drug abuse and HIV disease combined. Yet, despite these shocking facts, young people are still relentlessly initiating this addictive, lifelong habit. We provide inadequate guidance to our youth in how to deal with the manipulative influences of the tobacco companies, popular media and negative peer influences.

How do tobacco marketers take this deadly product and sell it as a pleasure? They use sophisticated methods to manipulate human beliefs (e.g., smokers deceive themselves into believing that tobacco relieves their stress, when in fact nicotine addiction adds to it).

So, what is the power of the tobacco industry's emotional appeals? They exploit human vulnerability by creating positive biases toward tobacco—associating images of pleasure, sexuality and/or attractive identities with smoking and targeting this association to an individual's needs, wants, desires, vanities, aspirations and/or fantasies in an implicit and meaningful way. They hook youth on tobacco during their vulnerable stages of development. They masterfully develop dynamic approaches with new angles on positive biases to influence health beliefs and to promote smoking behaviors. They produce spectacular results in the real world, without generating any hard evidence from randomized controlled trials about how marketing actually works.

In contrast, the scientific approach in health care is based on the premise of minimizing or removing biases in research studies: in effect, taking a neutral, factual and skeptical stance, in sharp contrast to tobacco marketers. The scientific community develops hard evidence from randomized controlled trials, but this evidence does not translate into significant results at a population-based level. For example, the smoking cessation guideline that uses the five A's model (ask, advise, assist, assess and arrange follow-up) relies on practitioners providing information and advice to patients. The impact of this guideline on cessation rates varies from 2-10%, depending on the duration of the intervention. But this guideline doesn't use sophisticated emotional appeals and negative biases against tobacco use, a strategy that goes against the grain of scientific impartiality of being bias-neutral. Because the factual evidence does not support it, the guideline provides little assistance in how practitioners can

- Work with adolescent smokers
- Help smokers in precontemplation
- Motivate patients who do not respond to the five A's approach

9

Many practitioners tire of or stop using this guideline protocol in any systematic way, for a variety of legitimate reasons. What we need are new, dynamic and innovative ways of engaging all smokers in the change process, using the best available evidence and state-of-the-art practices. In particular, we can use emotional appeals and biases that marketers use for tobacco initiation and apply them in the opposite direction to help patients work on the emotional aspects of tobacco cessation. But these techniques alone are not sufficient, because tobacco cessation is far more complex than its initiation. In addition to treating nicotine addiction, we need more sophisticated behavioral interventions. One approach (based on multiple methods) can be found in motivational practice. This approach provides practitioners with a wide range of interventions to address smoking cessation and other behaviors such as

- *Risk behaviors:* excessive alcohol use, illegal drug use, obesity, unhealthy diets, lack of exercise, unsafe sex and unwanted pregnancies
- *Disease management*: nonadherence to medication and treatment recommendations, suboptimal self-care of chronic diseases and failure to attend follow-up appointments
- *Preventive measures*: immunizations, mammogram and pap smears and injury prevention

WHAT IS MOTIVATIONAL PRACTICE?

This interdisciplinary book addresses how practitioners can learn to develop individualized interventions that meet patients' changing needs over time. The clinical approach of motivational practice builds on the shoulders of these trailblazers:

- Self-efficacy theory: A. Bandura[1-4]
- Transtheoretical model of change: J. Prochaska and C. DiClemente[5-7]
- Motivational interviewing: W. Miller and S. Rollnick[8;9]
- Self-determination theory: E. Deci and R. Ryan[10]
- Relapse prevention: G. Marlatt and J.Gordon[11]
- Solution-based therapy: S. De Shazer[12-15]
- Patient-centered approaches: M. Steward and colleagues[16]

No single theory, model or clinical approach has a monopoly on clinical effectiveness in predicting positive outcomes, but clearly some clinical approaches peak in popularity, and some fade over time as the field advances. The concept of self-efficacy has shown some durability but it has limitations (as described in Chapter 7). A systematic review (www.ncchta.org/fullmono/mon624.pdf) of interventions based on the stages of change model has questioned its effectiveness in promoting behavior change. Motivational interviewing has gained stature and popularity with a supportive foundation of evidence.

(For those interested in exploring different perspectives on evidence and the concept of translational research, go to www.MotivateHealthyHabits.com to download two chapters that address these issues in more detail.)

To assist you with the limitations of current evidence, this book incorporates state-of-the art clinical practices and learning processes that involve

- Using continuous innovation, testing and evaluation of individualized interventions
- Applying motivational principles for overcoming the knowledge-behavior gap (e.g., "I know what to do but I don't do it")
- Developing the art of dialogue (nonlinear, dynamic processes) to address cognitive-emotional dissonance (e.g., "I think I should change but don't feel like it") and so-called irrational behavior
- Incorporating learning portfolios (e.g., gathering personal evidence about developing motivational skills) into your continuing professional development

Consider exploring your professional role, mental maps (ways of thinking) and assumptions before developing your motivational skills. This premise may help you learn how to work more effectively and efficiently with patients. You may even have to unlearn some of your training-of-origin perspectives so that you can expand your repertoire of skills. This process can challenge your assumptions and evoke emotional reactions, such as ambivalence or even resistance to the introspective process.

Instead of imposing a concept/model/theory-driven worldview on patients, you learn how to work from the patients' worldviews and select theories and models that fit into their worldviews rather than the other way around—making patients fit into a particular mould. This learning process can help you develop individualized interventions that activate patients to become researchers of their own behavior change and learn new ways of acting in their best interest.

Do not quench your inspiration and your imagination;
do not become the slave of your model
—Vincent Van Gogh

May this quotation inspire your creativity and sustain your enthusiasm for lifelong learning on how to help patients change.

AN OVERVIEW OF WHAT YOU COULD LEARN

Section I explores how cultural, personal and professional issues affect the change process in patients. Scientific rationality lacks sophistication in addressing human irrationality and in dealing with otherwise knowledgeable patients who lack the critical factor: motivation. Chapter 1 highlights the limitations of the rational, scientific approach in providing health information and advice to patients about changing their unhealthy behaviors, and explores key concepts, models and ideas for addressing common, everyday situations. Chapter 2 offers a case study that contrasts the advice-giving or fix-it approach with a motivational one. The aim here is to highlight the merits of adopting a motivational role. Chapter 3 explores the implications for patient change based on which role you adopt—the fix-it, preventive or motivational one. Each of these roles is defined according to its characteristics, functions and boundaries to examine how they differ in helping patients change their behavior. Chapter 4 examines how assumptions can help or hinder the change process for the patient.

Section II is an overview for understanding and facilitating individual change. Using a Forces of Change model, you learn how both individual and systems factors can generate positive and negative forces for change (Chapter 5). More specific attention is then given to understanding the individual dynamics of resistance (Chapter 6) and motivation (Chapter 7) from different perspectives. These three chapters help you become familiar with the key theories, models and concepts that have shaped the development and practical applications of the six-step approach. To prepare for using the materials in Section III, Chapter 8 is an overview of the six-step approach with an example of a practitioner-patient partnership working toward behavior change and using this approach as a mental map for thinking about how to motivate behavior change.

Section III describes in detail the six-step, interdisciplinary approach for negotiating behavior change with patients. A chapter is devoted to each of the six steps, describing micro skills that you can use for addressing a broad range of health behaviors in health promotion (e.g., physical activity), disease prevention (e.g., smoking cessation, regular mammograms), chronic disease management (e.g., diabetes) and injury prevention (e.g., the use of car safety belts). Though you will become familiar with a wide range of micro skills used in this method, you still need to learn how to use these skills in an effective, patient-centered way.

Section IV specifically addresses tobacco use, excessive alcohol intake and self-care of diabetes. Consider doing an in-depth study of a specific behavior so that you can learn how to generalize this approach to other behaviors. You can also use these chapters when you get stuck with patients to identify new ideas for interventions.

An interdisciplinary note

I use the term *practitioner* to describe all professionals who help patients to change: physicians, physician assistants, nurse practitioners, nurses, psychologists, therapists, community and public health workers, social workers and allied health professionals. All members of your health care team can benefit from learning how to become motivational practitioners and can adopt a variety of roles when working with patients. In the examples and stories in this book, I have used the abbreviations FP, PP or MP (and Dr. F., Dr. P. or Dr. M) to represent the fix-it, preventive or motivational role for practitioners (and physicians).

In the text of this book, I have used the first person (we) and second person (you) to describe the fix-it and motivational roles, respectively. As practitioners, we all assume the fix-it role, but when it is not working, you can opt for adopting a motivational role. This personal style of writing sets a tone that aims to engage you in the change process in ways that you may replicate with your patients.

HOW TO USE THIS BOOK

Motivational skills are fundamental core competencies for all health care practitioners. Yet this topic is inadequately or poorly addressed in health care education. Instead, you are left to learn on the job. This book could have a cascade of positive benefits on your continuing professional development by

- Reducing your frustration in working with so-called resistant patients
- Enjoying engaging patients in dialogues about change over time
- Developing individualized approaches to meet patients' changing needs
- Enhancing patients' readiness to change
- Improving patient outcomes

Ideally, you would use a variety of ongoing learning opportunities to enhance your motivational skills over time: self-directed learning; online group learning (see www.MotivateHealthyHabits.com); longitudinal skills-based training opportunities in small groups led by supervisors or facilitators; direct observation with simulated and actual patients with feedback and evaluation; and in-depth learning experiences working with a small number of patients on behavior change over one to two years.

You can use this book to initiate the process of creating a learning portfolio. The story about the race between the turtle and hare is an apt analogy for understanding different ways of using the book. If you race through this book (like the hare), you may only gain a superficial understanding about individualizing interventions for patient care, and that limited understanding may constrain your ability to enhance motivational skills.

On the other hand, you can use the way of the turtle: take your time in reading this book and learn more from your journey as you go along. Experiment in applying new ideas and concepts in your clinical work and learn from those experiences. Introspective journaling can further enhance your continuing professional development. This process of higher learning (as described by Dr. Lonka in Foreword 2) can help you gain an in-depth understanding about how to enhance your ability to engage patients in change dialogues. However, many practitioners are reluctant to engage in such a learning process because it takes hard work to change (just like our patients).

To assist you with this learning process, each chapter begins with a question or brief statement that helps you focus on what you can learn from reading this chapter. Case examples and learning exercises are provided throughout to help you better understand key concepts, principles, strategies and interventions for motivating change. Questions are also posed at the end of each chapter with space given for writing a summary about your new learning and its potential impact on working with your patients. This book invites you to journal your learning process about changes in yourself and in your clinical work. Consider using the PARE improvement cycle as you read (and hopefully revisit) chapters of this book over time.

- **Prepare:** Set a flexible timetable for reading these chapters that gives you time to experiment in applying new ideas and concepts in your clinical work.
- **Act:** Consider highlighting areas with a yellow marker and making notes in the margins to help you write summaries for the next phases of the learning cycle.
- **Reflect:** Write a summary (in 200 words or so) about what you learned that was new for you. Write in the first person (I) about your internal reactions to the material rather than reiterating the text of the book (it).
- **Enhance:** Write down your ideas (in 100 words or so) about how your new learning could improve what you do with your patients.

These notes will help you gather personal evidence about your continuing professional development.[17] For example, your notes may refer to changes in your mental maps, your understanding about your assumptions and roles and the potential application of new ideas, metaphors, concepts, models and theories. You can add these notes to build your learning portfolio. Whether or not you are willing to make a commitment to this journaling process, you can still assess whether you gained any of the benefits mentioned on the previous page. Whatever you decide, this learning process needs to be considered within a much larger context.

AN ECOLOGICAL PERSPECTIVE

An ecological approach to engaging and activating individuals, families, organizations, communities and systems is needed to promote healthy habits and self-care of chronic diseases at multiple levels. Such an approach integrates macro (policy), meso (organizational) and micro (individual) strategies with multimodal methods to generate synergistic collaboration among the top-down (political and administrative), side-to-side (intersectoral) and bottom-up (grassroots) processes.[18] A brief description of these strategies provides a wider context to understand the complexities of disseminating motivational practice into health care and the contributions of this book toward this overarching goal.

MACRO STRATEGIES

Changes in political vision, leadership and public policies establish national organizations to

- Shift the health care agenda and resources from an acute cure paradigm toward health promotion, disease prevention and disease management
- Enforce national and international laws and policies to reduce risk behaviors (e.g., the Framework Convention on Tobacco Control)
- Align financial incentives to quality improvement initiatives in health promotion, disease prevention and disease management
- Develop clinical information technology systems to analyze how process improves outcomes at population-based levels
- Provide data about improvements in performance at organizational and practitioner levels
- Use marketing strategies to promote the transformation from a disease-producing to a health-promoting society
- Foster the development of intersectoral approaches, community mobilization and grassroots programs

MESO STRATEGIES

Changes in public policies provide the necessary learning resources to support the continuing professional and organizational development that is needed to enhance health promotion, disease prevention and disease management programs across health care settings, schools and work sites. Such programs enable practitioners to learn how to

- Contribute toward a continuous improvement of their comprehensive programs
- Change from the fix-it, advice-giving role to the motivational role
- Enhance their motivational skills over time
- Link up with community mobilization initiatives and grassroots movements

MICRO STRATEGIES

Changes in the organizational setting, teamwork, professional roles, workflow and clinical information systems are developed to

- Use a spectrum of methods (as described at the beginning of this section) and develop individualized interventions to meet patients' changing needs.
- Use a variety of delivery methods (e.g., individual encounters, group visits, telephonic support and online learning programs)

- Encourage the general public to systematically use mutual aid and self-help (MASH) approaches to behavior change, with or without professional support

Even with ideal political leadership and public policies supporting this ecological approach, individuals ultimately determine the impact of any systematic approach. The quality and effectiveness of the individualized interventions will determine the ultimate success of any program. We cannot wait until such ideal public policies exist before learning how to motivate patients to change their unhealthy habits.

REFERENCES

1. Bandura A. Self-efficacy: The exercise of control. New York: W.H. Freeman; 1997
2. Bandura A. Self-efficacy in changing societies. New York: Cambridge University Press; 1995
3. Bandura A. Social foundations of thought and action. Englewood Cliffs, NJ: Prentice Hall; 1986
4. Bandura A. Self-efficacy: Toward a unifying theory of behavior change. Psychological Review 1977;84: 191-215
5. Prochaska JO, DiClemente CC. Toward a comprehensive model of change. In: Miller WR, Heather N, eds. Treating addictive behaviors: Processes of change. New York: Plenum Press; 1986:3-276.
6. Prochaska JO, DiClemente CC. The transtheoretical approach: Crossing traditional boundaries of therapy. Homewood, IL: Dow Jones/Irwin; 1984
7. Prochaska JO, DiClemente CC. Transtheoretical therapy: Toward a more integrative model of change. Psychotherapy Theory, Research and Practice 1982;19: 276-288
8. Miller WR, Rollnick S. Motivational interviewing: Preparing people to change addictive behavior. New York: Guilford Press; 1991
9. Miller W, Rollnick S, Conforti K. Motivational interviewing, 2nd Edition: Preparing People for Change. New York: Guilford Press; 2002
10. Deci EL, Ryan RM. Intrinsic motivation and self-determination in human behavior. New York: Plenum Press; 1985
11. Marlatt GA, Gordon JR. Determinants of relapse: Implications for the maintenance of behavior change. In: Davidson P, Davidson S, eds. Behavioral medicine: Changing health lifestyles. New York: Brunner/Mezel, Inc.; 1980:410-452
12. De Shazer S. Words were originally magic. New York: W.W. Norton & Co.; 1994
13. De Shazer S. Putting difference to work. New York: W.W. Norton & Co.; 1991
14. De Shazer S. Clues: Investigating solutions in brief therapy. New York: W.W. Norton & Co.; 1988
15. De Shazer S. Keys to solutions in brief therapy. New York: W.W. Norton & Co.; 1985
16. Stewart M, Brown JB, Weston WW, et al. Patient-centered medicine: Transforming the clinical method. Thousand Oaks, CA: Sage Publications; 1995
17. Sweeney KG, MacAuley D, Gray DP. Personal significance: the third dimension. Lancet 1998;351: 134-136
18. Noncommunicable Diseases and Mental Health, World Health Organization. Innovative care for chronic conditions: Building blocks for action. Geneva, Switzerland, World Health Organization: 2002.

SECTION I

CONSIDER CHANGING YOURSELF
BEFORE HELPING OTHERS

Chapter 1 invites you to learn about improving your own health behaviors and transforming your professional role before learning how to help patients change. A case study in Chapter 2 contrasts how a fix-it and a motivational practitioner deal with the same patient. The purpose of this example is to emphasize the advantages of a new role rather than to illustrate the limitations of the traditional role for addressing behavior change. Chapter 3 describes a conceptual framework for better understanding how you can adapt your role to meet patients' needs. Chapter 4 explores how assumptions can either hinder or facilitate the change process for patients and their families. Over time, you can discover for yourself whether this premise (change yourself before helping others) helped you become a more effective and efficient motivational practitioner.

CHAPTER 1
WHEN GIVING HEALTH INFORMATION
AND ADVICE DOESN'T WORK

FOR REFLECTION

*What do you do when patients do not change their unhealthy behaviors
in response to your health information and advice?*

OVERVIEW

When we use only a hammer (provide advice), we treat patients' unhealthy behaviors as nails. Most patients and their behaviors, however, are more like nuts and bolts rusted together. Hammering away can damage the threads of the bolt, so the nut never comes off. With advice only, patients may become more resistant and less likely to consider change.

Do you keep hammering away, give up the advice-giving approach altogether, or do you learn from your clinical experiences about how to work with patients in alternative ways?

Mere knowledge about the negative consequences of risk behaviors is insufficient to motivate most patients to change. Even when individuals know what is good for them and have the skills to change, many do not. Resistant patients work against our attempts to help them change. Unmotivated ones are indifferent to change. Ambivalent patients have mixed thoughts and feelings about change.

Thus, most patients are not ready to change their unhealthy behaviors. They may or may not even be thinking about change.[1;2] Not surprisingly, health information and advice do not help most patients to change. We need to develop skills to help our patients work on changing over time.

This book invites you to consider learning about how you change yourself as you learn how to help patients change. It encourages you to consider

- Analyzing your health behaviors, professional roles and assumptions
- Internalizing the six-step approach (described in Sections II and III) as a mental map for working with patients over time
- Initiating the process of gathering a learning portfolio for your continuing professional development
- Learning micro skills to address tobacco use and excessive alcohol intake

If you are curious about why patients do or do not change, this book may assist you on a journey of lifelong learning about motivating health behavior change.

LIMITATIONS OF GIVING INFORMATION AND ADVICE

What is the impact of giving health information and advice to patients, in relation to the overall magnitude of unhealthy behaviors and their consequences? (Section IV in this book and the Web sites listed in the tables and footnotes provide additional evidence for using such interventions.[abcd]) Such approaches are the first step in helping *patients* change their unhealthy behaviors, but they benefit only 5-20% of patients.[3-10] Let's briefly focus on the tobacco issue again, because it is the single greatest preventable contributor to disease and premature death internationally. In community surveys conducted in the

---

a. For information about smoking, alcohol, dietary practices, physical activity, cardiovascular disease, diabetes and asthma, check out the Center for the Advancement of Healthy www.cfah.org and click on Publications.

b. For evidence about preventive and behavioral health interventions, check out the Cochrane Database of Systematic Reviews and the database of abstracts of reviews of effectiveness at www.update-software.com/cochrane/abstract.htm.

c. For information about clinical prevention guidelines for smoking and related health behaviors, check out the Agency for Healthcare Research and Quality www.update-software.com/cochrane/abstract.htm.

d. For evidence and approaches for improving chronic diseases, check out the Improving Chronic Illness Care Web site at www.improvingchroniccare.org.

United States, 40% of smokers are not thinking about quitting, and 40% of smokers are thinking about it.[11-14] Giving information and advice may be appropriate for only 20% of smokers who are ready to quit. This approach helps 2.3-12.8% of smokers to quit, depending on the time length of the session, the total number of sessions and the number of different clinicians involved in delivering interventions.[3]

Consider this fact in relation to the tobacco pandemic, as described in the Introduction. The report *Trust Us: We're the Tobacco Industry* helps us to understand how the tobacco industry contributed toward creating this pandemic.[e] To counteract these disease-promoting practices, the World Health Organization's Tobacco Free Initiative (http://www.who.int/toh) and the Framework Convention on Tobacco control aim to decrease global tobacco consumption. Yet in spite of our knowledge about this problem, tobacco use will remain the leading cause of death worldwide for the foreseeable future.

Giving information and advice does not always change behavior. Furthermore, this seemingly helpful approach can have negative consequences that may or may not be apparent.[15;16] For example, increases in depression, anxiety and overall disability occurred at three months after physicians advised patients to quit smoking, but this finding was not found with medication-related or dietary change advice.[15;16] Two examples highlight this issue from a practitioner and patient perspective:

> Dr. N., a general practitioner from Nepal, was treating a patient who was a smoker and a doctor. Dr. N. advised his patient to quit smoking on three separate occasions over time. The patient got fed up with Dr. N. and decided to see another doctor, a doctor who smoked cigarettes and would not advise him to quit smoking. Dr. N. felt rejected and wished that he could have been more helpful to his patient. He was interested in learning more about how to work with smokers in alternative ways.

> Mrs. D. was an overweight middle-aged woman who had diabetes. Her overweight endocrinologist repeatedly advised her to change her eating habits, to lose weight and to exercise more. She could not live up to her doctor's expectations and had resigned herself that she would need to rely on her medications to control her diabetes. Mrs. D. had mixed feelings about continuing to see the endocrinologist because he made her feel guilty, but she also respected him and depended on him for her ongoing care. Mrs. D. resented his lack of empathy, given that he was also overweight, and wished that he was better trained in how to understand her situation.

Michael Balint once stated that doctors are the most commonly prescribed drug in general practice.[17] This drug metaphor has merit in acknowledging the psychotherapeutic impact of the doctor, but its literal interpretation highlights how we fail to resolve

---

e. You can download the full report (html version) from www.ash.org.uk/html/conduct/html/trustus.html or the pdf format from tobaccofreekids.org/campaign/global/framework/docs/TrustUs.pdf.

behavior change issues effectively with our patients. Giving rational advice to patients about changing unhealthy behaviors is on a par with the placebo impact of 19th-century drugs. The use of this "drug" over and over again, when it is clearly not working, could be regarded as a form of medical error.

LIMITATIONS OF THE BEST EVIDENCE

In helping our patients change, we should always use the best available evidence from randomized controlled trials (RCTs). However, most behavioral RCTs conducted in primary care provide limited guidance in how to help patients change, because they use only one or two health information and advice-giving interventions with patients, with time-limited follow-up, for a year or so. Such rational interventions are the most frequently studied for tobacco cessation in primary care.[4;6;18-21] Doctors are encouraged to use these approaches routinely and repeatedly with all smokers at each visit, but this does not happen in practice.

Doctors prefer to give advice to patients who have smoking-related problems or who are ready to quit; conversely, they avoid confronting patients who do not fit into this group.[22-25] Such avoidance has some justification: patients react negatively or prefer not to get such advice.[26;27] For these and other reasons, the feasibility of implementing these guidelines has been questioned.[28]

Furthermore, rational interventions do not work for the majority of patients because they are simply not ready to take action. Evidence-based tobacco cessation guidelines tell us what works, but they don't tell us how to work with people when proven interventions fail. Something is missing in the conduct of RCTs in terms of dealing with the full spectrum of patients. RCTs rarely address the internal process of why change did or did not occur. They do not tell us the whole story about change, either from the practitioner's or the patient's perspective. Instead, they provide a very limited view for understanding human experience and behavior change.

With unhealthy behaviors, emotions often supersede reason. Patients frequently decide that the short-term emotional benefits (e.g., smoking to relax) are more important than the long-term quantifiable benefits (e.g., live longer). They make so-called "irrational" decisions. Recommendations from RCTs provide no guidance on how to deal with human emotions, perceptions and values. Scientific rationality lacks sophistication in dealing with human irrationality and otherwise knowledgeable patients who lack the critical factor: motivation.

ADOPTING NEW METAPHORS

Metaphors can help us understand better the gaps between scientific evidence and the complexity of dealing with individual patients' unhealthy behaviors. Here is a visual metaphor to illustrate the gaps in our understanding: RCTs are tiny square pegs in a large round hole. The hole (gaps in our understanding) simply gets bigger with each additional peg. No matter how many pegs are put into the hole, the gaps in our understanding will remain between rational evidence and the emotional complexity of issues affecting behavior change. Evidence-based medicine alone will never close all the gaps.

Metaphors that shape our professional behavior toward patients are embedded in our everyday language.[29] Here are some metaphors that make explicit our fix-it approach toward our patients: "Medical care is a high-tech machine in a competitive market manufacturing magic bullets [e.g., drugs] to cure diseases."[30;31] These mechanistic metaphors suggest objectivity, predictability, beating the competition, winning, cure, war, control and death.

Here, as a complementary worldview, are ecological metaphors that expand the narrow focus of medical care:[30] "Health care is an endangered plant in a threatened ecosystem that needs environmental restoration; in addition to the fix-it role, we adopt a motivational role and become 'gardeners': cultivating the soil, fertilizing the ground, and planting seeds." These organismic metaphors suggest subjectivity, unpredictability, sharing interdependence, collaboration, care, growth, nurture and quality of life. Changing the dominant metaphors in medical care, however, is a major paradigm shift and no simple task. Metaphors can act as weapons against change, as well as agents for change. The underlying value system of the mechanistic metaphors in health care that work against mainstreaming organismic ones are summarized in Table 1.1.

Table 1.1. Comparing Medical and Behavioral Worldviews and Value Systems

Quick-fix: Treating Diseases	Long Haul: Motivating Healthy Behaviors

1. Address complicated, decontextualized tasks
    Use "closed system" approach
	1. Address complex, contextualized tasks
	    Use "open system" approach

2. Focus on objectivity and entities	2. Focus on subjectivity and context

3. Use mechanistic thinking
    "Technicians using tools"
	3. Use organismic thinking
	    "Gardeners planting seeds"

4. Use reductionist and linear approaches
    Apply scientific rationality
	4. Use holistic and nonlinear approaches
	    Address human irrationality

5. Intervene in symptomatic phase
    Patients depend on their practitioners
	5. Intervene in asymptomatic phase
	    Patients start thinking about change

6. Control and cure diseases
    Practitioners save lives
	6. Support autonomy to influence behavior
	    Activate patients to take charge

7. Focus on harms, deficits and pathology	7. Address emotions, perceptions and values

8. Use high-tech treatments (drugs and surgery)
    Static, prescribed interventions
	8. Employ low-tech interventions (dialogue)
	    Dynamic, changing interventions

9. Produce dramatic results
    Immediate benefits
	9. Foster incremental change
	    Delayed benefits

THE NEED FOR A COMPLEMENTARY APPROACH

Modern drug research emphasizes purposeful nonvariation, that is, developing highly specific drugs to target particular enzymes, receptor sites or genes to treat and cure diseases. Unlike the development of drugs, purposeful variation is needed to design highly individualized behavioral interventions to enhance their potency and impact on patients. The "receptor site" is not only different for each patient but also for each of his or her unhealthy behaviors. In spite of the diversity of patient needs, we tend to fall into the trap of using the one-size-fits-all approach.

For this reason, the top-down, "from research to practice," rational choice model, while important in determining what works in some circumstances,[32] has a limited impact, because evidence-based guidelines don't teach practitioners how to attend to the diversity of emotions, perceptions and values that affect patients' health behaviors.[33] With the top-down approach, researchers often try to make patients fit a particular theory: in effect, a controlling method. The researcher is the principal investigator, and practitioners are coinvestigators ostensibly working with patients but in effect telling them what to do. The following quotation provides another perspective about the limitation of this approach.

> *Rational planning and decision-making are doomed to failure in the face of the remarkable complexity of human motivation, encompassing interlocking hurts, disappointments,, confusions, affections and aspirations.*[34]

We need to use a bottom-up, "from practice to research" approach if we are to help our patients close the large gap between evidence and practice and to work with the discrepancy between so-called rationality and their emotions. With the bottom-up approach, the patient is the principal investigator researching his or her health behavior change, and the practitioner is the coinvestigator working with researchers to select theories that fit the particular needs of the patient.

We should also move beyond hierarchy (the top-down, one-way-street approach) and toward partnerships if we want to develop innovative approaches to health care and behavior change. It is vitally important that researchers, theorists and practitioners collaborate in a two-way street to develop partnerships with patients. Patient-centered approaches can help to develop such partnerships and enhance the process and outcome of health care.[35;36] The motivational approach described in this book adds to the patient-centered concept, which addresses concerns, feelings, expectations and consequences relevant to episodes about their care and describes how to develop individualized interventions that help patients change their perceptions and values. To encourage such partnerships, this approach has been developed from state-of-the-art clinical practices (working with patients, students and health care practitioners), research evidence and different theories and models (described in Chapters 6 and 7) about health behavior

Carl Rogers, a seminal thinker about human psychology, captures an essential ingredient for motivating change—listening:

> *We think we listen, but very rarely do we listen with real understanding, true empathy. Yet listening, of this very special kind, is one of the most potent forces for change that I know.*[78]

In many instances, listening with empathy is a prerequisite for helping patients to change. Paolo Freire, a radical contemporary educator, builds on this fundamental principle by emphasizing another critical ingredient needed to work toward effective action:[79;80]

*Listening precedes **Dialogue,** which precedes **Action.***

Freire's aphorism highlights the need to engage patients in constructive dialogue about change in order to motivate them to action.

Motivational practitioners appreciate that each person is unique in what might motivate him or her to change. These practitioners use motivational principles (see Table 1.3) as a guide to engaging patients in the change process over time and work through the three phases of Freire's aphorism (listening, dialogue, action), whereas fix-it practitioners jump in at the action phase.

Table 1.3.

Motivational Principles
• Develop empathic relationships with patients
• Clarify roles and responsibilities for health behavior change
• Gain consent from patients to address behavior change
• Respect patients' autonomy—use influence, not control, to effect change
• Work at a pace sensitive to the patients' needs and their readiness to change
• Help patients explore and understand better their values and perceptions
• Help patients decide whether to change their values and perceptions
• Focus on strengths, successes and health, not weaknesses, failures and pathology
• Focus on solutions rather than on problems
• Enhance patients' confidence and competence to change (self-efficacy)
• Negotiate reasonable goals for change
• Help patients believe that healthy outcomes are possible
• Help patients increase their supports and reduce their barriers to change.
• Develop plans to prevent relapses and use so-called failures as learning opportunities

Attempts to force patients to act in healthy ways when they are not ready can sometimes have the opposite effect.[81;82] For example, if you are a parent, consider the last time that you gave strong, directive advice to your children (especially teenagers) about changing their behavior. Or recollect when you were a teenager and were told not to do something by your parents or teachers. Sometimes you did it anyway! Years later, you realized that their advice was right, but how did you feel about the advice at the time it was given? Controlling or threatening messages, such as providing highly directive advice—"Do this . . . you should . . . or else"—often proves counterproductive. Individuals may become even more resistant in response to such controlling advice. Strong unsolicited advice, even if logical, can bring out the rebellious teenager in all of us.

We must move beyond the idea of control,[83] that is, beyond trying to control our patients or having patients control themselves, to the idea of autonomy.[84] Patients are more likely to adopt healthy behaviors if they *want to* rather than if they *ought to* or *have to* change. Over time, patients are more likely to behave in *healthy* ways if we openly acknowledge their choice to engage in an unhealthy behavior rather than trying to make them change. Autonomy-supportive approaches (offering choices) are more effective in helping patients change than are coercive measures.[84] Examples of the distinctions between controlling and autonomy-supportive approaches are interspersed throughout this book.[85]

CONSIDER CHANGING YOURSELF

Consider taking a step back from changing patients' behaviors to focus on your own health behaviors, professional roles and assumptions. Learning from your attempts to change your personal and professional behaviors may help you empathize and work more effectively with your patients. This suggestion is important for another reason. Our health habits affect how we work with patients. Physicians with healthy behaviors (e.g., nonsmoking, low-risk drinking or abstinence, regular exercise) are more likely to counsel patients about the same behaviors.[86-90] In a few countries, an overall decline in the smoking rate was preceded by a decline in the smoking rate among physicians. Yet the smoking rate among health care professionals remains high in many countries. Perhaps the health care professions can indeed do a better job of helping its members develop healthier habits. No one, of course, is perfect. We all have something that we could do to improve our health (healthy diets, weight reduction and more exercise).

Mohandas K. Gandhi emphasized the importance of beginning with oneself when addressing change:

Be the change that you want to see in the world.

I have only three enemies. My favorite enemy, the one most easily influenced for the better, is the British Empire. My second enemy, the Indian people, is far more difficult. But my most formidable opponent is a man named Mohandas K. Gandhi. With him I seem to have very little influence.

An important take-home message is that you may find it easier to influence patients to change than to change your own family members, or even yourself.

The inner process of learning how to change your health behaviors and how to become a motivational practitioner can accelerate the outer process of expanding your depth and range of motivational skills and of developing individualized interventions to meet your patients' changing needs. This premise, however, can be threatening or seem irrelevant or unnecessary to some practitioners, so they avoid exploring personal or professional issues about self-change. As you read through the next section of this chapter, assess your internal reactions about the extent to which you have positive, negative or mixed responses to different aspects of this premise or this chapter. In what ways are your internal reactions similar or different from some of your patients?

Practitioner Example of Internal "Mixed" Reactions: A general practitioner from Bergen, Norway, felt that this chapter was persuasive about promoting healthy habits but also expressed concerns about practitioners "overdoing it" with their patients and acting as health care imperialists.

Commentary: These concerns speak to a crucial issue about the differences between autonomy-supportiveness and behaviorally controlling ways. This chapter introduces the motivational principle of autonomy-supportiveness, but some practitioners may not fully understand how to put this principle into practice and may unknowingly act in controlling ways that are antithetical to this principle. In effect, they fall into the trap of health care imperialism. At the other extreme, we fall into the enabling trap—acting as our patients' unconditional advocates to support their choice to do as they please, without setting any limits. As a middle way between these extremes, we can support patients' autonomy without either of us abandoning or imposing our health care values. Instead of becoming immobilized by this ethical dilemma, we can respect, explore and work with our differences in values with our patients, all, of course, with their explicit consent or implicitly based on mutual trust.

Now, if you wish, consider identifying a professional or personal issue that you want to change. Much can be learned from your attempt to unravel the individual and contextual factors that shape this behavior—doing so may help both you and your patients. Kurt Lewin succinctly captures the essence of this kind of learning opportunity:

If you want to understand something, try to change it.[91]

Personal Change: Your Health Behaviors and Life Situation

Personal health habits influence our professional behavior. Practitioners with unhealthy behaviors (e.g., lack of exercise, unhealthy diet and overeating, causing obesity) are less likely to counsel patients who have the same behaviors. This is yet another reason why it's important to address change by beginning with yourself. Learning Exercise 1.1 helps you reflect about changing yourself as a way to understanding yourself. Such self-understanding can help you become a more effective motivational practitioner with patients. Find out where you stand by completing the exercise.

Learning Exercise 1.1. Assess your overall health behaviors and life issues
   Complete the questionnaires for 10 Health Behaviors and 10 Life issues.
Circle N or Y for each health decision.
N = Not applicable to me.
Y = Yes. For each yes response, use this readiness-to-change" scale:
   1= not thinking about change 2 = thinking about change 3 = preparing to change

Health Behaviors and Life Issues

A Self-evaluation	Self-assessment		Readiness to change
1. Tobacco use	N	Y	1 2 3
2. Eating habits	N	Y	1 2 3
3. Weight	N	Y	1 2 3
4. Physical activity	N	Y	1 2 3
5. Alcohol use	N	Y	1 2 3
6. Illegal drug use	N	Y	1 2 3
7. Safe sex practices	N	Y	1 2 3
8. Contraception to prevent pregnancy	N	Y	1 2 3
9. Regular use of prescribed drugs	N	Y	1 2 3
10. Safety belt use and bicycle helmets	N	Y	1 2 3
11. Social relationships	N	Y	1 2 3
12. Job satisfaction	N	Y	1 2 3
13. Financial situation	N	Y	1 2 3
14. Work/family/social balance	N	Y	1 2 3
15. Professional/personal overfunctioning	N	Y	1 2 3
16. Physical and sexual abuse	N	Y	1 2 3
17. Emotional health	N	Y	1 2 3
18. Coping with stress	N	Y	1 2 3
19. Environmental health (work/home)	N	Y	1 2 3
20. Spiritual health	N	Y	1 2 3

- *For each health behavior and life situation of concern (those circled "Y"), complete the scale of your readiness to change. Look at each concern where you're not thinking about change or are thinking about it but are unsure what to do. **Questions to Ponder:** How long have you been thinking about change? What is holding you back? What is keeping your foot nailed to the floor in addressing change?*
- *Think about a recent time when someone did not follow your advice to address a health concern. **Question to Ponder:** How does your previous analysis of difficulties in changing your own behavior help you understand why it can be so difficult for someone else to change, especially when it is an issue that is not a concern for you personally?*
- *Think about the occasions when a health issue came up with someone you know: a patient, colleague, family member or friend. **Questions to Ponder:** How was your behavior in this interaction influenced by your own health choices? Can you see any positive or negative patterns in the ways that you interact with others, for better or worse?*

You may even need some additional assistance to address some behaviors such as lack of exercise, unhealthy diet or even overwork. If so, you may find it helpful to use *Motivate Healthy Habits: Stepping Stones to Lasting Change* (a self-guided change version of this book) to work on your behaviors.[92] Your personal experience of using it can then help you to help your patients learn how to use this guidebook with or without your ongoing support.

Professional Change: Roles, Perspectives and Mental Models

We need to incorporate new similes and metaphors into well-established ones. The mechanistic similes (hammer and nails, nuts and bolts) used at the beginning of this chapter only tell practitioners to stop using the fix-it role when health information and advice doesn't work. As previously noted, the machine and gardener metaphors characterize the fix-it and motivational roles respectively. Organic metaphors can help us move beyond the toolbox metaphors; it is not just a question of picking up a new tool. These metaphors more aptly capture how we need to work in addressing health behavior change with our patients. This process also involves professional change: changing your roles appropriately, learning about different perspectives on resistance and motivation and using mental maps for developing individualized interventions to meet your patients' changing needs over time.

Changing roles

An understanding about different roles (motivational, preventive and fix-it) lays the foundation for learning how to enhance your skills at motivating behavior change. (Chapters 2-4 present these three roles in detail and describe how different roles can have both positive and negative impacts on our work with patients.) A brief description about the distinctions between these roles will help you to understand why it is important to change your role before developing new skills.

The term *agent of change* is used figuratively to clarify different roles that you may assume in working with patients. Practitioner-centered advice is the agent of change for fix-it roles. Such advice is based on what practitioners think patients should be given, rather than on what patients may prefer or need. In a preventive role, education tailored to the needs of patients becomes the agent of change. In a motivational role, you work with, rather than against, indifferent or resistant patients. Your dialogue with patients becomes the agency of change. You use such dialogue (together with a motivational assessment) to help develop individualized interventions to meet patients' changing needs over time.

The fix-it role is more appropriate for treating diseases *caused by* risk behaviors (e.g., giving antibiotics for acute bronchitis) than it is for helping patients *change* risk behaviors (e.g., giving advice to quit smoking). If we remain in a fix-it role, we may persist in providing more information and advice to resistant, indifferent and ambivalent patients than they want. This situation can evoke mutual frustration in addition to possible anger and guilt and become such a negative experience that patients may avoid us or fail to seek appropriate care.

Learning about resistance and motivation
Patient resistance is a normal and expected phenomenon, but it is also a learning opportunity to understand why patients resist change in spite of our good intentions to help them. We are often on different wavelengths from our patients. Unless we change our wavelength, we cancel out each other's energy, so nothing happens but perpetual inertia and wariness. How can you motivate these patients to change? First, learn how to adapt your role to meet patients' needs. Different perspectives on resistance and motivation (Chapters 5-7) can help you learn how to work with resistance, rather than work against it. Then you are in a better position to help patients redirect their energy in healthy directions.

Internalizing the six-step approach as a mental map
A mental map is a framework or way of thinking derived from internalizing a model. You can use the six-step approach (summarized in Table 1.4 and explained in Chapters 8-14) as a mental map for negotiating about behavior change with patients. Even if you internalize this map, it does not mean that you are skillful in navigating the territory—in this case, the patient's world. Always keep in mind that the map is not the territory.[93] It is just a guide, but it can help you learn to negotiate an appropriate rate at which to work through the change process with your patients.[94] In addition, a mental map can help you learn how to use words, language and dialogue more effectively in working with your patients. With repeated practice in using this guide, you can become more effective over time in developing individualized interventions for your patients.

Table 1.4. Six-step Approach for Negotiating Change

Mental Map for Negotiating Change	Desired Impact on Patients
Step 1: Building a partnership Step 2: Negotiating an agenda	Helps patients move from not thinking about change to thinking about it.
Step 3: Assessing resistance and motivation Step 4: Enhancing mutual understanding	Helps patients move from thinking about change to preparing to change.
Step 5: Implementing a plan	Helps patients move from preparing to change to taking action.
Step 6: Following through	Helps patients move from taking action to maintaining change.

Patients have good reasons for their health decisions, but you may disagree with their logic. To work with the so-called irrationality, you need to work with patients at the level of their perceptions and values. A decision balance (used in Step 3) is a simple tool that can help you do this. This tool can help your patients organize their thoughts about staying the same (resistance) versus changing (motivation), and uncover what lies beneath their thoughts about change: emotions, perceptions and values. If you understand how their values affect their perceptions, and in turn their behaviors, you will at least understand their decision-making process. The example below illustrates how you can use this tool to understand so-called human irrationality when seeing your patients in your office.

Resistance to the Practice of Safe Sex: Mrs. S., a 45-year-old woman, came to her family physician (Dr. M.) for a follow-up to her HIV test. Two years ago, she remarried after being divorced for many years. She had recently moved back to her hometown after her husband broke his parole and was returned to jail. Mr. and Mrs. S. had regularly attended an HIV clinic because Mr. S. was HIV-positive. Even though Mrs. S. knew how to put a condom on her husband, he did not want to wear one. Fortunately, she remained HIV-negative even without practicing safe sex. The doctor at the HIV clinic had advised Mrs. S. to have an HIV test done every three months. Dr. M. ordered the HIV test and asked her if she would be willing to fill out a decision balance in order to better understand why she did not want to use condoms. Dr. M. saw another patient while Mrs. S. completed this task, and then returned to see what she had written.

Learning Exercise 1.2. Reflect on Mrs. S.'s decision balance
Reflect on the following questions as you read Mrs. S.'s decision balance.
- *How does she perceive her reasons to stay the same versus her reasons to change, based on how she thinks and feels?*
- *What does she feel about her husband?*
- *What does she feel about herself?*
- *How does she value her relationship as compared to herself and her own family?*

Then analyze her decision balance. The left column represents Mrs. S.'s reasons to stay the same, and the right column represents her reasons to change.

Mrs. S.'s Decision Balance about Safe Sex

Reasons not to use condoms (resistance)	Reasons to use condoms (motivation)
1. Benefits of not using condoms Not make him feel he is failing at being sexually competent. He feels secure that I'll stay with him.	2. Concerns about not using condoms Don't want HIV. Don't want my family hurt. Maybe people will think he doesn't care to protect me.
3. Concerns about using condoms He will have erection problems and it will make him sad. He will wish he were with his ex-girlfriend (who is HIV) so he won't have to use them.	4. Benefits of using condoms Won't get HIV so won't upset family. Won't get sick myself so I can take care of him when he gets sicker. Will feel that he cares enough about me and will not allow me to get sick.
Resistance Score = 9 Feeling score = 9 Think score = 6	Motivation Score = 4 Feeling score = 4 Think score = 8

Assessing Mrs. S.'s perceptions about her resistance and motivation: When Dr. M. reentered the room, he read what Mrs. S. wrote and first pointed to the left-hand column of her decision balance. He asked her to use a scale from 0 to 10 (0 = not important and 10 = very important) to rate her overall reasons for not using condoms. Mrs. S. gave a resistance score of 9. Dr. M. then asked to rate her reasons for using them. She gave a motivation score of 4. Dr. M. asked her whether her scores were based on her feelings or her thoughts. Mrs. S stated that her scores were based on her feelings. Dr. M. then asked her to rate her overall reasons to stay the same versus her reasons to change based on what she thought about it. Mrs. S. gave 6 for her resistance score and 8 for her motivation score. This process helped her understand much better how much her heart ruled her head in making decisions. Emotionally, she felt that she should stay the same, but rationally she thought she should protect herself.

Assessing Mrs. S's emotions and values: Looking over her decision balance again, Dr. M. reflected back to Mrs. S. that she must really love her husband. Mrs. S. smiled in total agreement and expressed devotion to her husband, stating that she wanted to care for him when he gets terminally ill. Dr. M. asked her how she valued her relationship with her husband in comparison to herself and the relationship to her own family. Mrs. S. loved her husband so much that she was willing to sacrifice her life for him, but admitted to having mixed feelings when thinking about her own children from her first marriage. Her adult children did not know about her current situation. Mrs. S. stated she came from an abusive family and has suffered from chronic low self-esteem since childhood.

This example demonstrates how you can begin to engage patients in dialogue about change and to develop individualized interventions during a 15-minute appointment. Over time, effective interventions can assist your patients in deciding whether to change their values and perceptions in ways that motivate them to take charge of changing their behavior. The six-step approach described in Section III can help you learn how to use words, language and dialogue more effectively with your patients. With repeated practice in using this approach, you could become a more effective and efficient motivational practitioner.

CONTINUING PROFESSIONAL DEVELOPMENT

A continuing professional development (CPD) curriculum on motivating health behavior change must revisit topics at increasing levels of complexity to foster lifelong learning, enrich professional development and improve clinical performance. Such a dynamic curriculum could help us develop skills at self-directed learning as well as provide opportunities for small group learning, individual supervision and/or a longitudinal relationship with a mentor throughout our formal education and career. Given that such ideal curricula are rare, however, it is important to take charge of your own CPD. Whatever your level of clinical experience, you can use this book to prepare for and design a learning plan for your ongoing professional development.

Taking Charge of Your Professional Development

Even if you were not trained in how to motivate behavior change, you can use self-directed learning methods, ideally working with patients over time. Section IV in this book describes how you can develop skills for initiating dialogues with patients in addressing specific behaviors. If available, workshops can also help you enhance your motivational skills. Dr. S.'s written evaluation of such a workshop captures the merits of such training:

> Although it has been 15 years since I have done any role-playing, I found it extremely captivating. Afterward, I found that I was immediately applying in the office what I had learned in role-playing. I became consciously aware of resistance during patient interviews and was more apt to closely examine patients' agendas, as well as their perceptions. Patients appeared extremely gratified. My frustration level was also considerably diminished. These have been the gifts:
>
> - Seeing the therapeutic relationship as a worthy goal in and of itself
> - Seeing where someone is at along the change continuum and using that to respect the patient's autonomy and our own humble role as advisers
> - Finding out what people want and how they see things rather than working with what I think they want and how I think they see things
> - Being sensitive to resistance helps me change my approach to patients

With training and practice, you can become more effective, deliberate and purposeful in helping patients work through the change process. At first, this process will take more time and even slow you down, but in time you will expand your range and depth of motivational skills. However, you can develop a learning plan for continuing professional development so that you can monitor your progress, whatever your starting point or level of clinical experience, on your journey from a novice to a master. Becoming a master is not a destination but a journey without end.

YOUR SUMMARY

Reflect: write a note (in 200 words or so) summarizing how this chapter helped you understand better the potential benefits of exploring your own health behaviors, professional roles and assumptions, as you learn about how to develop motivation skills. Which aspects of this premise, if any, evoke some resistance in you? What have you learned that was new for you?

_____
_____
_____
_____
_____
_____
_____
_____
_____
_____
_____
_____
_____
_____
_____
_____
_____
_____
_____
_____
_____
_____
_____

Enhance: write down your ideas about how your new learning could improve your interactions with patients. Add your notes to your learning portfolio.

_____
_____
_____

37. Botelho RJ, Novak SJ. Dealing with substance misuse, abuse, and dependency. Primary Care 1993;20(1): 51-70

38. Botelho RJ, Skinner HA. Motivating change in health behavior: Implications for health promotion and disease prevention. Primary Care (Saunders) 1995;22: 565-589

39. Botelho RJ, Skinner HA, Williams GC, et al. Patients with alcohol problems in primary care: Understanding their resistance and motivating change. In: Stuart MR, Lieberman IJA, eds. Primary care: Clinics in office practice. Philadelphia: W.B. Saunders Company; 1999:279-298

40. Harackiewicz JM, Sansone C, Blair LW, et al. Attributional processes in behavior change and maintenance: Smoking cessation and continued abstinence. Journal of Consulting and Clinical Psychology 1987;55: 372-378

41. Ockene JK, Kristeller J, Goldberg R, et al. Increasing the efficacy of physician-delivered smoking interventions: A randomized clinical trial [see comments]. Journal of General Internal Medicine 1991;6: 1-8

42. Currie CE, Amos A, Hunt SM. The dynamics and processes of behavioral change in five classes of health-related behavior-findings from qualitative research. Health Education Research 1991;6: 443-453

43. Ryan RM, Plant RW, O'Malley S. Initial motivations for alcohol treatment: Relations with patient characteristics, treatment involvement, and dropout. Addictive Behaviors 1995;20: 279-297

44. Williams GC, Grow VM, Freedman ZR, et al. Motivational predictors of weight loss and weight-loss maintenance. Journal of Personality and Social Psychology 1996;70(1): 115-126

45. Williams GC, Rodin GC, Ryan RM, et al. Autonomous regulation and long-term medication adherence in adult outpatients. Health Psychology 1998;17: 269-276

46. Perz CA, DiClemente CC, Carbonari JP. Doing the right thing at the right time? The interaction of stages and processes of change in successful smoking cessation. Health Psychology 1996;15: 462-468

47. Patrick K, Sallis J, Long B, et al. A new tool for encouraging activity: The physician and sports medicine 1994;22

48. Calfas KJ, Long BJ, Sallis JF, et al. A controlled trial of physician counseling to promote the adoption of physical activity. Preventive Medicine 1996;25: 225-233

49. Long BJ, Calfas KJ, Wooten W, et al. A multisite field test of the acceptability of physical activity counseling in primary care: project PACE. American Journal of Preventive Medicine 1996;12: 73-81

50. Sutton S. Can "stage of change" provide guidance in the treatment of addictions? A critical examination of Prochaska and DiClemente's model. In: Edwards G, Dare C, eds. Psychotherapy, psychological treatments and the addictions. New York: Cambridge University Press; 1996

51. Farkas AJ, Pierce JP, Gilpin EA, et al. Is stage-of-change a useful measure of the likelihood of smoking cessation? Annals of Behavioral Medicine 1996;18: 79-86

52. Prochaska JO, Velicer WF. On models, methods and premature conclusions. Addiction 1996;91: 1281-1283

53. Farkas AJ, Pierce JP, Zhu SH, et al. Addiction versus stages of change models in predicting smoking cessation. Addiction 1996;91: 1271-1280

54. Joseph J, Breslin C, Skinner HA. Critical perspective on the transtheoretical model and the stages of change. In: Tucher J, Donovan D, Marlatt A, eds. Changing addictive behavior: Moving beyond therapy assisted change. New York: Guilford Press; 1999:160-190

55. Bien TH, Miller WR, Tonigan JS. Brief interventions for alcohol problems: A review. Addiction 1993;88: 315-335

56. Ershoff DH, Quinn V, Boyd NR, et al. The Kaiser Permanente prenatal smoking-cessation trial: When more isn't better, what is enough? American Journal of Preventive Medicine 1999;17: 161-168

57. Miller WR, Sovereign RG, Krege B. Motivational interviewing with problem drinkers: II. The drinker's check-up as a preventative intervention. Behavioral Psychotherapy 1988;16: 251-268

58. Stephens RS, Roffman RA, Simpson EE. Treating adult marijuana dependence: A test of the relapse prevention model. Journal of Consulting and Clinical Psychology 1994;62: 92-99

59. Baer JS, Marlatt GA. Maintenance of smoking cessation [published erratum appears in Clinical Chest Medicine 1992 Mar;13(1):ix]. Clinical Chest Medicine 1991;12: 793-800

60. Smith DE, Heckmeyer CM, Kratt PP, et al. Motivational interviewing to improve adherence to a behavioral weight-control program for older obese women with NIDDM. Diabetes Care 1997;20: 52-54

61. Brown JM, Miller WR. Impact of motivational interviewing on participation in residential alcoholism treatment. Psychology of Addictive Behaviors 1993;7: 211-218

62. Allsop S, Saunders B, Phillips M, et al. A trial of relapse prevention with severely dependent male problem drinkers. Addiction 1997;92: 61-73

63. Project MATCH Research Group. Matching alcoholism treatments to client heterogeneity: Project MATCH posttreatment drinking outcomes. Journal of Studies on Alcohol 1997;58: 7-29

64. May WW. Findings from Project MATCH: Fact or artifact? Behavioral Health Management 1998;January/February: 38-39

65. Matching alcoholism treatments to client heterogeneity: Project MATCH three-year drinking outcomes. Alcoholism, Clinical and Experimental Research 1998;22: 1300-1311

66. Saunders B, Wilkinson C, Phillips M. The impact of a brief motivational intervention with opiate users attending a methadone programme. Addiction 1995;90: 415-424

67. Heather N, Rollnick S, Bell A, et al. Effects of brief counseling among male heavy drinkers identified on general hospital wards. Drug and Alcohol Review 1996;15: 29-38

68. Woollard J, Beilin L, Lord T, et al. A controlled trial of nurse counseling on lifestyle change for hypertensives treated in general practice: Preliminary results. Clinical and Experimental Pharmacology and Physiology 1995;22: 466-468

69. Butler CC, Rollnick S, Cohen DA, et al. Motivational consulting versus brief advice for smokers in general practice: A randomized trial. British Journal of General Practice 1999;49: 611-616

70. Berg-Smith SM, Stevens VJ, Brown KM, et al. A brief motivational intervention to improve dietary adherence in adolescents. The Dietary Intervention Study in Children (DISC) Research Group. Health Education Research 1999;14: 399-410

71. Lowman C, Allen J, Stout RL. Replication and extension of Marlatt's taxonomy of relapse precipitants: Overview of procedures and results. The Relapse Research Group. Addiction 1996;91: S51-S71

72. Carroll K. Relapse prevention as a psychosocial treatment: A review of controlled clinical trials. Experimental and Clinical Psychopharmacology 1996;4: 46-54

73. Botelho RJ. Negotiating partnerships in healthcare: Contexts and methods. In: Suchman AL, Botelho RJ, Hinton-Walker P, eds. Partnerships in healthcare: Transforming relational process. Rochester, NY: University of Rochester Press; 1998:19-49

74. Bartlett's Familiar Quotations. 14th, rev. and enl. ed. Boston: Little, Brown and Co.; 1968

75. Miller WR, Rollnick S. Motivational interviewing: Preparing people to change addictive behavior. New York: Guilford Press; 1991

76. Rollnick S, Mason P, Butler C. Health behavior change: A guide for practitioners. Edinburgh, Scotland: Churchill Livingstone; 1999

77. McGinnis JM, Foege WH. Actual causes of death in the United States. Journal of the American Medical Association 1993;270: 2207-2212

78. Rogers CR. A way of being. Boston: Houghton Mifflin; 1980

79. Freire P. Education for critical consciousness. New York: Seabury Press; 1973

80. Wallerstein N, Bernstein E. Empowerment education: Freire's ideas adapted to health education. Health Education Quarterly 1988;15: 379-394

81. Brehm JW. A theory of psychological reactance. New York: Academic Press; 1966

82. Brehm SS, Brehm JW. Psychological reactance: A theory of freedom and control. New York: Academic Press; 1981

83. Shapiro DH, Jr., Schwartz CE, Astin JA. Controlling ourselves, controlling our world. American Psychologist 1996;51: 1213-1230

84. Deci EL, Ryan RM. Intrinsic motivation and self-determination in human behavior. New York: Plenum Press; 1985

85. Williams GC, Deci EL, Ryan RM. Building healthcare partnerships by supporting autonomy: Promoting maintained behavior change and positive healthcare outcomes. In: Suchman AL, Botelho RJ, Hinton-Walker P, eds. Partnerships in healthcare: Transforming relational process. Rochester, NY: University of Rochester Press; 1998:67-87

86. Lewis CE, Clancy C, Leake B, et al. The counseling practices of internists. Annals of Internal Medicine 1991;114: 54-58

87. Wells KB, Lewis CE, Leake B, et al. Do physicians preach what they practice? A study of physicians' health habits and counseling practices. Journal of the American Medical Association 1984;252: 2846-2848

88. Schwartz JS, Lewis CE, Clancy C, et al. Internists' practices in health promotion and disease prevention. A survey [see comments]. Annals of Internal Medicine 1991;114: 46-53

89. Frank E, Rothenberg R, Lewis C, et al. Correlates of physicians' prevention-related practices. Findings from the Women Physicians' Health Study. Archives of Family Medicine 2000;9: 359-367

90. Frank E, Breyan J, Elon L. Physician disclosure of healthy personal behaviors improves credibility and ability to motivate. Archives of Family Medicine 2000;9: 287-290

91. Lewin K. Field theory in social science. New York: Harper Torchbooks; 1951

92. Botelho RJ. Motivate healthy habits: Stepping stones to lasting change. Rochester, NY; 2004

93. Bateson G. Mind and nature: A necessary unity. New York: E.P. Dutton; 1979

94. Botelho RJ. A negotiation model for the doctor-patient relationship. Family Practice 1992;9: 210-21

CHAPTER 2

CONTRASTING THE FIX-IT AND MOTIVATIONAL ROLES

FOR REFLECTION

How do fix-it and motivational practitioners differ in helping their patients change?

OVERVIEW

The fix-it role is most effective in treating injuries and diseases caused by risk behaviors, providing instant gratification for the patient and rewards for the practitioner, if it is successful. In this role, we typically wait until patients have developed complications before advising them to change their behavior. This approach has a limited impact on patients, however, and is often frustrating for them and for us. The purpose of this chapter is to compare this traditional method with a new approach to behavior change and to highlight some differences in how these two roles affect the process and outcome of health care. This comparison deliberately focuses on the limitations of the fix-it role, which is effective in addressing immediate medical problems, and emphasizes the strengths of the motivational role, which is helpful in addressing health behavior change over time. The purpose of this comparison is to enhance your understanding about how different roles work for different health issues.

Practitioners can adopt a variety of roles when they relate to patients and their families. In the more traditional role, a directive, "take charge" approach is appropriate in situations requiring technological and pharmacological (fix-it) treatments, such as emergency care or the cure of acute diseases. This approach, however, may be ineffective or even counterproductive in helping some patients deal with chronic conditions and risk behaviors. A clinical example will compare how a fix-it practitioner (Dr. F.) and a motivational practitioner (Dr. M.) dealt with the same patient (Mr. B.) to address the need for drug adherence. Using the six-step approach (described in Chapter 8) as a guide in both cases, this example will describe how Dr. F. and then Dr. M. related differently to Mr. B based on the role each adopted.

Drug adherence is used in this example because only 50% of patients take medications as prescribed[1-4] or are sufficiently adherent to long-term medications (greater than two weeks' duration) for them to be clinically effective.[5-7] There is a great need for strengthening the scientific basis for increasing drug adherence.[1:8-11] We need to learn how to work with patients over time to improve long-term drug adherence.

CLINICAL EXAMPLE

Mr. B. is a 75-year-old man who returned to his physician about five months late for a follow-up appointment. He was two months late in renewing his antihypertensive prescription. He thought his blood pressure was high because he was not feeling well and wanted to go back on his medications to feel better.

EXAMPLE OF THE FIX-IT PRACTITIONER

Dr. F.	Commentary
Dr. F. felt annoyed that Mr. B. had not kept the follow-up appointment on time. On reviewing the chart before going into the examination room, Dr. F. noticed that Mr. B.'s father had died of a stroke. Dr. F. was determined to persuade Mr. B. to take his medications regularly.	Dr. F. assumed a paternalistic position.
On entering the room, Dr. F. immediately warned Mr. B. about the consequences of drug non-adherence and insisted that he take his medications regularly.	Dr. F. immediately took control of the agenda
Mr. B. became defensive, stating that he disliked the drug side effects. Inwardly, he felt childlike and embarrassed about not taking the medications Dr. F. had prescribed.	Mr. B. deferred to Dr. F.

Dr. F. informed Mr. B. that not all his side effects were due to the medications, and told him to take them.

Dr. F. educated Mr. B. by stating that he needed to take the medications in spite of some drug side effects (implement a plan using practitioner-centered values).

After Dr. F. again reinforced the need for Mr. B. to take his medications on a continuing basis, Mr. B. admitted that he did not think it was always necessary to take medications, particularly when he felt well. Mr. B. then placated Dr. F. by stating that he would try to take his medications on a regular basis, but he did not give his full commitment to this goal.

When Dr. F. failed to follow up on Mr. B.'s additional reason for not taking his medications, Dr. F. missed an opportunity to enhance mutual understanding about Mr. B.'s reasons for his non-adherence to long-term medications. Instead, Dr. F. tried to make Mr. B. stick to the plan.

Dr. F. asked Mr. B. to come back in two weeks.

Dr. F. again took a paternalistic position by setting up an appointment (follow-through) without checking whether it was convenient for Mr. B.

EXAMPLE OF THE MOTIVATIONAL PRACTITIONER

Dr. M.

Commentary

Dr. M. noted that Mr. B. had missed his last appointment and was late in refilling his prescription. When Dr. M. asked Mr. B. about taking his medications, Mr. B. admitted that he often skipped them because of the side effects. Dr. M. then asked Mr. B. whether he had any other reasons for not taking his medications.

Because Mr. B. openly admitted that he did not take his medications due to their side effects, Dr. M. was able to follow up and encourage Mr. B. to talk about his other reasons for not taking his medications continuously.

Although Dr. M. was not convinced that all Mr. B.'s symptoms were due to drug side effects, he did not share this opinion with Mr. B.

Dr. M. decided instead to address the drug sideeffect issue first and then to gather more assessment information about Mr. B.'s drug non-adherence.

Dr. M. first clarified with Mr. B. that some of his symptoms also occurred when he was not taking the medications. Dr. M also discovered that Mr. B. would restart the medications when he felt unwell.

Dr. M. and Mr. B. began to develop more of a shared understanding about his symptoms and use of medications.

Dr. M. then asked if there were any other reasons Mr. B. was not taking his medications.

Dr. M. allowed Mr. B. to provide more information about his drug non-adherence

Mr. B. stated that he did not feel it was necessary to take medications when he felt well. When he felt well, he thought his blood pressure was normal.

(assessment). It became clear that Mr. B. and Dr. M. had different perceptions about the benefits for Mr. B. of taking the medications when he was feeling well.

Dr. M. explained to Mr. B. that he could have a stroke whether he felt well or unwell, but he was more likely to have a stroke when not taking his medications. Then Dr. M. asked Mr. B. in a non threatening manner whether he understood this information.

To enhance mutual understanding about this issue, Dr. M. provided individualized information to Mr. B.

Although he told Dr. M. that he understood this information, Mr. B. had difficulty believing it. Dr. M explained again that if Mr. B. wanted to prevent a stroke, he also needed to take his medications when he felt well.

Dr. M. focused on implementing a plan that emphasized continuous rather than episodic adherence.

Dr. M. asked Mr. B. whether Mrs. B. was concerned about him and asked him to decide whether he wanted to bring his wife with him next time.

Dr. M. allowed Mr. B. to take charge by letting him decide whether he would want his wife to come to the next appointment. This is in contrast to telling the patient to bring his wife in or inviting his wife without knowing whether the patient wanted this or not.

After some reflection, Mr. B. thought the suggestion was a good idea. Dr. M. then asked when would be a convenient time for the next appointment. Mr. B. said he would bring his wife with him in three to four weeks, because they were going to a wedding in two weeks.

Mr. B. decided with Dr. M. when to return for a follow-up, rather than have the doctor alone decide.

Although the description of the patient encounter with Dr. M. is longer than that of Dr. F., the difference in the duration of the clinical encounter was only about one to two minutes. Dr. M. used his encounter time more efficiently because the dialogue process was more engaging, effective and complex than Dr F.'s interaction. Conversely, Dr. F. used the sequence of the problem-solving activities with Mr. B. in a less coherent and purposeful manner than Dr. M. did.

COMPARING THE PROCESS OF EXPLORING RISK PERCEPTIONS

Fix-it role	Motivational role
Dr. F. and Mr. B. perceived, thought and felt differently about the risks of not taking the medications. Mr. B. stopped taking them when the side effects bothered him. He felt that avoidance of the side effects was worth more than the benefits of taking the medications, particularly when he felt well. Dr. F. did not explore this issue.	Dr. M. helped Mr. B. to rethink his belief that all his symptoms were due to drug side effects. He also helped Mr. B. better understand that he was just as likely to have a stroke when feeling well as when feeling unwell, and that taking his medications could help to prevent a stroke regardless of how well he felt. Mr. B. began to think that it might be worth tolerating the drug side effects for the benefits of taking the medications.

Many factors can affect how practitioners and patients perceive the pros and cons of health behavior change: agendas and priorities about health care issues; perceptions about risks, harms (concerns) and benefits; attributions; coping styles; spirituality (issues related to values, meanings, purpose, connection); and cultural influences. Drs. F. and M. used their authority and expertise differently in addressing the patient's perceptions. To facilitate the sharing of professional and lay expertise, practitioners need to identify pertinent differences so that they can negotiate toward a common understanding about the risks, harms, and benefits associated with an unhealthy behavior.

Dr. M. used his assessment skills to help Mr. B. reconsider his perceived benefits and concerns (risks and harms) about drug adherence by allowing him to voice his lay expertise about how he evaluated the risks, harms, and benefits associated with drug nonadherence. When Mr. B. stated that he did not take his tablets when he felt well, because he associated feeling well with having no risks, Dr. M. worked from Mr. B.'s perspective, using it as the starting point for change. Dr. M. used their respective expertise synergistically to enhance the prospects of improving health care outcomes. This kind of encounter is described as a meeting between "experts." [12]

In contrast, Dr. F. used his own perspective as a starting point for change. He used his authority to impose his perceptions and values on Mr. B., without fully understanding his patient's perspective.

COMPARING IMMEDIATE IMPACT

Fix-it role

Mr. B. felt that Dr. F. did not appreciate his concerns about the drug side effects or believe that Mr. B. did not feel the need to take the medications continuously, in spite of Dr. F.'s recommendations. Mr. B. did not feel that he could share what he thought about this issue with his doctor.

Motivational role

Dr. M. helped Mr. B. to think about the drug side effects differently. Furthermore, Dr. M. moved Mr. B. from thinking that he could not have a stroke when feeling well (and therefore not have to take his medications) to the possibility that he might have a stroke even when feeling well. This was despite the fact that Mr. B. still had difficulty in accepting the idea that he could have high blood pressure (and could have a stroke) when he felt fine.

Dr. M. had an immediate impact on Mr. B., who changed from not thinking to thinking about how drug non-adherence affected his health. This transition was an important intermediary step toward the ultimate goal of changing his behavior. After his visit with Dr. M., Mr. B. came to feel some ambivalence about change. In contrast, after his appointment with Dr. F., Mr. B. did not feel ambivalent about his behavior.

Consequently, the immediate impact for Dr. M. and Dr. F. was different. First, Dr. F. left the encounter feeling unconvinced that Mr. B. would take his medications regularly. In contrast, Dr. M. better understood the challenge that Mr. B. faced in terms of deciding whether to adhere more consistently to his drug regimen. Second, Mr. B.'s emotional response was negative with Dr. F. and positive with Dr. M. Third, Dr. M. began to address a discrepancy between Mr. B.'s risk behavior (not taking blood pressure tablets when feeling well) and some aspect of his self-interest (avoiding a stroke). Dr. M. thus helped Mr. B. to confront himself and reflect about his own behavior, rather than being directly confronted by his practitioner (as happened with Dr. F.). Over time, this autonomy-supportive approach can encourage patients to take responsibility for change.

COMPARING OUTCOMES ON THE QUALITY OF FOLLOW-UP ENCOUNTERS

Fix-it role

Mr. B. did not keep his follow-up appointment. Dr. F. phoned and spoke to his wife about the missed appointment, and Mrs. B. made another appointment. Mr. B. resented the fact that that Dr. F. had spoken to his wife about his health problems. Mr. B. remained unconvinced that he needed to take medications when he felt well and knew that his blood pressure was normal.

Motivational role

Mr. and Mrs. B. both attended the follow-up appointment. Dr. M. reiterated to Mr. B. and his wife the rationale for taking the medication: to prevent a stroke even when he was feeling well. Mrs. B. expressed some anger toward her husband about not taking his medication, and said she was pleased that Dr. M. had invited her to the meeting.

46

When Mr. B. went to his next appointment, his wife accompanied him, but he did not want her to accompany him into the exam room. Dr. F. again told Mr. B. that the benefits of taking the medications were more important than the concerns about the side effects. Mr. B. felt annoyed by that remark, as well as misunderstood. In an attempt to clarify his position on medications, Mr. B. retorted that he didn't take the medications when he was feeling well because he could tell when his blood pressure was down. Dr. F. quickly corrected Mr. B. by telling him that he could not reliably judge his own blood pressure. Mr. B.'s response was "Really?" This ambiguous remark did not alert Dr. F. that he had not convinced Mr. B.

Because Mr. B. seemed to resent the way in which his wife expressed anger about his drug non-adherence, Dr. M. then reframed Mrs. B.'s expression of anger as a measure of how much she was concerned about Mr. B. and how her intent was to help him avoid having a stroke. Mr. B. became less defensive and more willing to talk about taking the medications on a regular basis, but he wanted to be in charge, and he did not want his wife to remind him unless he forgot the medications by the end of the day. He was also willing to let his wife buy a pill box so that he could monitor his use of medications by himself. He was beginning to take more responsibility for changing his behavior.

Dr. M. was more effective than Dr. F. in helping Mr. B. become more invested in making the follow-up appointment. Furthermore, Dr. M. introduced a different perspective by helping Mr. B. to view his wife as caring about him rather than being angry with him. Together, Mr. and Mrs. B. reached a new understanding about how to work together.

COMPARING OUTCOMES ON MR. B.'S MOTIVATION AND FAMILY INVOLVEMENT

Fix-it role

Mr. B. felt that he should take his medications, but only because Dr. F. had told him he should. His wife also nagged him about taking his tablets. He was annoyed by his pressure, because he felt that neither his wife nor Dr. F. understood his position.

Motivational role

Both Mr. B. and his wife were concerned that he could have a stroke, even when he was feeling well. He had discussed this concern with his wife after his last appointment and had become even more concerned about avoiding a stroke. He seemed committed to taking his medications on a more regular basis.

With Dr. F., Mr. B. felt pushed to change (extrinsic motivation) and resented his wife's involvement in his health care. In contrast, Dr. M. helped Mr. and Mrs. B. together reach a greater understanding about the risk of a stroke and the benefits of adherence, even when Mr. B. was feeling well. Furthermore, Dr. M. enlisted Mrs. B. as an asset rather than a barrier to support change. Mr. B. began to feel a need to take the medication on a regular basis (intrinsic motivation).

YOUR SUMMARY

Reflect: write a summary about what you have learned that was new for you.

_____
_____
_____
_____
_____
_____
_____
_____
_____
_____
_____
_____
_____
_____
_____
_____
_____
_____
_____
_____
_____
_____
_____
_____
_____

Enhance: write down your ideas about how your new learning could improve your interactions with patients. Add your notes to your learning portfolio.

_____
_____
_____
_____
_____
_____
_____
_____
_____
_____
_____
_____
_____
_____
_____

REFERENCES

1. Haynes RB, McKibbon KA, Kanani R. Systematic review of randomised trials of interventions to assist patients to follow prescriptions for medications [published erratum appears in Lancet 1997 Apr 19;349(9059):1180]. Lancet 1996;348: 383-386
2. Rudd P, Byyny RL, Zachary V, et al. Pill count measures of compliance in a drug trial: variability and suitability. American Journal of Hypertension 1988;1: 309-312
3. Sackett DL, Snow JC. The magnitude of compliance and noncompliance. In: Haynes RB, Taylor DW, Sackett DL, eds. Compliance in health care. Baltimore: Johns Hopkins University Press; 1979:11-22
4. Botelho RJ, Dudrak R. Home assessment of adherence to long-term medication in the elderly. Journal of Family Practice 1992;35: 61-65
5. World Health Organization. Adherence to long-term therapies: Evidence for action. 2003. Geneva, Switzerland, World Health Organization
6. Dwyer MS, Levy RA, Menander KB. Improving medication compliance through the use of modern dosage forms. Journal of Pharmacy Technology 1986;2: 166-170
7. Epstein LH, Cluss PA. A behavioral medicine perspective on adherence to long-term medical regimens. Journal of Consulting and Clinical Psychology 1982;50: 950-971
8. DiMatteo MR, DiNicola DD. Achieving patient compliance: The psychology of the medical practitioner's role. New York: Pergamon Press; 1982
9. Horwitz RI, Horwitz SM. Adherence to treatment and health outcomes. Archives of Internal Medicine 1993;153: 1863-1868
10. Becker MH, Maiman LA. Sociobehavioral determinants of compliance with health and medical care recommendations. Medical Care 1975;13: 10-24
11. Williams GC, Rodin GC, Ryan RM, et al. Autonomous regulation and long-term medication adherence in adult outpatients. Health Psychology 1998;17: 269-276
12. Tuckett D, Boulton M, Olson C, et al. Meetings between experts: An approach to sharing ideas in medical consultations. London: Tavistock; 1985
13. Botelho RJ. Negotiating partnerships in healthcare: Contexts and methods. In: Suchman AL, Botelho RJ, Hinton-Walker P, eds. Partnerships in healthcare: Transforming relational process. Rochester, NY: University of Rochester Press; 1998:19-49

CHAPTER 3

ADAPTING YOUR ROLE TO PATIENTS' NEEDS

FOR REFLECTION

What different roles can you adopt to best meet your patients' particular needs?

OVERVIEW

You are more likely to help patients change if you adapt your role to meet their changing needs over time. The fix-it role is effective and highly appropriate in addressing injuries and diseases caused by risk behaviors. In this role, we typically wait until patients have medical complications before advising them to change. The fix-it approach is based on the assumption that patients will only change when they are sick. This advice-giving approach, even if repeated over time, is of limited effectiveness. But you can intervene earlier and identify at-risk patients before such complications occur. In the preventive role, you educate and provide advice in patient-centered ways. When this tailored approach does not work or loses its effectiveness, you can adopt a motivational role and develop an individualized approach whether or not your patients have any complications. The motivational role helps you work more effectively with so-called resistant patients over time than using the fix-it or preventive role.

Personal background and formal education powerfully shape our professional role. The professional role that we adopt in turn shapes how we talk and act with patients. Understanding the fix-it, preventive and motivational roles, preferably early in our careers, can help us make better decisions about when it is appropriate to adopt different roles with patients. Unfortunately, most of us have been predominantly trained to adopt a fix-it role. Familiarity with this role can blind us to alternatives, so that we fail to develop an appreciation of the challenge of adopting different roles with patients. A classic question (modified from anthropology) highlights the challenge of developing self-awareness about roles and assumptions:

How can a fish see water?

Professional training can be like water to the fish. We may not be fully aware of how our role limits our capacity to work more effectively with patients. It is important to have an in-depth understanding of them because it can assist with the process of using limited contact time efficiently with patients.[1-3] The fix-it, preventive and motivational roles are described in terms of

- Characteristics: how you can recognize different roles
- Functions: what you do in each role
- Boundaries: what your respective responsibilities are with your patients
- Outcomes: the impact your role has on patients

Role characteristics help to set parameters around role functions, which describe your tasks in working with patients, and role boundaries, which shape how you and your patients have shared or separate responsibilities for different health care issues. Both role functions and role boundaries affect the emotional tone (positive vs. negative) and distance (overinvolvement vs. underinvolvement) in your relationship with patients.[4-7] These categories (characteristics, functions, boundaries) are used to describe a continuum of roles. A greater understanding of this continuum may help you adopt the right role to meet your patients' needs, because different roles can have a positive and a negative impact on patients.

Learning Exercise 3.1: Anchor your learning
   The purpose of the exercise is to anchor your learning to a particular experience in working with someone. If you have not previously been asked questions about role functions and boundaries, take a moment now to reflect about these questions before reading about individual role characteristics. This may prepare you better for making some important distinctions between different kinds of roles.

Identify a patient (family member or friend) who resists changing his or her behavior. Reflect on the following questions:

1. *Role functions: What are your tasks in working with this patient? How can you try to make or help the patient change?*
2. *Role boundaries: What are your responsibilities, your patient's responsibilities and your shared responsibilities in addressing different health care issues?*
3. *How do you feel about what has happened or could happen?*

In the following discussion, the fix-it, preventive and motivational practitioners (or doctors) are given the following abbreviations—FP, PP and MP (or Dr. F., Dr. P. and Dr. M.), respectively—to represent the different roles described in this book.[2;3]

ROLE CHARACTERISTICS

FIX-IT ROLE

When we adopt the fix-it role, we address risk behaviors as we would treat diseases. Typically, we wait until patients have developed medical complications from their unhealthy behaviors. We then feel a sense of urgency that patients should change their behaviors immediately, almost as if it were an emergency. In our enthusiasm to help patients, we may impose our own values and perceptions about health and disease on them.

We can adopt two kinds of fix-it roles: traditional versus nontraditional. In the traditional role, we provide authoritarian advice to our patients in a paternalistic and controlling style, even when patients are not yet ready to think about change. We use words such as *must*, *ought* or *should* to instruct patients to change. Even if we do not use these words, we may still imply that patients should change. We neglect to acknowledge the patient's choice to change or not to change. Needless to say, most patients do not respond favorably to this kind of fix-it approach, as was seen in the case of Mr. B. and Dr. F. in Chapter 2.

We can also adopt a different kind of fix-it role and provide authoritative advice to patients in a nonthreatening and noncoercive manner. We may not fully understand our patients' perspectives, but we do explicitly acknowledge a patient's right to stay the same. Even with this kind of nontraditional approach, many patients still do not change their behavior.

In both kinds of fix-it roles, we educate our patients in practitioner-centered ways by focusing on the negative consequences of their risk behaviors. In effect, practitioner-centered education and advice becomes the *agency of change*.

> **Fix-it role:** Dr. F. advised Mr. D. in an authoritative, directive manner that he must lose weight to control his diabetes and hypertension. Mr. D. responded well to this advice. He lost 50 pounds the following year, controlled his

noninsulin-dependent diabetes by diet alone, kept his hemoglobin A1c within the normal range and reduced his antihypertensive regimen from two tablets to one tablet a day. He resented it when Dr. F. lectured him about the dangers of smoking and advised him to quit. After leaving his last appointment, he was particularly annoyed, and complained to his girlfriend that Dr. F. did not understand him.

Commentary: Dr. F. worked well in a fix-it role when advising Mr. D. to lose weight. Mr. D. appreciated the advice and lost weight because he disliked taking more tablets and feared diabetes because of the effect that it had had on his father. Mr. D. felt positive about Dr. F.'s help. When Dr. F. continued this same approach and advised Mr. D. to quit smoking, Dr. F. was unaware that Mr. D. was annoyed and felt misunderstood.

PREVENTIVE ROLE

When adopting preventive roles, you work with patients before risk behaviors have caused complications.[2;3;8-10] You relate to patients in egalitarian ways. With a limited understanding of their perspective, you use your expertise authoritatively and provide patient-centered education and a rationale for change, but you do not tell patients that they should change. Instead, you support the patient's autonomy to decide what to do. In effect, tailored educational messages become the *agent of change.*

Preventive role: The nurse practitioner (PP) on Dr. F.'s team saw Mr. D. about his smoking problem. She adopted a preventive role after receiving training in a new smoking cessation program developed by the U.S. Agency for Health Care Quality. (This evidence-based smoking cessation program uses the five A's model: ask, advise, assess assist and arrange follow-up). PP assessed the patient's smoking history in more detail and came to better understand how Mr. D. struggled with his addiction to nicotine. She then told him how to use the nicotine patch. Mr. D. tried it, but one morning, he forgot to put the patch on and started smoking during a work break. Mr. D. was under a great deal of work stress and felt that this was not a good time to try and quit again. PP was unsure about how to motivate Mr. D. to try again, but encouraged him to do so soon. She then referred him to a health educator who was recently trained in a motivational approach to behavior change.
Commentary: The preventive role worked better than a fix-it role because Mr. D. felt that the PP understood his difficulties in quitting. Even though PP reached an impasse with Mr. D., she left him thinking about the challenge of quitting, rather than feeling annoyed about being misunderstood.

Although the preventive role is helpful, you may still feel unfulfilled if you are unable to get a commitment to change, particularly from resistant patients who are at high risk for complications. This unfulfilled feeling can arise in part because your expectations exceed the limitations of a preventive role. A motivational role may help you work more effectively in such situations and set more realistic expectations.

MOTIVATIONAL ROLE

An essential characteristic of a motivational practitioner is the capacity for self-awareness: understanding how culture, values, beliefs and attitudes affect roles and assumptions in our clinical encounters (see Figure 3.1).

Figure 3.1. Factors Affecting Our Roles and Assumptions

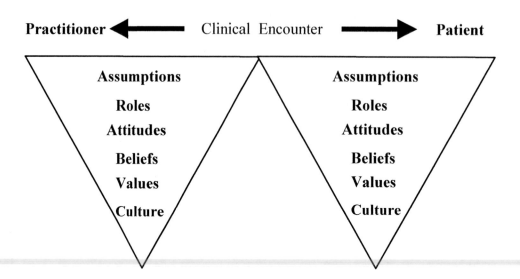

Motivational roles are particularly appropriate when patients do not respond to health information and advice. This role can help you learn how to engage patients in the process of change on an ongoing basis, without evoking destructive reactions from them. Part of this process involves you and your patients learning about, respecting and working with your differences in perceptions and values about behavior change.

To understand your differences, you should ask patients about the benefits and concerns of engaging in a risk behavior and of changing their behavior. In this way, you relate to patients in flexible and autonomy-supportive ways in order to use your influence more effectively. Your dialogues with patients are two-way, educational processes. You generate meaningful dialogues that catalyze the change process. In effect, dialogue becomes the agency of change in helping you develop individualized interventions for patients. This process in turn helps patients shift their values and perceptions about behavior change so they become motivated to change.

This is easier said than done. Given your differences with your patients, you have to *be* with someone before you can effectively *do* something together. *Being* means that you reflect about yourself and your patients without trying to do something; in other words, you learn about, and appreciate, your differences.

Reflection-in-action involves both being and doing: you simultaneously try to understand yourself and your patients while helping them change.[11] In other words, you reflect about how your actions affect patients in the moment and make instantaneous adjustments to work effectively with them.

This does not always happen. Impasses commonly occur with patients. When they do, time-outs after patient encounters and reflection-on-action can help you work through such impasses.[11] This process can then help you generate ideas about how to respond and act in new ways.

Motivational role: After receiving training in how to adopt a motivational role, the health educator (MP) on Dr. F.'s team encouraged Mr. D. to view his work stress from a different perspective by stating, "I understand why you may think that this is the worst time to try to quit smoking, but in fact it may be the best time to try again soon." Mr. D. looked puzzled and asked why. MP continued, "Well, work stress is one of your most likely reasons to start smoking again. If you can quit at a time of high work stress, you are more likely to avoid a relapse when you are under a lot of stress again." Mr. D. was silent, and MP did not say anything either. Mr. D. then agreed that it was a good point, and that he needed to think about it more. MP asked Mr. D. whether he would like to come back to talk about work stress and quitting again. Mr. D. stated he would come back in two weeks.

Commentary: The health educator provided a different perspective on the same issue (used a reframing intervention) to help Mr. D. reflect about whether to set a quit date on account of work stress. Furthermore, MP did not push Mr. D. to set a quit date, but let him decide whether and when to return for a follow-up appointment.

Although different practitioners were used in these three examples, everyone on the health care team needs training in how to adapt their role to meet patients' needs. The key questions are

- Which role is most appropriate for this patient in a particular situation?
- How can the health care team best work together in helping patients change?

Role characteristics can help you understand different ways of interacting with your patients. The characteristics assigned to each role are not fixed; you can blend them in ways that achieve favorable outcomes. Their purpose is to help you understand the spectrum of role characteristics and become more deliberate, explicit and conscious about the kind of roles that you can adopt in working with patients (see Table 3.1).

Table 3.1. Spectrum of Role Characteristics

Fix-it Roles	Preventive Roles	Motivational Roles
Agents of curative medicine	Agents of public health	Agents of behavioral science
Focus on diseases	Focus on risks and harm	Focus on benefits, risks & harm
Paternalistic relationship	Egalitarian relationship	Flexible partnership
Practitioner-centered education	Patient-centered education	Educational exchange
Authoritarian advice	Authoritative advice	Dialogue
Nonspecific interventions	Tailored interventions	Individualized interventions
Impose their values and perceptions about health and disease onto patients	Understand patients' values and perceptions about risk behaviors	Help patients change their values and perceptions about health behavior change

ROLE FUNCTIONS

Only the fix-it and motivational roles are described in this and the next section because they represent the two ends of a role continuum. To help you understand how your stance and functions in working with patients are very different when adopting these roles, compare the role functions in Table 3.2. This can help you understand distinct ways of addressing behavior change: working with or against patients.

FIX-IT ROLE

In this role, we try to make patients change by forming a coalition with the risk behavior against the patient (see Figure 3.2). In effect, our focus on behavior change becomes more important than our relationship with the patient. Such relationships take on an adversarial tone in spite of good intentions to improve the patient's health.

Figure 3.2. Coalition against the Patient (Jeopardized Relational Connection)

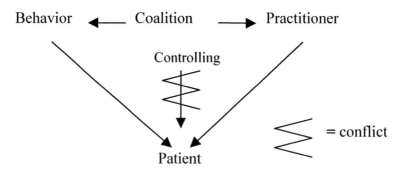

We may threaten, scare and/or confront patients to force them to change by stressing the anticipated complications from their risk behaviors. We set a gold standard or ideal goals for patients and give them directives on how to achieve these goals. Some patients may respond favorably to this approach because this is what they want from us.

MOTIVATIONAL ROLE

In this role, you establish an alliance with your patients to address risk behaviors so that they feel supported in working toward change (see Figure 3.3). You help patients understand their health values and perceptions about behavior change. Consequently, they feel as though they have an ally or coach who understands their perspective. You educate them about the risks of their behaviors in respectful, nonthreatening and meaningful ways. In effect, you help patients confront themselves about the need for behavior change.

You can also invite patients to consider changing their health values and perceptions about behavior change. A dynamic tension can then develop between providing nondirect support to patients and encouraging them to change. But if you push too hard or too fast, patients may resist.

You negotiate with patients about what they think are achievable goals. Using an approach of risk and harm reduction, patients can take intermediary steps toward their goals. You encourage patients to find their own solutions before offering your ideas about how they can achieve their goals.

Figure 3.3. Alliance with the Patient (Potential Partnership)

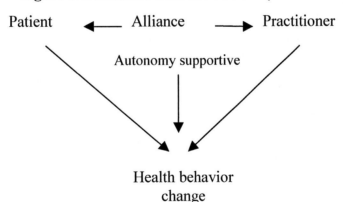

There is an important distinction between direct and indirect confrontation. In the fix-it role, you directly confront patients about the risks and consequences of their unhealthy behaviors. You work against resistance and try to break down patients' rationalizations for engaging in these behaviors. In the motivational role, you work indirectly, addressing the inconsistencies in their rationalizations and offering new perspectives, to help patients confront themselves about the need for behavior change. Chapters 11-12 discuss how you can work with patients in this way.

ROLE BOUNDARIES

You and your patients have both separate and shared responsibilities for addressing health behavior change and the medical aspects of risk behaviors. These responsibilities shape the role boundaries for the fix-it and motivational roles (see Table 3.2). For example, you may take full responsibility for dealing with the clinical issues (e.g., treatment of gastritis associated with alcohol use); the patient may take full responsibility for the social consequences (e.g., driving while intoxicated); and you and your patient may share responsibility for dealing with the psychological issues (e.g., depression leading to an increased use of alcohol). However, these issues are not usually addressed explicitly.

FIX-IT ROLE

When adopting a fix-it role, we may overstep the boundaries of our responsibilities and try to make patients change their behavior. We may fall into this trap for several reasons:

- Deep commitment and a sense of caring for our patients' well-being
- Desire to help patients avoid the complications of risk behaviors
- Inadequate training in handling time-pressured situations
- Unrealistically high expectations about acting as a catalyst for change

Consequently, in the fix-it role, we tend to take on either too much or too little responsibility for our patients. At one extreme, we are highly conscientious in our work and become idealistic rescuers. We get emotionally overinvolved with our patients; we try to do most of the work for them. Over time, we run the risk of becoming professionally burned out and of ending up at the other extreme, as nihilistic minimalists. We can then become underinvolved with our patients or disengage from them altogether. Disillusioned and pessimistic about them, we may end up reacting in negative ways (e.g., scapegoating, blaming or punishing).

MOTIVATIONAL ROLE

In the motivational role, you develop an appropriate involvement with your patients that is flexible to both of your respective needs, responsibilities and goals. In brief, you develop a shared understanding of how you will work together over time. This understanding can help to avoid practitioner overinvolvement and minimize patient resistance.

ROLE OUTCOMES

As a consequence of role characteristics, functions and boundaries, practitioners experience different outcomes when adopting fix-it and motivational roles (see Table 3.2). In the fix-it role, success is measured only in terms of behavior change. If we remain in this role long after it is clear that health information and advice-giving are not working for the patient, we may experience negative feelings such as anger, frustration, anxiety, despondency and pessimism. Furthermore, patients may feel a sense of obligation to change, without being ready to.

If patients do not change, we may run the risk of expressing our emotions inappropriately, for example, blaming our patients and getting into arguments with them. Or we may fail to recognize our anger toward our patients and simply disengage from them. Patients may also experience similar negative emotions. For example, they may get so frustrated or angry that they discontinue the relationship with us.

Negative emotions arising from patient encounters may remind us of the need to adopt a motivational role. If we do not change our role, these negative emotions can build up inside, and we run the risk of professional dissatisfaction or even burnout. At some level, we try to make change happen, even when the patient is not ready. When adopting a motivational role, your success is measured in terms of increasing patients' readiness to change over time. You are more likely to evoke positive emotions with your patients and help them become intrinsically motivated to change. Consequently, you find your clinical work increasingly enriching and rewarding.

Table 3.2. Contrasting Role Functions, Boundaries and Outcomes

Fix-it Roles	Motivational Roles
Role Functions Form coalitions against patients Threaten, scare and confront patients Set ideal goals for change Give directives on how to change	**Role Functions** Form alliances with patients Help patients confront themselves Negotiate about goals for change Help patients find their own solutions
Role Boundaries Either get overinvolved or disengage Tend to work too much or too little, depending on their own needs Assume too much or too little responsibility for promoting behavior change	**Role Boundaries** Maintain appropriate involvement Work appropriately, taking into account their needs and their patients' needs Help patients take responsibility for motivating change
Outcomes Evoke negative emotions toward patients Argue with patients Make patients feel obliged to change Run the risk of professional burnout	**Outcomes** Evoke positive emotions toward change Engage patients to work on change Enhance intrinsic motivation Enhance professional satisfaction

YOUR CHOICE ABOUT ROLES

Given the demands for increased productivity and performance with limited resources in health care (the constant challenge of doing more with less), a major issue is the additional time that may be needed to adopt a motivational role with patients. In some countries, practitioners may have 60 to 100 patients per day, with an average of three to six minutes per encounter. This makes the practitioner's dilemma of changing roles even more challenging. We need to work smarter, not harder. Such circumstances may call for using alternative approaches, for example: having patients fill in the decision balance while waiting to see the practitioner; using community workers to help with patients before and after the seeing the practitioner; and organizing individual and group sessions led by lay counselors.

Whatever your setting, it may help to work through your own decision balance (see Chapters 1 and 11 for examples of how to complete a decision balance) about whether to adopt a motivational role, particularly when the fix-it role is not working. This may help you better understand your own resistance to change and your perceptions about the advantages and disadvantages of these two roles.

Table 3.3 provides an example of a completed decision balance, weighing the pros and cons of each role. The list is not exhaustive, and you can certainly add many more items, particularly about organizational issues. The short-term, professional demands and needs to treat diseases are usually given a much higher priority than the long-term goal of reducing the prevalence of risk behaviors. In an analogous fashion, patients face a similar dilemma: short-term benefits outweighing the long-term gain of improved health.

Table 3.3. Comparing the Fix-it and Motivational Roles

Reasons for Staying in the Fix-it Role	Reasons for Adopting the Motivational Role
Advantages of the Fix-it Role Very quick—takes one to three minutes Standardized intervention Often designed as single interventions Works with some patients and issues Easy to learn	Disadvantages of the Fix-it Role Patients may not want advice Wastes time if used repetitively Practitioners become bored with this approach Repeated advice generates frustration Patients may avoid practitioners
Disadvantages of the Motivational Role Takes more patient time Need to work with people over time Takes time to develop complex skills Often takes time to get results Need ongoing training	Advantages of the Motivational Role Individualized interventions Doing the effective thing Expands repertoire of skill Enhances professional satisfaction Lifelong learning

Regrettably, most educational and clinical organizations lack appropriately trained personnel, adequate reimbursement and infrastructures (such as data management systems and information technology) to develop comprehensive behavior change and disease management programs. Furthermore, you may find that your educational and/or clinical organizations do not understand the importance of making these role distinctions. For these reasons, you may lack support for your continuing professional development as a motivational practitioner. This situation may affect your decision about whether to learn how to adopt a motivational role.

These role descriptions can help your educational and/or clinical organizations appreciate the benefits of enhancing practitioner and patient satisfaction in addressing health behavior change issues. As a result, your organization may decide to support your development as a motivational practitioner. Some organizations even go a step further by developing quality assurance programs to identify practitioners who have poor patient satisfaction ratings and suboptimal performance in addressing behavior change. They then provide these practitioners with self-directed learning methods and training sessions to help them develop their patient skills.

As a step further, health care organizations can integrate continuous improvement methods into training and clinical aspects of their comprehensive behavior change and disease management programs.[12-15] With appropriate support, the whole health care team can continuously improve their ability to work as motivational practitioners. This approach has the potential of enhancing the team's overall performance in reducing the prevalence of risk behaviors in cost-effective ways.[16]

YOUR SUMMARY

Reflect: write a summary about what you have learned that was new for you.

_____
_____
_____
_____
_____
_____
_____
_____
_____
_____
_____
_____
_____

_____

_____

_____

_____

_____

_____

_____

_____

_____

_____

Enhance: write down your ideas about how your new learning could improve your interactions with patients. Add your notes to your learning portfolio.

_____

_____

_____

_____

_____

_____

_____

_____

_____

_____

_____

_____

_____

_____

REFERENCES

1. Australian Government Pub. Service. Appendix 2 The role of the medical practitioner as an agent for disease prevention. Looking forward to better health. Vol. 3. The workshops and consultations: Reports to the Better Health Commission. Canberra, Australia: Australian Government Pub. Service; 1986:201-212
2. Demak MM, Becker MH. The doctor-patient relationship and counseling for preventive care. Patient Education & Counseling 1987;9: 5-24
3. Calnan M. Examining the general practitioner's role in health education: A critical review. Family Practice 1988;5: 217-223
4. Linklater D, MacDougall S. Boundary issues. What do they mean for family physicians? Canadian Family Physician 1993;39: 2569-2573
5. Rourke JT, Smith LF, Brown JB. Patients, friends, and relationship boundaries. Canadian Family Physician 1993;39: 2557-2564
6. Gabbard GO, Nadelson C. Professional boundaries in the physician-patient relationship. Journal of the American Medical Association 1995;273: 1445-1449
7. Yeo M, Longhurst M. Intimacy in the patient-physician relationship. Committee on Ethics of the College of Family Physicians of Canada. Canadian Family Physician 1996;42: 1505-1508

8. Johns MB, Hovell MF, Ganiats T, et al. Primary care and health promotion: A model for preventive medicine. American Journal of Preventive Medicine 1987;3: 346-357

9. Anonymous. Education for health. A role for physicians and the efficacy of health education efforts. Council on Scientific Affairs. Journal of the American Medical Association 1990;263: 1816-1819

10. McClellan W. The physician and patient education: A review. Patient Education & Counseling 1986;8: 151-163

11. Schon D. The reflective practitioner. New York: Basic Books; 1983

12. Berwick DM. A primer on leading the improvement of systems. British Medical Journal 1996;312: 619-622

13. Berwick DM, Nolan TW. Physicians as leaders in improving health care: A new series in Annals of Internal Medicine [see comments]. Ann Intern Med 1998;128: 289-292

14. Wagner EH, Austin BT, Von Korff M. Organizing care for patients with chronic illness. Milbank Quarterly 1996;74: 511-544

15. Taplin S, Galvin MS, Payne T, et al. Putting population-based care into practice: Real option or rhetoric? JABFP 1998;11: 116-126

16. Thompson RS, Taplin SH, McAfee TA, et al. Primary and secondary prevention services in clinical practice: Twenty years' experience in development, implementation, and evaluation. JAMA 1995;273: 1130-113

CHAPTER 4

BECOMING AWARE OF ASSUMPTIONS

*How do different assumptions from practitioners, patients and their families
help or hinder the prospects of promoting patient behavior change?*

OVERVIEW

Many training programs do not provide adequate time, preparation, and opportunities to reflect on and understand implicit assumptions that affect the practitioner-patient-family relationship. This chapter may help you become aware of how assumptions either facilitate or hinder the process of motivating patients to change. Culture, values, beliefs and attitudes powerfully shape the assumptions that you and your patients make about behavior change. Both you and your patients can benefit from identifying how assumptions can positively and negatively affect your relationship in working together. Facilitating assumptions enhance the prospect of motivating patients to change. Stumbling-block assumptions are self-limiting, self-defeating and/or self-fulfilling prophecies.

Each person entering a human service profession should begin by examining her or his underlying assumptions about the human condition.

George Albee, *The Scientist Practitioner* (December 1991)

This quotation highlights the need to understand our assumptions when working with patients. The following exercise poses questions that may help you identify implicit assumptions that may facilitate or hinder the change process for your patients.

Learning Exercise 4.1: Think about a challenging patient

Think about a particular patient whom you find challenging to work with in terms of changing a risk behavior. Reflect on the questions below.

Practitioner-focused Questions:
- *What are your assumptions that help or hinder the change process for this patient?*
- *Why do you think the patient engages in this behavior?*
- *What do think you should do about it?*
- *What do you think the patient should do about it?*
- *What feelings do you have about the prospect of change, and why do you feel that way?*

Patient-focused Questions:
- *What are the patient's and family's assumptions that help or hinder the prospects for change?*
- *What is the patient's thinking about why he or she engages in this behavior?*
- *What do the patient and family think he or she should do about it?*
- *What do they think you should do about it?*
- *What feelings do they have about the prospects for change, and why do they feel that way?*

Take a moment to write down or make a mental note about your assumptions. The next exercise may help clarify whether you are making assumptions that hinder change (stumbling-block assumptions) or ones that help change (facilitating assumptions). Both you and your patients can benefit from clarifying whether these assumptions hinder or facilitate your work together. You will be more effective if you work with patients in ways that change stumbling-block assumptions to facilitating assumptions.

RANGE OF ASSUMPTIONS

Contrasting a fix-it and a motivational practitioner working with the same patient will illustrate how stumbling-block and facilitating assumptions affect the process and outcome of care. In the following example, commentaries will be made about such assumptions from three perspectives: practitioner, patient, and family.

PRACTITIONER'S ASSUMPTIONS

In a fix-it role, such as the one Dr. F. takes below, we are often too time-pressured to recognize whether our assumptions are creating stumbling blocks.

How Dr. F.'s stumbling-block assumptions affected Dave: Mrs. W., a single parent, brought her 15-year-old son, Dave, to see the doctor because Dave had started smoking marijuana. Dave clearly did not want to be there. Dr. F. and Mrs. W. both assumed that Dave was going to be a victim of his drug use, drop out of school and run into trouble with the law. Dr. F. tried to scare Dave into not using marijuana by telling him it could lead to more dangerous drug addictions and trouble with the law. When Dr. F. asked Dave why he smoked marijuana, Dave stated that he could study better at school. Dr. F. thought Dave's reasoning was ridiculous and that it was hopeless trying to deal with him. When Dr. F. asked Mrs. W. what concerned her about Dave's future, she expressed concerns similar to those of Dr. F. Mrs. W. also felt frustrated and hopeless about trying to stop her son from ruining his life. Dr. F. recommended to Dave that he see a counselor. Dave was not keen on this idea.

In a motivational role, you are more likely to make facilitating assumptions about yourself, your patients and their families. Acting on these assumptions, you can model for patients and family members how to develop their own facilitating assumptions. Let's see how Dr. M. behaves in the same scenario.

How Dr. M.'s facilitating assumptions affected Dave: Dave clearly did not want to be there, and Dr. M.'s immediate concern was about being triangulated into a conflict between mother and son. Dr. M. listened to Mrs. W. express concerns that her son might become a victim of drug use, drop out of school and run into trouble with the law. Dr. M. acknowledged her concerns and then thanked Dave for coming to the appointment. Dr. M. asked Dave why he decided to come with his mother. Dave said he wanted her to get off his back because he felt he was old enough to do what he liked. In his interactions with both Dave and his mother, Dr. M. validated both of their perspectives without taking sides or approving of Dave's use of marijuana.

Mrs. W. then stated that she didn't want Dave and his friends smoking marijuana in her home. She felt very strongly that they should stop. When Dr. M. asked Dave why he smoked marijuana, he said that he wanted to be part of the in crowd, that he could study better, that it was fun and that he didn't want to be regarded as a nerd by his peer group. Dr. M. paraphrased what Dave said by stating, "Either you smoke marijuana, or you're a nerd?" Dave agreed. Dr. M. planted a seed of an idea by asking Dave whether he thought he had more than two choices. Dr. M. next asked Dave if marijuana was indeed improving his grades in school. Dave looked to his mother and replied, "Not really, but I'm more calm at school." Dr. M. suggested that Dave might need to do something else to reduce his stress and keep his grades up.

Dr. M. proceeded to ask Mrs. W. what she thought needed to be done. Mrs. W. stated that she felt that Dave should be in counseling and that he should stop using all drugs because she was afraid he would get in trouble with the law or get shot in a drug deal. Dr. M. asked Dave what he thought needed to be done. Dave said that he didn't think he needed counseling, and he wanted his mother to get off his back.

Dr. M. said that he was impressed by how much Dave and his mother cared for one another, even though they had a difference of opinion on this particular subject. He suggested that perhaps they should go to counseling together to work out their differences. They decided to think about this option. When Mrs. W. repeated her concerns about her son getting into trouble, Dr. M. suggested that perhaps by being too protective, Mrs. W. might be making her son do things that she did not want him to do. In the presence of Dave, Dr. M. encouraged Mrs. W. to separate the things that she could and could not control. For example, she could make it absolutely clear to her son and any of his friends that no drugs should be used or kept in the house and that she was prepared to call the police to inspect her house if she ever suspected drug use in it. Dr. M. mentioned that she certainly should try to stop Dave from using drugs in her house and in school and encourage him not to use drugs elsewhere, but that ultimately only Dave could decide whether to use them. Dr. M. also suggested to Mrs. W. that Dave's father might help them sort through this problem. Mrs. W. hadn't told her ex-husband about Dave's drug use. After some reflection, she thought this was a good idea, since her ex-husband had been in recovery for many years. Dave seemed uncomfortable with this idea but did not raise any objections.

Dr. M. then asked Dave what his father thought about the current situation. Dave did not know because he had stopped visiting his father about eight months ago because of friction with his father's new girlfriend, who had tried to get Dave to go to church. Dave resented her trying to tell him what to do, so he stopped seeing his father.

Mrs. W. and her son were ambivalent about counseling, because they had reservations about the possible need for it. Mrs. W. and her son wanted to think about whether to set up a follow-up appointment to discuss what to do further.

Learning Exercise 4.2: Reflect about your assumptions

Circle a letter to state whether you disagree or agree with the assumptions listed in Table 4.1. This exercise can help you reflect about your assumptions that you make with patients.

SDA = *Strongly disagree*
D   = *Disagree*
N   = *Neither agree nor disagree*
A   = *Agree*
SA   = *Strongly agree*

Table 4.1. Reflecting about Your Assumptions

Assumptions	Circle Your Response
About Ourselves *We can make patients change their behaviors.*	SDA DA N A SA
We can motivate patients if we understand their reasons not to change.	SDA DA N A SA
It is a waste of time trying to help patients who do not want to change.	SDA DA N A SA
About Our Patients *Patients are poor decision makers and too weak-willed to change.*	SDA DA N A SA
Patients can find the time, energy and motivation to change.	SDA DA N A SA
Patients are not willing to take the responsibility for change.	SDA DA N A SA
About the Patient's Family Members *Most families believe that the patient is incapable of changing.*	SDA DA N A SA
Most families can support the patient in ways that facilitate change.	SDA DA N A SA
Most families typically only nag the patient to change.	SDA DA N A SA

After completing this task, reflect about whether you think that your response to these statements can help or hinder the change process.

PATIENTS' ASSUMPTIONS

Patients also make assumptions that can either hinder or facilitate the change process. You can work with patients to help them transform their stumbling-block assumptions into facilitating ones (see Table 4.2), thereby facilitating the change process. Many patients make assumptions that facilitate the change process and change their risk behavior without even consulting their practitioner.

Dave's perspective about Dr. F. and Mrs. W.: Dave assumed that Dr. F. would agree with Mrs. W.'s concerns and recommendation that he see a counselor. He also assumed that Dr. F. would take a male parental role and try to coerce him into changing his behavior. Dave asserted that smoking marijuana was not putting his health at risk and that, in fact, it was improving his school performance. Dave assumed that his mother and Dr. F. were not capable of understanding why he smoked marijuana. In contrast to the fears of his mother and Dr. F., Dave did not think that he would get into trouble with the law. He resented Dr. F. for siding with his mother.

Dave's perspective about Dr. M. and Mrs. W.: Dave's previous experience with Dr. M. was that he took a neutral position in dealing with most family problems, since Dr. M. had helped his mother and his alcoholic father go through a separation when Dave was nine years old. (His father has been in recovery for over four years.) Dave assumed that Dr. M. would not side entirely with his mother against him, that he would try to understand Dave's side of the story and that he would help Dave and his mother deal with their conflicts. Dr. M. took a stand that there was a struggle between Dave's need for independence and his mother's need to protect. Dave did not feel criticized for his use of marijuana, but he did feel that his doctor probably did not approve of it. He began to think that his mother was trying to help him, but not in a very effective way.

Table 4.2. Patient's Perspective:
Stumbling-Block Assumptions　　　Versus　　　Facilitating Assumptions

About Myself (the Patient)	
I think that the short-term benefits of unhealthy behaviors outweigh their long-term risks.	*I can change my perceptions and values about health behavior change.*
I lack will power, confidence and/or the ability to change.	*I can motivate myself to change and develop the confidence and/or ability to change.*
About My Practitioner	
My practitioner cannot understand the challenge of changing my "risk" behavior.	*My practitioner can help me feel positive for thinking more about change.*
My practitioner makes me feel guilty, ashamed or humiliated for engaging in risk behaviors.	*My practitioner can help me view lapses and relapses as learning opportunities.*
About My Family Members	
My family members cannot understand why I do what I do.	*My family members will respect the pace at which I work through the change process.*
My family members only interfere, make the situation worse and/or are unhelpful.	*My family members will support me in a variety of ways to help me change.*

Family's Assumptions

Family members can also make stumbling-block assumptions that hinder their understanding of behavioral change (see Table 4.3).

Mrs. W.'s perspective about Dr. F. and her son—Mrs. W. wanted Dr. F. to get her son into counseling. She viewed Dr. F. as an ally and wanted him to behave like a father toward her son. She wanted her son to shape up now and wanted Dr. F. to get her son off drugs.

Family members can also make facilitating assumptions that can lead to a greater understanding of unhealthy behavior.

Mrs. W.'s perspective about Dr. M. and her son: Mrs. W. assumed that Dr. M. would try to get her and her son to work together in a different way. She assumed that Dr. M. would try to understand Dave's side of the story, a task she had difficulty doing. She was amazed by Dr. M.'s suggestion about contacting her ex-husband because she had stopped talking to him except about issues related to visitation. After talking with Dr. M., she thought her ex-husband might help Dave avoid repeating what had happened to his dad.

Table 4.3. Family's Perspectives:
Stumbling-block Assumptions   versus   Facilitating Assumptions

About Ourselves (as Family Members)	
At all costs, we must make him or her change.	*Nagging him or her will not help him or her change.*
We feel incapable of helping him or her change.	*We can enhance his or her prospects of changing.*
About Our Family Member (the patient)	
He or she just has to pull himself/herself together to change.	*He or she can work to accelerate the pace of change.*
He or she deserves our rejection if there is no change.	*He or she will inform us about what kinds of support are needed at different times.*
About Our Family Member's Practitioner	
The practitioner can "fix" him or her.	*The practitioner can help him or her become more receptive to the possibility of change.*
The practitioner will work with us to make him or her change.	*The practitioner will work with our family's strengths.*

By acting in autonomy-supportive ways, you let patients decide for themselves whether, why, when and how to change their risk behaviors. For example, you ask patients for their consent to discuss their risk behaviors and thereby help to establish collaborative alliances. With this approach, patients are more likely to cooperate with you, to feel as though they can freely choose what they want to do and to assume responsibility for developing a plan for change.

By acting in controlling ways, you are more likely to evoke patient resistance and decrease their intrinsic motivation to change. If patients do change, they are more likely to do so for external reasons: "I stopped smoking because my health care practitioner told me to." Patients with intrinsic or autonomous motivation are more likely to maintain behavior change than are those with extrinsic or controlled motivation.

YOUR SUMMARY

Reflect: write a summary about what you have learned that was new for you.

_____
_____
_____
_____
_____
_____
_____
_____

_____
_____
_____
_____
_____
_____
_____
_____
_____
_____
_____
_____
_____
_____

Enhance*: write down your ideas about how your new learning could improve your interactions with patients. Add your notes to your learning portfolio.*

_____
_____
_____
_____
_____
_____
_____
_____
_____
_____
_____

SECTION II

UNDERSTANDING INDIVIDUAL CHANGE

Section II describes how theory and research evidence can provide insights into and guide your work with patients. To enhance your understanding of behavior change, Chapters 5-7 address how

- Four vectors affect the force of change toward a positive or negative outcome
- Different perspectives can each contribute toward insights about resistance
- Theories and models provide different ways of understanding motivation

Chapter 8 provides an overview of the six-step approach using the Ladder of Change as a conceptual framework for helping you address the large gaps between the best theories and research evidence and the complexity of working with individual patients over time. This framework can help you work with some of the limitations of applying scientific evidence to individual patients.

CHAPTER 5
FORCES OF CHANGE

FOR REFLECTION

Change can be threatening, involve risk and create discomfort.

OVERVIEW

The Forces of Change model provides a framework to help you think about how to intervene to help patients change. The individual vectors for and against change are motivation and resistance; the system vectors for and against individual change are supports and barriers. Motivation and supports generate a positive force toward healthy outcomes, while resistance and barriers generate a negative force toward unhealthy outcomes. The relative strengths of these opposing forces influence whether individuals engage in healthy or unhealthy behaviors. Your challenge is to understand these opposing forces of change so that you can help patients reduce the negative force and increase the positive force for change.

Opposing vectors working at individual and system levels affect the forces of change for patients, practitioners and health care organizations. Multiple factors can affect the strength of these opposing vectors and can arise from

- Individuals (e.g., personal histories of the patient and practitioner that shape values, beliefs, attitudes, perceptions, roles and assumptions)
- Relationships (e.g., patient-practitioner dialogue)
- The context (e.g., psychosocial situations for patients and the organizational milieu of the health care setting for practitioners)

A central tenet of systems theory is that all these factors interact to influence organizational and individual behavior.[1] The Forces of Change model embodies both systems theory and the concept of reciprocal determinism: the dynamic and simultaneous interaction between a person and the environment (systems) in which the behavior is performed.[2]

THE FORCES OF CHANGE MODEL

Four vectors generate positive and negative forces for change (see Figure 5.1). Resistance and motivation are the individual vectors. Barriers and supports are the system vectors.

Figure 5.1. Forces of Change Model

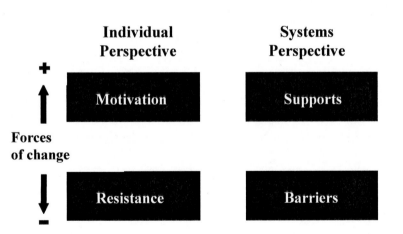

Positive (healthy) forces of change occur when motivation is greater than resistance and when supports are greater than barriers. Conversely, negative (unhealthy) forces against change occur when resistance is greater than motivation and when barriers are greater than supports. The overall challenge is to help patients reduce the negative force and increase the positive force for change. When barriers and supports are difficult to change, patients need assistance in how to differentiate and separate from an unhelpful environment (social, family and/or work situation). An understanding of these vectors can, in turn, help you in selecting and testing whether interventions help patients change their behavior.

LEVERAGE POINTS AND EFFORT

Leverage points and effort are concepts that can help you think about how to use the Forces of Change model more effectively with patients. You need to create leverage points when working with patients: finding out what is important to them and linking it to behavior change. Effort refers to the amount of input you provide to facilitate change. For example, at a high leverage point, a small amount of your effort leads to a big change. Conversely, at a low leverage point, a large amount of your effort leads to a small change. In the absence of a leverage point, your effort does not lead to any change; it may also be a sign that patients need to be sure of your support before addressing the issue of behavior change, as in the case of concomitant psychiatric illnesses. Or your efforts may work in the opposite direction: the more effort you put in, the less patients put in. Sometimes patients become more needy and inappropriately dependent on you.

Leverage points may occur at an individual and/or systems level. If change does not occur working at an individual level (by reducing resistance and increasing motivation), you may be more effective working at a systems level. Conversely, if change does not occur when working at a systems level (by reducing barriers and increasing supports), you may be more effective working at an individual level.

The challenge is first to work on a particular vector that will help the patient change the quickest—reducing resistance, enhancing motivation, reducing barriers and increasing supports. Second, you need to identify what are the best leverage points for facilitating change. Finally, to assess the impact of your efforts, you need to consider what are reasonable goals for a particular patient, given the complexity and challenges of the change process. For example, if you fail to enhance patients' motivation, you might first try to help them reduce their resistance. In such situations, success can be measured in terms of the extent to which patients become more open to the possibility of change.

The following example illustrates how you can use the Forces of Change model in practice:

> Mrs. O. has diabetes and is chronically tired from working as a waitress and housewife (reasons for resisting change). She has three small children, takes little time for herself (barriers for change) and places a higher priority on taking care of her family rather than herself (reasons for resisting change). Dr. M. explained that diabetic complications could interfere with her ability to carry out her caretaking role (attempting to reduce her resistance to change) and that better control of her diabetes could increase her energy (attempting to increase her motivation to change). Mrs. O. agreed to work on reducing her hemoglobin A1c.

Dr. M. also suggested a biomedical solution to help Mrs. O. take better care of her diabetes. With her permission, he enrolled her in a program that implanted an insulin pump with a flexible insulin regimen to accommodate her irregular meals. (This individual intervention aims to make it easier for patients to enhance their motivation and reduce their risks of complications.) However, Mrs. O. was depressed and fed up with checking her blood glucose levels (reasons for resisting change). She did not adjust her dose of regular insulin in a consistent manner. Furthermore, her low family income also reduced how often she checked her glucose levels, since she had to make copayments for the strips to test her blood glucose (barrier for change). Table 5.1 identifies some of the factors that affect Mrs. O.'s ability to take care of her diabetes.

Dr. M. first treated Mrs. O.'s depression to increase her energy so that she might check her blood glucose levels regularly (attempting to reduce resistance to change). With only a partial response to the maximum dose of an antidepressant, she still felt tired. He then arranged a family meeting to see if Mrs. O.'s husband and children would help more with the domestic chores (increase supports for change) so that she could take better charge of her diabetes.

Table 5.1. Factors Affecting the Forces of Change

Forces of Change	Individual Factors	Systems Factors
Positive	Motivation Wants to avoid complications Wants a more flexible insulin regimen	Supports Husband wants her to take better care of her diabetes Women's support group for diabetes (but stopped going after several months)
Negative	Resistance Fatigue Depression	Barriers Does all of domestic chores for the family Works as waitress and goes off her diet while on the job

Table 5.1 can help you identify leverage points within any of the four vectors. Your task is to create leverage points for change and to select appropriate interventions based on your knowledge of the patient's situation, needs and preferences. In this instance, the major barrier to promoting self-care of diabetes was Mrs. O.'s overfunctioning role as a wife and caretaker and her family's lack of involvement in domestic chores. (In other circumstances, the intervention might involve a referral to a social worker to reduce another barrier: the copayment costs for test strips.) In addition, Mrs. O.'s temptations to eat unsuitable food at work needs to be addressed as well. The key issue is to identify high leverage points that promote change.

The rest of this chapter explores further how supports and barriers can promote and hinder change. Chapters 6 and 7 address the issues of individual resistance and motivation in more detail. These chapters will also help you better understand how patients can change their behavior, even when there are barriers and/or a lack of support.

SUPPORTS AND BARRIERS TO CHANGE (SYSTEM VECTORS)

System factors either generate supports or barriers that can influence individual behavior. They are important determinants for avoiding, initiating or perpetuating risk behaviors. For example, teenagers whose parents and peers smoke (barrier) are much more likely to smoke than teenagers who have nonsmoking parents and friends (support). Smoking parents and peers provide ready access to cigarettes and act as role models in developing a smoking habit. As adults, smokers are also more likely to marry smokers; these partners are more likely to smoke about the same number of cigarettes and quit at the same time.[3] Conversely, smokers who are married to nonsmokers or ex-smokers are more likely to quit or remain abstinent.[4]

The National Longitudinal Study on Adolescent Health explored this association of risk behaviors with individual, school and family factors.[5] The results showed that parent-family connectedness and perceived school connectedness (supports) were protection against the following risk behaviors: emotional distress; suicidal thoughts and behavior; violence; the use of alcohol, cigarettes and marijuana; and age of sexual debut. Access to substances at home (a negative family factor or barrier), on the other hand, was associated with the use of cigarettes, alcohol and marijuana among all students. Working more than 20 hours a week (a barrier) was also associated with cigarette, alcohol and marijuana use.

Individual factors, such as appearing older than most other children in the class, were likewise associated with substance use and early age of sexual activity among both junior and senior high school students. In this study, individual factors explained the greatest variance in risk behaviors, accounting for 7-10% in substance abuse, as compared to the school factor (4.3-5.7%) and the family factor (6.1-8.6%).

Interpretation of these findings requires some caution, however,[6] since they were only weakly associated with risky behaviors. Interventions that enhance these factors are at best of moderate effectiveness; consequently, because these factors account for only a small amount of the variance, their impact is limited. Therefore, while it is important to develop interventions that can reduce the initiation of risk behaviors using all three factors (parent-child, child-teacher and individual factors), other interventions are needed to help children increase their resistance against developing unhealthy behaviors and enhance their motivation to engage in healthy behaviors.

Individual, family, social and cultural factors can influence the acquisition, maintenance and avoidance of risk behaviors when they generate supports for the patient. When such factors are lacking or negative, they can act as a barrier to patient change.[7] The distinction between these kinds of situations is important if you are to understand these etiological factors.

For example, negative family interactions can act as a barrier in treating psychiatric conditions such as schizophrenia and depression.[8] A factor known as high expressed emotion, which measures family hostility and perceived criticism, is used to predict relapses of depression and schizophrenia. Interventions that enhance positive social support from the family, however, have not been shown to improve outcomes. With psychiatric illness, the data support the proposition that psychoeducational programs that reduce negative family interactions (a barrier) are far more effective in helping prevent relapses than trying to provide positive support to improve health care outcomes.

A similar study found that higher levels of perceived family criticism were indirectly associated with higher rates of risk behaviors.[9] For example, families who nag their relatives who smoke actually lessen the odds of their quitting; in other words, negative family interactions and social influences can demotivate patients to consider quitting, or even increase the number of cigarettes they smoke. Family and social support may help some smokers quit.[10] Yet, interventions aimed at enhancing social and family support have either limited or no impact in helping patients achieve higher smoking cessation rates. Thus, you are more likely to have a positive impact if you help families stop nagging the patient than if you try to enhance family support.[11] On the other hand, patients may not take advantage of family support because they lack motivation to change or the family does not provide the right kind of support to make a difference.

SUPPORTS FOR CHANGE

Supports are resources that patients can use to initiate, change and/or maintain a behavior. Such supports include resourceful social and family networks and the availability of and access to community resources such as Alcoholics Anonymous, patient advocacy groups and different kinds of health care professionals. Supports are also a major determinant of health and disease.[12]

Social support consists of at least three distinct concepts.[13-15] First, social support is a structure or network of people (taking into account an individual's marital status and the number and frequency of contact with others) around the individual who may or may not provide support.[16] Second, functional social support is the amount and nature of financial, instrumental and emotional assistance provided by the individual's network.[17] Third, subjective assessment of the global quality of one's social support, sometimes referred to as perceived social support, is important.[18] How individuals perceive the level of their social support is a better predictor of subjective (psychological adjustment, depression and functional status) and objective health measures (coronary occlusion, hypertension, mortality, natural killer cell activity) than either structural or functional social supports.[19] Studies about preventing risk behaviors in youth, for example, show that positive support is associated with lower rates of developing risk behaviors. In a model that described 40 assets (both individual and systems factors) that may or may not have been available to youths, the number of risk behaviors per youth decreased as the number of assets increased.

Research about the effectiveness of interventions is needed to clarify what kind of social supports can best help individuals change their risk behaviors. For example, with diabetes, positive supportive family behaviors are fairly separate dimensions from negative family behaviors.[20] Perceived social support and higher levels of family function are correlated with better adherence and glycemic control in adolescents with insulin-dependent diabetes.[21-24] This correlation is much less clear among adults with type 1 and type 2 diabetes. In addition, social support has different effects in men and women with type 2 diabetes.[25] Women satisfied with their social support achieve better glucose control than women who are less satisfied. In contrast, men satisfied with their social support have poorer glucose control than men who are less satisfied with their social support. This finding raises an interesting gender issue regarding the positive and negative effects of satisfactory social support. It also raises the issue of how well intended family support may hinder rather than help.[26]

While family support predicts adherence with several regimen tasks,[20;21;21;23;27;28] diabetic-specific measures of family support are stronger predictors of self-care of diabetes than are more global measures of social and family functioning.[29;30] Family members may need to learn specific skills in how to enhance patient motivation rather than simply provide general encouragement. Yet in type 2 diabetes among the elderly, peer support groups may promote adherence to diet and exercise regimens.[31;32] Thus, positive social support needs to be tailored to the specific behaviors and the particular needs of patients according to their age and gender.

With respect to smoking, naturally occurring partner support helps with early maintenance of abstinence from smoking in women.[33] Abstinence is associated with positive interactions (reinforcement and cooperative participation) and a lack of negative interactions (nagging and policing behaviors) from partners.[34] However, an intervention study that aimed to enhance partner support failed to increase smoking cessation.[35] Other studies have had similar findings.[36-40] The effects of social support and relapse prevention as an adjunct to a televised smoking cessation program did increase smoking cessation rates. The training for smokers and their partners increased the ratio of positive to negative interactions by decreasing unhelpful behaviors (nagging, policing).[41] Thus, there is a need to develop more effective ways of helping family members provide the kind of support that enhances smoking cessation rates. My self-guided change book, *Motivate*

Healthy Habits: Stepping Stones to Lasting Change, also helps family members provide specific support and individualized interventions to one another.[42]

BARRIERS TO CHANGE

Barriers are factors external to individuals that impair their ability to initiate and maintain healthy behaviors. Dealing with these conditions can help patients achieve their goals for change and improve their health. These conditions include competing domestic demands; transportation difficulties; financial difficulties and/or poverty; inadequate health care coverage; situational temptations, reinforcements and inducements not to adhere to recommendations; negative peer pressure; compliance to group norms or subcultures; unsafe work, school, family and/or housing situations; and institutional and bureaucratic factors.[43] Again using diabetes as an example, many factors can impede patients from putting ideal recommendations into action.[23;44-47] Helping patients develop strategies to overcome these barriers may enhance self-care of their diabetes.[48]

FAMILY INVOLVEMENT

Supports and barriers can make individual behavior change more or less difficult for patients. As part of the process of developing positive family support, family members can be trained to help patients take charge of their health. Mutual aid and self-help (MASH) guidebooks, videotapes and/or small group training can encourage family members to assume a supportive role in helping patients decide whether to change. Such training shows promise in assisting family members to provide the right kind of positive support to help their relatives change risk behaviors. Families are an untapped resource; they vastly outnumber health care professionals. To enhance the public health impact of motivational approaches, the involvement of family members can greatly increase the number of individuals who can deliver motivational interventions. The development of MASH programs for family members and the use of lay health facilitators in telephone counseling are new supports in reducing the prevalence and incidence of risk behaviors.

Even with lowered barriers and increased supports to change, individuals may still engage in risk behaviors, because their resistance to change is greater than their motivation to change. If patients cannot reduce their barriers and enhance their supports to change themselves, your challenge in working with them becomes even more of an individual issue—helping them to separate from and differentiate situations that perpetuate the risk behavior. You need to focus your time, attention and effort on influencing individual vectors (motivation and resistance) that can influence change.

YOUR SUMMARY

Reflect: write a summary about what you have learned that was new for you.

_____
_____
_____
_____
_____
_____
_____
_____
_____
_____
_____
_____
_____
_____
_____
_____
_____
_____
_____
_____
_____
_____
_____
_____
_____

Enhance: write down your ideas about how your new learning could improve your interactions with patients. Add your notes to your learning portfolio.

_____
_____
_____
_____
_____
_____
_____
_____
_____
_____
_____
_____

REFERENCES

1. Bertalanffy LV. General systems theory—A critical review. In: Buckley W, ed. Modern systems research for the behavioral scientist: A sourcebook. Chicago: Aldine; 1968

2. Bandura A. Self-efficacy: The exercise of control. New York: W.H. Freeman; 1997

3. Venters MH, Jacobs DR, Luepker RV, et al. Spouse concordance of smoking patterns: The Minnesota heart survey. American Journal of Epidemiology 1984;120: 608-616

4. Price RA, Chen KH, Cavalli SL, et al. Models of spouse influence and their applications to smoking behavior. Social Biology 1981;28: 14-29

5. Resnick MD, Bearman PS, Blum RW, et al. Protecting adolescents from harm. Findings from the national longitudinal study on adolescent health. Journal of the American Medical Associationi 1997;278: 823-832

6. Klein JD. The national longitudinal study on adolescent health [editorial]. Journal of the American Medical Association 1997;278: 864-865

7. Rook KS. The negative side of social interaction: Impact on psychological well-being. Journal of Personality and Social Psychology 1984;46: 1097-1108

8. Goldstein MJ, Strachan AM, Wynne LC. Relational problems related to a mental disorder or general medical condition. In: Widiger TA, Frances AJ, Pincus HA, et al., eds. DSM-IV sourcebook. Washington, DC: American Psychiatric Association Press; 1998:531-567

9. Fiscella K, Campbell TL. Association of perceived family criticism with health behaviors. Journal of Family Practice 1999;48: 128-134

10. Morgan GD, Ashenberg ZS, Fisher EB, Jr. Abstinence from smoking and the social environment. Journal of Consulting and Clinical Psychology 1988;56: 298-301

11. Antonuccio DO, Boutilier LR, Ward CH, et al. The behavioral treatment of cigarette smoking. Progress in Behavior Modification 1992;28: 119-181

12. House JS, Landis KR, Umberson D. Social relationships and health. Science 1988;241: 540-545

13. Berkman LF, Oxman TE, Seeman TE. Social networks and social support among the elderly: Assessment issues. In: Wallace RB, Woolson RF, eds. The epidemiologic study of the elderly. New York: Academic Press; 1992:196-212

14. Cohen S. Psychosocial models of the role of social support in the etiology of physical disease. Health Psychology 1988;7: 269-297

15. Weinberger M, Hiner SL, Tierney WM. Assessing social support in elderly adults. Social Science and Medicine 1987;25: 1049-1055

16. Fischer A, Jackson R, Stueve C, et al. Networks and places: Social relations in the urban setting. New York: The Free Press; 1977

17. Kaplan HB, Cassel J, Gore S. Social support and health. Medical Care 1977;15: 47-58

18. Barrera M, Sandler IN, Ramsay TB. Preliminary development of a scale of social support: Studies on college students. American Journal of Community Psychology 1981;9: 435-443

19. Penninx B. Social support in elderly people with chronic diseases: Does it really help? Amsterdam: Brenda W.J.H. Penninx; 1996

20. Glasgow RE, Toobert DJ. Social environment and regimen adherence among Type II diabetic patients. Diabetes Care 1988;11: 377-386

21. Schafer LC, Glasgow RE, McCaul KD, et al. Adherence to IDDM regimens: Relationship to psychosocial variables and metabolic control. Diabetes Care 1983;6: 493-498

22. Anderson BJ, Auslander WF. Research on diabetes management and the family: A critique. Diabetes Care 1980;3: 696-702

23. Hanson CL, Henggeler SW, Burghen GA. Model of associations between psychosocial variables and health-outcome measures of adolescents with IDDM. Diabetes Care 1987;10: 752-758

24. Hanson CL, Henggeler SW, Burghen GA. Social competence and parental support as mediators of the link between stress and metabolic control in adolescents with insulin-dependent diabetes mellitus. Journal of Consulting and Clinical Psychology 1987;55: 529-533

25. Hartwell SL, Kaplan RM, Wallace JP. Comparison of behavioral interventions for control of Type II diabetes mellitus. Behavior Therapy 1986;17: 447-461

26. Anderson BJ. Involving family members in diabetes treatment. In: Anderson BJ, Rubin RR, eds. Practical psychology for diabetes clinicians. Alexandria, VA: American Diabetes Assoc.; 1996:43-50

27. Wilson W, Ary DV, Biglan A, et al. Psychosocial predictors of self-care behaviors (compliance) and glycemic control in non-insulin dependent diabetes mellitus. Diabetes Care 1986;9: 614-622

28. Heiby EM, Gafarian CT, McCann SC. Situational and behavioral correlates of compliance to a diabetic regimen. Journal of Compliance in Health Care 1989;4: 101-116

29. Connell CM, Fisher EB, Houston CA. Relationships among social support, diabetes outcomes, and morale for older men and women. Journal of Aging and Health 1992;4: 77-100

30. Kaplan RM, Hartwell SL. Differential effects of social support and social network on physiological and social outcomes in men and women with type 2 diabetes mellitus. Health Psychology 1987;6: 387-398

31. Glasgow R. Compliance to diabetes regimens: Conceptualization, complexity, and determinants. In: Cramer JA, Spilker B, eds. Patient compliance in medical practice and clinical trials, 1st ed. New York: Raven Press; 1991: 209-224

32. Wilson W, Pratt C. The impact of diabetes education and peer support upon weight and glycemic control of elderly persons with noninsulin-dependent diabetes mellitus (NIDDM).American Journal of Public Health 1987;77: 634-635

33. Coppotelli HC, Orleans CT. Partner support and other determinants of smoking cessation among women. Journal of Consulting and Clinical Psychology 1985;53: 455-460

34. Mermelstein R, Lichtenstein E, McIntyre K. Partner support and relapse in smoking-cessation programs. Journal of Consulting and Clinical Psychology 1983;51: 465-466

35. Ginsberg D, Hall SM, Rosinski M. Partner support, psychological treatment, and nicotine gum in smoking treatment: An incremental study. The International Journal of the Addictions 1992;27: 503-514

36. Malott JM, Glasgow RE, O'Neill HK, et al. Co-worker social support in a worksite smoking control program. Journal of Applied Behavior Analysis 1984;17: 485-495

37. Orleans CT, Schoenbach VJ, Wagner EH, et al. Self-help quit smoking interventions: Effects of self-help materials, social support instructions, and telephone counseling. Journal of Consulting and Clinical Psychology 1991;59: 439-448

38. McIntyre-Kingsolver K, Lichtenstein E, Mermelstein RJ. Spouse training in a multicomponent smoking-cessation program. Behavior Therapy 1986;17: 67-74

39. Couples who smoke: A comparison of couples training versus individual training for smoking cessation. Behavior Therapy 1986;17: 620-625

40. Glasgow RE, Klesges RC, O'Neill HK. Programming social support for smoking modification: An extension and replication. Addictive Behaviors 1986;11: 453-457

41. Gruder CL, Mermelstein RJ, Kirkendol S, et al. Effects of social support and relapse prevention training as adjuncts to a televised smoking-cessation intervention. Journal of Consulting and Clinical Psychology 1993;61: 113-120

42. Botelho RJ. Motivate Healthy Habits: Stepping Stones to Lasting Change. Rochester, NY: MHH Publications; 2004

43. Glasgow R. Social-environmental factors in diabetes: Barriers to diabetes self-care. Eugene: Oregon Research Institute; 1989: 335-349

44. Sims DF. Barriers to adherence. Diabetes Care 1979;2: 524-525

45. Glasgow RE, McCaul KD, Schafer LC. Barriers to regimen adherence among persons with insulin-dependent diabetes. Journal of Behavioral Medicine 1986;9: 65-77

46. Irvine AA, Saunders JT, Blank M, et al. Validation of scale measuring environmental barriers to diabetes regimen adherence. Diabetes Care 1990;13: 705-711

47. Anderson L, Jenkins C. Educational innovations in diabetes: Where are we now? Diabetes Spectrum 1994;7(2): 90-124

48. Glasgow RE, Easkin EG. Issues in diabetes self-management. In: Shumaker S, Schron E, Ockene J, et al., eds. The handbook of health behavior change. New York: Springer Publishing Co.; 1997

CHAPTER 6

UNDERSTANDING RESISTANCE

FOR REFLECTION

What is your understanding of the word **resistance?**
What assumptions do you make about patient resistance?

OVERVIEW

Patient resistance is an expected and normal part of the change process.[1] Different concepts and models provide different ways of understanding it. These different perspectives can also help you understand how you may unintentionally contribute to such patient resistance. A surefire way to evoke resistance is to advise patients to change when you assume they are ready but they are not. For example, a simple, open-ended question about smoking may inadvertently evoke resistance in some patients. You need to recognize both the subtle and blatant forms of resistance in order to work effectively with patients. Otherwise, your relationship with them will feel like a tug-of-war. The following aphorism about patient autonomy captures the rationale for working with rather than against resistance.

> *Patients become more willing to consider change if you acknowledge their choice to behave in "unhealthy" ways and if they think that you really understand their reasons to stay the same.*

86

Human motivation is familiar to us all, but often perplexing to understand. Consider our fear of flying. Airplanes are one of the safest forms of travel; indeed, the most dangerous aspect is driving to and from the airport. In North America, the lifetime risk of death from flying is about 1 in 5,092, whereas the odds of dying in a motor vehicle accident are 1 in 81 (U.S. National Safety Council). Dramatic airline crashes, such as the September 11 terrorist actions, can have a profound impact on turning off many people to flying. In contrast, the local news almost every day carries stories about fatal car crashes, yet our propensity for car travel is rarely altered, in spite of the greater odds of dying in a car accident than in an airline crash. What truly motivates our travel behavior? Emotions, such as fear, are often more important than the facts about the actual risks in shaping our behavior.

Understanding what causes patient resistance can be equally perplexing.[3] Consider the case of a practitioner who confronts a patient, Mrs. C., about her repeated intoxication and alcohol dependence. She rejects the idea that she has a drinking problem and claims she drinks for social and relaxation purposes. Her practitioner labels her as being in denial and confronts Mrs. C. more aggressively by trying to persuade her that excessive drinking is a problem for her. She again denies that she drinks too much and claims that all her friends drink a lot. Mrs. C. and her practitioner are locked in a dance (confrontation-resistance-confrontation-resistance), with neither partner able to change their step. The practitioner becomes more frustrated and blames Mrs. C. She becomes angrier outwardly but feels scared inside. She does not keep her follow-up appointments, and a year later her medical records are transferred to another practice. Mrs. C. also highlights how resistance occurs in any interactions when the need for change challenges the status quo.

Resistance is a normal process—an attempt to maintain homeostasis (the familiar) rather than to risk change (the unknown). The example of Mrs. C. highlights a human tendency to accentuate the emotional benefits of a behavior (e.g., drinking to relieve stress) and to downplay the factual risks of harm from that behavior (e.g., alcohol-related problems). The following quotation captures how our emotional needs alter our perceptions of benefits, risks and harm.

> *We see what we want to see. Our perceptions fly straight out of our deepest needs.*
> —Carol Shields, *The Stone Diaries*

As practitioners, we place a premium on maximizing health-enhancing and health-risk-avoiding behaviors, such as exercising and eating nutritious food to maintain fitness and appropriate weight, and using safe sex practices. Even without saying *"I'm the expert and you need to do as I say,"* we may still be tempted to take a know-it-all stance with the patient. Knowingly or unknowingly, we impose our values on him or her. If we fall into this trap of "health care imperialism,"[4] we run the risk of blaming the patient for not changing. Many of our patients have different values and perceptions about health behaviors from us. They may not place such a high value on their health or may have priorities that override their health priorities. These differences are powerfully influenced by life experiences, gender, age, diversity in ethnicity, race, educational level and socioeconomic status. The following exercise may help you understand how your well-meaning intentions may contribute to resistance.

> *Learning Exercise 6.1: Think of a resistant patient*
> *Think of a challenging patient (family member, student or colleague) who resisted your advice to change his or her behavior.*
> *1. In what ways did this person demonstrate resistant behavior?*
> *2. Consider how your approach may have evoked this resistance.*
> *3. How did you feel about and respond to his or her resistance?*
>
> *Now replay the interaction in your mind. Freeze-frame the interaction at the point when you first detected resistance on the part of this person. Now think of different ways of handling this situation.*

Patient resistance arises from the differences between how you and your patients think, perceive and feel about the benefits and risks of a particular behavior. Understanding this resistance will provide you with invaluable information about patients and help you to motivate change. As such, it can be viewed as a force to work with and redirect rather than as a force to be ignored, disregarded or broken down.

UNDERSTANDING PATIENT RESISTANCE

Resistance and denial provide different ways of explaining human behavior. When patients are resisting change, they are either ignoring or minimizing the risks and harm of their unhealthy behaviors. In contrast, denial implies that the patient either does not recognize the health risks, even when informed about them, or refutes the validity of evidence of a health risk: "That won't happen to me."

Denial involves predominantly unconscious processes. For example, consider a patient who was admitted to the intensive care unit for a myocardial infarction and was in a state of denial about his heart attack, despite being informed about the diagnosis. He did push-ups at his bedside the day after his attack because he wanted to prove to himself and others that he could get back to work as soon as possible, keep his business going and provide for his family. Or consider a patient who denied that he was under a great deal of stress and therefore did not see any connection between stress and his excessive alcohol use. In contrast, a resistant patient (who is not in denial) acknowledges that alcohol relieves his stress but feels that the benefits outweigh the risks.

When you encounter resistance, it is a clear signal that you need to change your approach and gain a better understanding about why patients do not want to change. This process may help patients lower their resistance so they become more receptive to the possibility of change. To do this effectively, it helps to understand patient resistance from different perspectives.

PRACTITIONER'S STYLE

How often have you found yourself in the situation where the harder you try to persuade a patient to change a health behavior, the more the individual balks? Both parties are pushing with increasing intensity, but from opposite directions. Consider the following example involving an advice-giving practitioner (Dr. F.):

> Dr. F. tried to persuade Mr. G., who had end-stage emphysema, to stop smoking in order to reduce his risk of dying. However, Mr. G. greatly enjoyed his cigarette smoking—indeed, more than almost anything else. Again and again, Dr. F. tried various ways of convincing Mr. G. to quit. Dr. F. upped the ante several times and at one point almost got into a shouting match with Mr. G. Mr. G., however, viewed his smoking as an important way to enhance his quality of life, even if it shortened it. The more pressure he felt from Dr. F., the more strongly Mr. G. felt about his right to smoke. Increasingly, Dr. F. did not enjoy working with Mr. G., who for his part felt more and more reluctant to make appointments with Dr. F.
>
> **Commentary:** This dynamic of resistance helps to highlight the problem between Dr. F. and Mr. G. As Dr. F. escalated his attempts to convince or persuade the patient to stop smoking, Mr. G became more attached to his smoking.

Reactance theory provides a way of understanding this universal experience to counter the pressure that is put on you.[5] This theory emphasizes the importance that individuals place on having the freedom to choose without coercion or threat to their autonomy. Any threat to or loss of a perceived freedom can provoke a person to protect or restore that freedom. This helps explain why patients may cling to a choice or a risk behavior in the face of increasing pressure from a practitioner or family member to change. Ironically, the attractiveness of the choice or risk behavior can actually increase if people feel that their freedom (right of choice) is being threatened. The principle of this theory is that the amount of reactance will increase as a direct function of the number of freedoms threatened.

Other illuminating insights on the dynamics of motivation and resistance have been gained from therapy process research. In one study, therapists switched every 12 minutes between either a directive-confrontational style or a supportive-reflective style in a study of family therapy.[6] Interestingly, the client's behavior mirrored the therapist's approach. When the therapist adopted a directive-confrontational style, client resistance increased. Conversely, when the therapist used a supportive-reflective style, client behaviors reflecting resistance decreased.

In another study, two therapist styles were evaluated with problem drinkers.[7] Patients were randomly assigned to three situations: (1) directive-confrontational counseling, (2) client-centered counseling or (3) waiting-list control. The directive-confrontational therapist style yielded significantly more resistance from clients, who were more likely to argue, interrupt and diverge from the focus of therapy. In comparison, problem drinkers who received client-centered counseling were more likely to exhibit positive behavior; in fact, the client's behavior strongly correlated with the therapist's style. For instance, the more the therapist confronted, the more likely the client would argue. Of particular importance was the finding that therapist behavior was predictive of the patient's drinking status one year following treatment. The more the therapist confronted the problem drinker, the more the client drank one year later. Both these research studies demonstrate that the practitioner's style can reliably influence the level of patient resistance.[6;7]

"PROBLEMS" AS "SOLUTIONS"

You may mistakenly assume that a patient shares your perspective about a risk behavior, seeing it as you do—in a negative light. The following example highlights how patients may view a risk behavior as a solution, not a problem; in other words, they have a positive perspective.

> Mr. B. had poorly controlled high blood pressure in spite of taking his medications regularly. He drank at least four beers a day and did not regard himself as having a drinking problem. In contrast, FP, a nurse practitioner, was convinced that Mr. B.'s poor blood pressure control was caused by his alcohol intake. Even when FP educated Mr. B. about this fact, he seemed to disregard this explanation. Annoyed by his response, FP asked why he did not believe that alcohol was causing his high blood pressure. Mr. B. explained that alcohol helped him deal with family stress caused by difficulties relating to his teenage stepdaughter. He also claimed that alcohol helped him lower his high blood pressure. In contrast to FP's professional opinion, Mr. B. thought his blood pressure would be even higher if he did not have a few drinks to relax.

Different Perceptions about Benefits

As demonstrated above, you and your patients can have different perceptions about the benefits of risk behaviors (see Figure 6.1 for benefits continuum).

Figure 6.1. Benefits Continuum

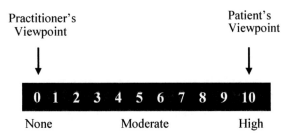

Using the same example of the smoker, Mr. G., mentioned earlier, MP, a nurse, took an alternative approach during consultations with Mr. G. about his cigarette smoking.

In contrast to Dr. F., who had great difficulty seeing anything positive about the patient's "self-destructive" smoking behavior, MP appreciated the fact that Mr. G. was not concerned about prolonging his life. MP respected Mr. G.'s decision and knew that he enjoyed smoking. She understood why he saw smoking as a benefit. However, as a result of asking a series of questions regarding what Mr. G. saw as the benefits and concerns about his smoking, MP discovered that the patient intensely disliked the prospect of being hospitalized for his emphysema. He wanted to avoid this at all costs. With this new information about the patient, MP explored, in a nonconfrontational way, whether Mr. G. might be prepared to cut down on his smoking to avoid being hospitalized. He agreed to cut down from more than a pack of cigarettes a day and set a goal of five cigarettes a day. He achieved this goal and was not admitted into a hospital for over a year.

This autonomy-supportive approach assisted Mr. G. in moving from a point where he would not even consider changing his cigarette smoking (precontemplation stage) to a point where he was giving serious thought to the idea of cutting down on his smoking (contemplation stage).

Different Perceptions about Risk and Harm

Another way to understand resistance is to assess the extent to which you and your patient agree about the risks of a behavior. One way is to use a behavioral risk continuum (see Figure 6.2). For various reasons, you and your patients are likely to assess and perceive risks differently and to be at different points on the risk continuum. This is because many patients minimize their personal susceptibility to a given behavior (e.g., getting a sexually transmitted disease [STD] from unprotected sex) due to an "optimism bias"[8]—"I am less vulnerable to the health consequence; it is more likely to happen to someone else than to me."

Figure 6.2.
Behavioral Risk Continuum

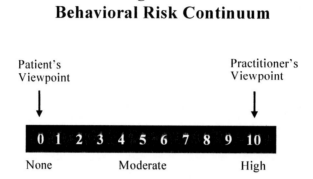

Once aware of this difference, you can work with patients to achieve a shared understanding about risks. This is important because resistance is greater as the differences in risk perception between you and your patient increase. This awareness is clearly illustrated in the following comments by a physician regarding his approach in dealing with patients who have drinking problems:

> *Diagnosis of alcohol problems involves more than just assigning a name to the patient's problems or offering treatment; it involves "the creation of the idea that it is a problem." This requires a willingness by doctor and patient alike to engage in a possibly lengthy process of negotiation until a shared understanding of the problem is reached.*[9]

Mismatches in Readiness for Change

Figure 6.3 measures the degree of mismatch between you and your patient and the likelihood of patient resistance. Your task is to work from where patients are coming from and then use appropriate interventions to help them change.

Figure 6.3.
Readiness for Change Continuum

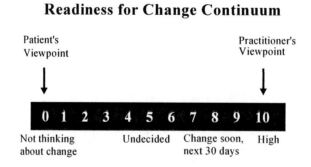

EVOKING PATIENT RESISTANCE

A wide range of behaviors may evoke patient resistance (see Table 6.1). Even a nonjudgmental, neutral question may trigger a negative reaction. The ways patients interpret the intentions of your comments, questions and even your attitude can provide invaluable diagnostic insight about the perceptual filters through which they interact with you and others. The patients' values, beliefs and attitudes all shape these filters.

Table 6.1.

Triggers for Patient Resistance	
Asking questions	Musts and shoulds
Giving advice	Lecturing
Making suggestions	Judging
Giving recommendations	Moralizing
Persuading with "logic"	Criticizing
Providing instructions	Interpreting
Offering solutions	Analyzing

Your challenge is to use your insight about patient resistance in ways that help them change their perceptions about their risk behaviors and thereby become more motivated to change. Pay particular attention to how your interviewing approach can powerfully affect patients' receptivity or resistance to the possibility of change.[10]

HOW DO PATIENTS RESIST CHANGE?

You may trigger patient resistance in subtle and/or obvious ways (see table 6.1).[11]

Table 6.2

Signs of Patient Resistance
• *Exhibiting nonverbal cues of negative emotions*: discomfort, flushing, fidgeting
• *Ignoring you:* inattention, no answer, nonresponse, cutting off
• *Evading issues:* interrupting, talking
• over, sidetracking, using humor to deflect
• *Deflecting issues:* giving rationalizations, placating others
• *Pseudo-agreeing:* making implied or halfhearted agreements to change
• *Projecting:* blaming others, holding others responsible for their actions
• *Rebelling:* arguing, challenging, disagreeing, being oppositional
• *Offending others:* discounting, discrediting, being hostile
• *Giving up:* resignation, unwillingness to try, defeated

All these tactics are indications that the patient is not ready for change or is unwilling to change. Such cues can help remind you to change your approach—for example, slow the pace of change, or use open-ended questions followed by reflective listening, and/or interrupt interactions that cause frustration or anger. This approach enables patients to tell their story about why they may not want to change, how they feel about it and how they perceive the benefits, risks and harms of changing. Also, this information gives you invaluable leads for negotiating an appropriate pace of change with patients.

GO WITH RESISTANCE

Patient resistance can occur even in skillfully conducted interviews. When patients are not ready for change, it can feel like a tug of war. If you pull, so does the patient, but in the opposite direction. The art of going with resistance means that you do not pick up the rope in the first place, but if you do, let go of it slowly. This will help avoid oppositional maneuvering.

Work toward understanding where patients are coming from. When you understand why patients resist change, they often become more willing to consider the possibility of change. After understanding each other's differences, you can then help patients decide whether they would like to redirect their energy in a healthier manner. This approach can help both you and your patients reduce the frustration and begin to work together.

When resistance is encountered, you will recognize it and be able to address it early by changing your approach to one that is more likely to engender cooperation. Eventually, you may even come to regard dealing with resistance as an intriguing challenge. If you become hooked on dealing with it, however, you run the risk of becoming a resistance junkie!

YOUR SUMMARY

Reflect: write a summary about what you have learned that was new for you.

_____
_____
_____
_____
_____
_____
_____
_____
_____
_____
_____
_____
_____
_____
_____
_____
_____
_____
_____
_____
_____
_____
_____
_____
_____

Enhance: write down your ideas about how your new learning could improve your interactions with patients. Add your notes to your learning portfolio.

_____
_____
_____
_____
_____
_____
_____
_____
_____
_____
_____
_____
_____

REFERENCES

1. Anderson C, Stewart S. Common resistances in ongoing treatment. In: Anderson C, Stewart S, eds. Mastering Resistance. 1995: 151-206

2. Deci EL, Ryan RM. Intrinsic motivation and self-determination in human behavior. New York: Plenum Press; 1985

3. Botelho RJ, Skinner HA, Williams GC, et al. Patients with alcohol problems in primary care: Understanding their resistance and motivating change. In: Stuart MR, Lieberman IJA, eds. Primary care: Clinics in office practice. Philadelphia: W.B. Saunders Company; 1999: 279-298

4. Lupton D. The imperative of health: Public health and the regulated body. London, England: Sage Publications, Ltd.; 1995

5. Brehm SS, Brehm JW. Psychological reactance: A theory of freedom and control. New York: Academic Press; 1981

6. Patterson GA, Forgatch MS. Therapist behavior as a determinant for client noncompliance: A paradox for the behavior modifier. Journal of Consulting and Clinical Psychology 1985;53: 846-851

7. Miller W, Benefield RG, Tonigan JS. Enhancing motivation for change in problem drinking: A controlled comparison of two therapist styles. Journal of Consulting and Clinical Psychology 1993;61: 455-461

8. Weinstein ND. Unrealistic optimism about susceptibility to health problems: Conclusions from a community-wide sample. Journal of Behavioral Medicine 1987;10: 481-500

9. Thom B, Tëllez C. A difficult business: Detecting and managing alcohol problems in general practice. British Journal of Addiction 1986;81: 405-418

10. Butler C, Rollnick S, Stott N. The practitioner, the patient and resistance to change: Recent ideas on compliance. Canadian Medical Association Journal 1996;154: 1357-1362

11. Miller WR, Rollnick S. Motivational interviewing: Preparing people to change addictive behavior. New York: Guilford Press; 1991

CHAPTER 7

UNDERSTANDING MOTIVATION

FOR REFLECTION

What is your understanding of the word **motivation?**
What assumptions do you make about patient motivation?

OVERVIEW

Selected concepts, models, theories and clinical approaches are highlighted to provide different perspectives on motivating behavior change. The concepts of self-efficacy and outcome expectancy address whether patients have the confidence and ability to change and whether they think they can achieve their goals for change, respectively. Self-determination theory addresses why patients change, that is, what kinds of motives are more likely to maintain change for life. The transtheoretical model (stages of change) helps to understand patients' readiness to change. Motivational interviewing and relapse prevention approaches help patients initiate and maintain change, respectively.

From a lay perspective, motivation is viewed as the reason humans feel and behave as they do. Individuals accomplish significant acts because they are "motivated." From a professional perspective, patients are often labeled as "unmotivated" when they fail to achieve a certain standard of behavior, such as maintaining abstinence following alcoholism treatment or not being able to quit cigarette use. Both of these perspectives are simplistic.

Your conceptual understanding of motivation influences how you work with patients. This chapter provides different perspectives on motivation.[1,2] Motivation arises from forces within individuals (e.g., energy, direction, needs, drives) as well as situational and environmental factors (e.g., supports, barriers and positive and negative incentives). A broader understanding of this concept may help you expand your repertoire of options in how you can help your patients. The Likelihood-of-Action Index (described at the end of this chapter) summarizes the different motivational factors that increase the prospects of change. This index can also help you and your patients understand better about the complexity of initiating and maintaining change.

CONCEPTS, MODELS, THEORIES AND CLINICAL APPROACHES

Selected concepts, models, theories and clinical approaches are briefly described to generate different perspectives on motivating behavior change.

SELF-EFFICACY AND OUTCOME EXPECTANCY

The concept of efficacy[3-6] has been used to address a variety of behaviors,[7-9] such as breast self-examination for cancer screening.[10] Self-efficacy is a person's expression of confidence that he or she has the capability necessary to achieve a behavioral goal.

Perceived efficacy can affect every phase of personal change—whether people even consider changing their health habits, whether they can enlist the motivation and perseverance needed to succeed should they choose to do so, and whether they adequately maintain the changes they have achieved.[11]

Outcome expectancy is distinct from self-efficacy. Outcome expectancy is the individual's belief that a given behavior (e.g., a low-calorie diabetic diet and physical exercise) will produce a particular outcome (e.g., normal glucose levels and weight reduction for diabetics). Patients may have high self-efficacy about sticking to a low-calorie diabetic diet and exercise program but doubt that these lifestyle changes will produce the desired change (40-pound weight loss and normalized blood glucose levels). With a low outcome expectancy, they may not even bother making any lifestyle changes.

A limitation of self-efficacy is that this concept does not adequately address why people decide to change. Individuals can have high self-efficacy ("I can do it"), yet their reasons for action can be governed by external and/or internal controlling forces ("I have to change because my doctor or family wants me to" or "I should [or ought to] change"). In other words, a personal sense of volition and free choice is lacking.

SELF-DETERMINATION THEORY

Deci and Ryan developed self-determination theory as a comprehensive approach for understanding human motivation.[12;17] They distinguish between three different aspects of motivation: energy, direction and motives. Energy arises innately from within the individual and/or is generated by interaction with others, the environment or a situation. Energy may also be generated by the degree of discrepancy between an individual's current state (e.g., poor physical fitness following an injury) and a highly valued goal (e.g., winning a 10-kilometer race).

Direction determines toward what, or away from what, an individual will move. The prospect of training with several highly competitive athletes may compel a runner to join an elite track club in order to enhance his chance of winning the 10K race. Conversely, some individuals avoid athletics but may have high energy to pursue other hobbies and interests, like playing a musical instrument.

Motives help to explain why patients take action (or not). They may have a blend of motives (indifferent/controlled/autonomous) that can change over time.[12]

- *Indifferent motives—"I don't care if I live or die."* Many factors may account for such indifference: stress, depression, environmental barriers and aversive social influences. You need to address these factors first before trying to motivate these patients.
- *External (controlled) motives—"I'm only changing because my family wants me to."* For example, a patient may comply with taking his blood pressure medication because he does not want to upset his wife and doctor. In other words, the patient is not exercising his genuine choice, but is being controlled by others. Relapse occurs when any external reinforcement is removed.
- *Introjected (controlled) motives—"I ought to quit smoking."* These individuals act more out of a sense that they should, must or ought to change their behavior. Outwardly, they may appear to have autonomous motives (see below), but inside they feel conflicted, anxious or guilty because they are ambivalent about change. They initiate and maintain change provided that they continue to internally prompt themselves. They relapse when this internal reinforcement stops.

- *Integrated (autonomous) motives—"I love to exercise. It makes me feel great."* With autonomous motives, individuals experience a true sense of volition about their behavioral choice. The initiation and maintenance of behavior change is self-regulated, driven by the patient's values and freely chosen motives, as opposed to being influenced by other people's value system. They do not change because of introjected motives or a sense of duty.

Figure 7.1 depicts how patients come to the clinical encounter with you bearing different dispositions and shows how their interpretation of your messages can produce these different motives. Patients may also be at more than one point on this continuum and move back and forth along it; they may experience different kinds of motives concurrently, but to different degrees. Furthermore, their profile can change over time with different risk behaviors. For this reason, you should assess patients' overall profile of motives. It helps to understand what are the predominant motives for change, because a person is more likely to change for autonomous reasons than for controlled ones[13;14]

Thus, your behavior can influence patients' motives. If you act in autonomy-supportive ways ("It's up to you whether to change or not, but may I help you improve your health?"), you are more likely to help patients develop autonomous motives for change.[12] Unfortunately, some patients may even interpret your autonomy-supportive message as controlling because they have been brought up in controlling situations. They have not been encouraged to exercise autonomy.

If you act in controlling ways with your patients, you are more likely to stifle their sense of autonomy and to generate indifference or controlled motives. Such a paternalistic position ("I'm the expert and you should follow my advice") can make patients feel pressured or even coerced to change. Consequently, they may oppose you and become more resistant.

Controlling systems, like totalitarian regimens, dictatorships and rigid hierarchies (work, family, social networks) can demotivate people. Such circumstances can make people lose their individual initiative and exhibit passivity, inertia and/or indifference. Conversely, patients who have autonomous motives often disregard controlling messages and circumstances, in part because they have been brought up in autonomy-supportive systems. Autonomous motives are also more robust against relapses than controlled (introjected and external) motives.[12;14]

Figure 7.1. Self-determination Theory

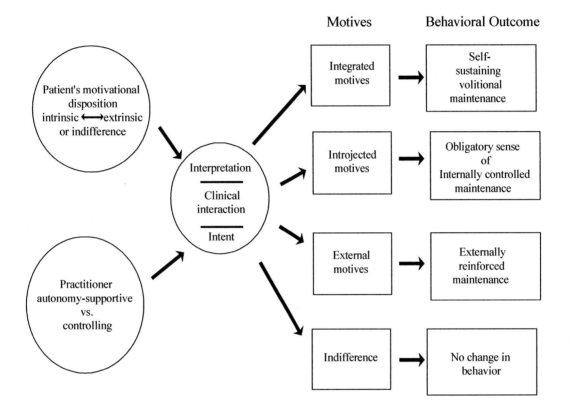

TRANSTHEORETICAL MODEL (stages of change)

According to this model, patients progress through five stages of change: precontemplation, contemplation, preparation, action and maintenance.[15] The definitions for the Stages of Change are provided in Table 7.1.

Table 7.1.

Stages of Change Model
Precontemplation: has no intention of taking action within the next six months
Contemplation: intends to take action within the next six months
Preparation: intends to take action within the next 30 days
Action: has changed overt behavior for less than six months
Maintenance: has changed overt behavior for more than six months

The decision balance (see Table 7.2) provides an example for understanding the pros and cons of change. The pros and cons affect the patients' readiness to change. Patients perceive or assess the pros and cons differently at each stage of change.[16-18]

Table 7.2. The Pros and Cons of Change

Reasons to smoke	Reasons to quit
Benefits of quitting Reduces stress	Concerns about smoking Lung cancer
Concerns about quitting Gain weight	Benefits of quitting Save money
Cons (resistance)	**Pros** (motivation)

In the precontemplation stage, the cons outweigh the pros. Some precontemplators may be largely unaware of the risks (e.g., heart disease) of a particular behavior (e.g., smoking). Even if they are aware of the risks and harm, they minimize the pros for change and maximize the cons against change. Other precontemplators, such as some die-hard smokers, are fully aware of the risks but totally disregard them.

The pros and cons equalize in the contemplation stage. Patients become ambivalent because their reasons to change (pros) and their reasons to stay the same (cons) are equally compelling.[19] While they are concerned about their health, chronic contemplators may think about changing a lifestyle behavior for many years before taking action. In the preparation stage, patients perceive the reasons to change (pros) as outweighing the reasons to stay the same (cons). They will set a date to change in the near future (within a month or so).

In the action stage, patients do something to achieve their goal. These goals may range from making short-term, incremental changes to adopting the ideal recommendations for the long term. A smoker has a variety of options. The ideal goal is quitting, with or without pharmacological treatments. An alternative option is gradually cutting down over a period of time before setting a quit date.

Patients move into the maintenance stage when they have achieved their goal for six months or more. A lapse at this stage is a temporary setback, such as smoking a couple of cigarettes over a few days, whereas a relapse is complete reversion to a previous pattern of behavior, such as smoking a pack of cigarettes daily. When patients relapse, they need to restart the process of change at an earlier stage.

Most people do not progress in a linear fashion through these stages. Relapses are common, especially with addictive behaviors. People often recycle through the stages several times before achieving a long-term goal. For example, cigarette smokers may take three to seven serious quit attempts before they achieve long-term abstinence.[20]

Most people are not in the action stage.[21] Yet, many prevention and behavior change initiatives, such as the five A's (ask, advise, assess, assist and arrange follow-up) approach to smoking cessation,[22] are directed at the action stage. The Stages of Change model provides a useful framework for understanding how individuals change over time. In the next chapter, you will see how the Ladder of Change combines the stages of change with the six-step approach to provide some guidance in developing appropriate interventions.

MOTIVATIONAL INTERVIEWING

Motivational interviewing, developed by Miller and Rollnick,[23] has sparked considerable interest among practitioners and researchers. Motivation is not regarded as an individual trait that is difficult to change but as a state that is changeable and influenced by the practitioner's interviewing style.[24] They advocate for taking a nonconfrontational stance with patients and describe five basic strategies for enhancing the patient's motivation and commitment to change.[23]

1. Express empathy through listening rather than telling
2. Develop discrepancy between where the patient is now (i.e., risk behavior) and where he or she wants to be
3. Avoid argumentation; do not convince patients by the force of your argument
4. Roll with resistance rather than meet patient resistance head-on
5. Support self-efficacy, instill hope and support patients' belief that they can change

Motivational interviewing (summarized in Table 7.3) is divided into two major phases.[23] First, you use motivational enhancement strategies for patients who are in the precontemplation and contemplation stages of change. Such an approach helps resistant and ambivalent patients become more receptive to the possibility of change. Second, you then use strategies to strengthen their decision and commitment to change. After patients have changed, you can use relapse prevention strategies to help them maintain change.[25]

Table 7.3. Strategies for Motivation Enhancement

A. Build Motivation for Change	B. Strengthen Commitment to Change
1. Ask open-ended questions	1. Recognize readiness for change
2. Listen reflectively	2. Discuss a plan
3. Affirm the patient	3. Communicate free choice
4. Summarize	4. Discuss consequences of action/inaction
5. Present personal feedback	5. Give information and advice
6. Handle resistance	6. Deal with resistance
7. Reframe statement	7. Make a plan
8. Elicit self-motivational statements	

Source: Miller and Rollnick (1991)[23]

More recently, Rollnick and colleagues published a guide for practitioners based on motivational interviewing principles.[26]

RELAPSE PREVENTION

When an individual first attempts to change a behavior, the most likely outcome is relapse, not successful maintenance. More than 25 years ago, a review of treatment programs for habitual smokers, heroin addicts and alcoholics found that approximately 66% of all participants relapsed by the 90-day follow-up.[27] These programs focused more on initiating behavioral change than on maintaining change over time.[27] This created a revolving door of treatment and relapse. Many patients lacked self-efficacy in preventing relapses. This led to the development of relapse prevention programs.

The relapse prevention approach draws heavily on the concept of self-efficacy and was developed to enhance patient self-efficacy in treating addictions, with abstinence as its primary goal.[4:5] Relapse prevention is based on four assumptions:[28]

1. Different processes govern the action and maintenance stages of behavior change
2. Relapse risks are complex and involve individual, situational, physiological and sociocultural factors
3. Relapse is a part of an ongoing process of recovery and should not be equated with treatment "failure"
4. Relapse prevention is most successful when patients are empowered to act confidently as their own therapist in implementing treatment process

Marlatt and colleagues have developed cognitive-behavioral strategies and self-management skills (such as coping strategies) to address the determinants of relapse (see Table 7.4) [25] Relapse prevention has been extended to address a range of health behaviors and outcome goals consistent with a harm-reduction philosophy.[28;29;30-32] An analysis of high-risk situations can help practitioners select appropriate strategies.[33]

Table 7.4. Determinants of Relapse

Intrapersonal
1. Negative emotional states
2. Negative physical states
3. Positive emotional states
4. Testing personal control
5. Urges and temptations
Interpersonal
6. Interpersonal conflict
7. Social pressure
8. Positive emotional states

Individuals work through assignments that involve progressively handling more risky situations in their natural environment. For instance, a high-risk situation (e.g., a cocktail party) can threaten problem drinkers' sense of perceived control. They have to make a judgment (efficacy expectation) about their ability to cope with this situation. If they cope successfully, this will increase their self-efficacy in dealing with other future risk situations. Conversely, if they do not cope adequately, this leads to an increase in fear about such situations and a decrease in their self-efficacy.

LIKELIHOOD-OF-ACTION INDEX

The Likelihood-of-Action Index (see Table 7.5) summarizes 10 factors that can help individuals change. In addition to concepts, models and theories described in the chapter, this index also includes (1) two factors (marked with asterisks) from the Health Belief Model, (2) the emotional aspects of changes (factor 6 that is part of motivational interviewing and motivational practice) and (3) supports and barriers (see Chapter 5).

Table 7.5. Likelihood-of-Action Index

People are more likely to change their risk behaviors if they
1. Assess their health risk as serious*
2. Feel personally susceptible to the risk*
3. Have the confidence and ability to change
4. Believe that their action will reduce this risk
5. Perceive that the pros are greater than the cons to change
6. Do the emotional work to change
7. Want to change for freely chosen reasons
8. Develop strategies to prevent lapses and relapses
9. View relapses as learning opportunities
10. Reduce barriers and increase support to change

Derived from the Health Belief Model[34]

The likelihood of action increases as a function of both the presence and intensity of theses factors. In the following example, these factors were initially absent.

Ms. H. is a 30-year-old woman. She knew that unprotected sex put her at risk for sexually transmitted disease (STD) (including HIV). She did not feel personally susceptible to this risk, however, because she was in a long-term relationship with the same partner. She was quite confident that her partner was not having other sexual relationships. Even when Ms. H. contracted an STD (chlamydia infection), she downplayed her risk of getting the AIDS virus. She did not show up for a six-month follow-up for a repeat HIV test. Her boyfriend never used condoms because he also minimized his personal risk of getting HIV. He avoided the idea of getting the HIV blood test because of a needle phobia. It was only after Ms. H. learned that her girlfriend had contracted HIV (factor 1) that she went for the HIV test (factor 2). She also insisted that her boyfriend now use a condom (factor 3).

The Likelihood-of-Action Index can also help your patients understand better the complexity of initiating and maintaining change.

YOUR SUMMARY

Reflect: write a summary about what you have learned that was new for you.

_____

_____

_____

_____

_____

_____

_____

_____

_____

_____

_____

_____

_____

_____

_____

_____

_____

_____

_____

_____

_____

_____

_____

Enhance: write down your ideas about how your new learning could improve your interactions with patients. Add your notes to your learning portfolio.

_____

_____

_____

_____

_____

_____
_____
_____
_____
_____
_____
_____

REFERENCES

1. Botelho RJ, Skinner HA, Williams GC, et al. Patients with alcohol problems in primary care: Understanding their resistance and motivating change. In: Stuart MR, Lieberman IJA, eds. Primary care: Clinics in office practice. Philadelphia: W.B. Saunders Company; 1999: 279-298

2. Skinner HA. What motivates people to change? Promoting health through organizational change. San Francisco: Benjamin Cummings; 2001: 113-146

3. Bandura A. Social foundations of thought and action. Englewood Cliffs, NJ: Prentice Hall; 1986

4. Bandura, A. Moving into forward gear in health promotion and disease prevention. 1995. Presented at Meeting of Society of Behavioural Medicine

5. Bandura A. Self-efficacy: The exercise of control. New York: W.H. Freeman; 1997

6. Bandura A. Self-efficacy: Toward a unifying theory of behavior change. Psychological Review 1977;84: 191-215

7. Mischel W. Toward a cognitive social learning reconceptualization of personality. Psychological Review 1973;80: 252-283

8. Mischel W, Shoda Y. A cognitive-affective system theory of personality: Reconceptualizing situations, dispositions, dynamics, and invariance in personality structure. Psychological Review 1995;102: 246-268

9. Maibach E, Murphy DA. Self-efficacy in health promotion research and practice: Conceptualization and measurement. Special Issue: Measurement in health education research. Health Education Research 1995;10: 37-50

10. Miller SM, Shoda Y, Hurley K. Applying cognitive-social theory to health-protective behavior: Breast self-examination in cancer screening. Psychological Bulletin 1996;119: 70-94

11. Bandura A. Self-efficacy mechanism in physiological activation and health-promoting behavior. In: Madden J, ed. Neurobiology of learning, emotion, and affect 4th ed. New York: Raven Press; 1991:

12. Deci EL, Ryan RM. Intrinsic motivation and self-determination in human behavior. New York: Plenum Press; 1985

13. Williams GC, Grow VM, Freedman ZR, et al. Motivational predictors of weight loss and weight-loss maintenance. Journal of Personality and Social Psychology 1996;70. No. 1: 115-126

14. Deci EL, Ryan RM. A motivational approach to self: Integration in personality. In: Dienstbier R, ed. Nebraska symposium on motivation: Vol 38. Perspectives on motivation. Lincoln, NE: University of Nebraska Press; 1991

15. Prochaska JO, DiClemente CC, Norcross JC. In search of how people change: Applications to addictive behaviors. American Psychologist 1992;47(9): 1102-1114

16. Prochaska JO, Velicer WF, Rossi JS, et al. Stages of change and decisional balance for 12 problem behaviors. Health Psychology 1994;13(1): 39-46
17. DiClemente CC, Prochaska JO, Fairhurst SK, et al. The process of smoking cessation: An analysis of precontemplation, contemplation and preparation stages of change. Journal of Consulting and Clinical Psychology 1991;59(2): 295-304
18. Velicer WF, DiClemente CC, Prochaska JO, et al. Decisional balance measure for assessing and predicting smoking status. Journal of Personality & Social Psychology 1985;48: 1279-1289
19. Prochaska JO. Strong and weak principles for progressing from precontemplation to action based on twelve problem behaviors. Health Psychology 1994;13 (1): 47-51
20. Prochaska JO, DiClemente CC. Toward a comprehensive model of change. In: Miller WR, Heather N, eds. Treating addictive behaviors: Processes of change. New York: Plenum Press; 1986:3-27
21. Velicer WF, Fava JL, Prochaska JO, et al. Distribution of smokers by stage in three representative samples. Preventive Medicine 1995;24: 401-411
22. Glynn TJ, Manley MW. How to help your patients stop smoking: A National Cancer Institute Manual for Physicians [NIH Publication No. 89-3064]. Bethesda, MD: U.S. Department of Health and Human Services; 1989
23. Miller WR, Rollnick S. Motivational interviewing: Preparing people to change addictive behavior. New York: Guilford Press; 1991
24. Miller WR. Motivation for treatment: A review with special emphasis on alcoholism. Psychological Bulletin 1985;98(1): 84-107
25. Marlatt GA, Gordon JR. Relapse prevention: Maintenance strategies in addictive behavior change. New York: Guilford Press; 1985
26. Rollnick S, Mason P, Butler C. Behavior Change: A Guide for Practitioners. London: Churchill Livingstone; 1999
27. Hunt WA, Barnett LW, Branch LG. Relapse rates in addiction programs. Journal of Clinical Psychology 1971;27: 455-456
28. Dimeff LA, Marlatt GA. Relapse prevention. In: Miller H, ed. Handbook of alcoholism treatment approaches. Allyn & Bacon; 1995:
29. Brownell KD, Marlatt GA, Lichtenstein E, et al. Understanding and preventing relapse. American Psychologist 1986;41: 765-782
30. Marlatt GA, Tapert SF. Harm reduction: Reducing the risks of addictive behaviors. In: Baer JS, Marlatt A, McMahon R, eds. Addictive behaviors across the lifespan. Newbury Park, CA: Sage Publications; 1993: 243-273
31. Marlatt GA. Harm Reduction: Pragmatic strategies for managing high-risk behaviors. New York: Guilford Press; 1998
32. Laws DR. Relapse prevention with sex offenders. New York: Guilford Press; 1989
33. Annis HM, Davis CS. Relapse prevention. Alcohol Health & Research World 1991;15: 204-212
34. Rosenstock IM. Historical origins of the health belief model. Health Education Monographs 1974;2: 328-335

CHAPTER 8

OVERVIEW OF THE SIX-STEP APPROACH

FOR REFLECTION

*How can you negotiate with patients and motivate them
to work through the change process?*

OVERVIEW

The six-step approach to change[1] is a mental map to help you negotiate with your patients to take charge of their health over time. This model can help you assess where your negotiations with patients were particularly effective, as well as where and why they broke down. The Ladder of Change provides a conceptual framework that combines the six-step approach with the Stages of Change model: precontemplation, contemplation, preparation, action and maintenance. Each rung on the ladder represents a stage of change—starting with the bottom rung, which represents the first stage of change, and going up. The six-step approach helps patients move up the Ladder of Change.

Negotiation means different things to different people.[2-6] For many, negotiation is associated with conflicts and adversarial relationships, leading to win/lose or lose/lose situations. On the other hand, practitioners can negotiate with patients in ways that lead to win/win situations.

With the authoritarian, fix-it role, we are more likely to use an idealistic (either/or and right/wrong) approach to behavior change. For example, abstinence from alcohol is the only option for a heavy drinker, and all other options are unacceptable. With such a dichotomous perspective on health care options, patients either pass or fail in terms of achieving the ideal goal. If we unilaterally set ideal goals and try to make patients achieve them, they often fail to follow our advice. In effect, we set ourselves up to lose by insisting that patients should change before they are ready. If we react negatively (anger or frustration) toward these patients, we can even convert a win/lose into a lose/lose situation. Patients may react negatively toward such advice and fail to return to see us again. In this situation, no one wins.

When adopting a pragmatic, motivational role, you recognize patients' negative emotions as cues that you may be trying to make change occur prematurely. The win/win art of negotiation can help you work toward a common goal with your patients rather than work against one another (win/lose). Using the six-step approach, you first begin by assessing where patients are coming from before negotiating about behavior change. As you enhance mutual understanding with patients, you help them reduce their resistance and enhance their motivation to change so that they can move up the Ladder of Change. This process prepares patients to take at least some steps toward behavior change. Even if patients start to think more about change, it is the beginning of a win/win situation.

The half-empty/half-full glass metaphor highlights the difference between the idealistic and pragmatic approach. With the ideal approach, we view patients from a deficit perspective: how far away they are from achieving the ideal goals. With the pragmatic approach, we view patients from an achievement perspective: how far along they are in making progress toward goals, however modest.

SIX STEPS

Many influences have shaped the development of the six-step approach for negotiating about behavior change.[7-17] You can use these steps to assess where your negotiations with patients were particularly effective as well as where and why they broke down.

- **Step 1.** Building a partnership: developing empathy, clarifying roles and responsibilities and using relational skills effectively
- **Step 2.** Negotiating an agenda: using preventive or problem-focused approaches to negotiate a shared agenda

- **Step 3.** Assessing resistance and motivation: asking about patients' readiness to change, their reasons for staying the same (resistance) and their reasons for change (motivation), and their levels of resistance and motivation.
- **Step 4.** Enhancing mutual understanding: understanding and addressing how you and your patients have differences in perceptions and values about reasons for staying the same and for changing; in other words, reducing patients' resistance, increasing their motivation and thereby helping them to take charge of their health
- **Step 5.** Implementing a plan for change: negotiating an appropriate plan with your patients based on your mutual understanding; for example, thinking more about change, preparing to change and taking baby steps or giant leaps toward change
- **Step 6.** Following through: negotiating about the need and timing for future clinical encounters

You can implicitly move back and forth between these six steps, particularly when dealing with multiple problems in a clinical encounter. If and when necessary, you can explicitly negotiate with patients about shifting from one step to another. If you get stuck working with a patient at a particular step (e.g., implementing a plan), you need to return to an earlier step before developing an action plan.

THE LADDER OF CHANGE

The Ladder of Change serves as a guiding framework for negotiating about behavior change (see Figure 8.1). The six steps make up the rungs of the ladder. The spaces between the rungs of the ladder represent the five stages in a patient's readiness to change, beginning at the bottom with precontemplation and moving upward to contemplation, preparation, action and, finally, maintenance. Relapse occurs when the patient slips down the ladder. You can use this framework to help patients step up the rungs of the ladder at a pace that suits them.

Figure 8.1. The Ladder of Change

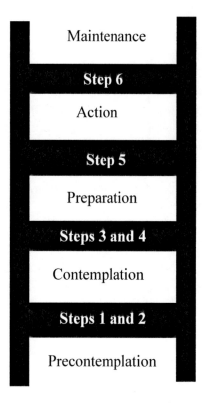

The following discussion outlines how the six-step approach and the stages of change combine to form a Ladder of Change that will help you individualize your approach to your patients.

Using Steps 1 and 2: Helping patients recognize and address a health issue
You can build an effective partnership and negotiate a shared agenda to help patients move from *not thinking* about a risk behavior (precontemplation) to *thinking* about behavior change (contemplation).

Using Steps 3 and 4: Helping patients take charge of their health
You can help patients move from *thinking* about to *preparing* for change (the preparation stage). When you conduct a motivational assessment, you help patients think more deeply about their reasons to change and not to change, and to understand better their resistance and motivation to change. When you try to enhance mutual understanding about their need for behavior change, you work to reduce patients' resistance and increase their motivation so that they take charge of their health.

Using Step 5: Helping patients change their behavior

After enhancing mutual understanding, you help patients move from *preparing to change* to *changing their behavior* (the action stage). You negotiate with patients about the goals and the dates for change and help them select and implement an appropriate plan of action.

Using Step 6: Helping patients maintain change

After patients have made a change, you can organize follow-up appointments and help them develop contingency plans to prevent relapses (the maintenance stage).

Each step includes a variety of strategies and interventions. These options can help you develop an individualized approach with all your patients so that they take charge of their own health over time.

A PRACTICAL APPLICATION

An example will illustrate the practical application of the six steps in helping a patient work through the five stages of change to reach the top of the ladder of change. In this case study, both the patient's husband and the practitioner worked together with the patient to encourage change.

NOT THINKING ABOUT CHANGE (precontemplation)

Patient unconcerned about her poor diabetic control: Mrs. D., a 70-year-old woman with mild obesity and adult-onset diabetes for the past 15 years, had just attended her 50th wedding anniversary reception, a large family gathering for over 100 guests. She thoroughly enjoyed the celebration, which was as memorable as her wedding 50 years ago. She paid no attention to her diet, drank a fair amount of alcohol and did not bother checking her blood glucose because she knew that it would be high despite her taking oral hypoglycemic medication. Her husband did not say anything throughout the celebration because he did not want to detract from her enjoyment of the occasion.

Commentary: Mrs. D. was not concerned about normalizing her blood glucose levels. Nor was she afraid of dying from diabetes. She had enjoyed her life and planned to continue to enjoy it on her own terms. From her perspective on achieving normal blood glucose levels, if she were to fill out a decision balance, she would view the reasons for staying the same as far outweighing the reasons to change. In contrast, her husband was concerned because he wanted his wife to be healthy and around for as long as possible. From his perspective about his wife, he viewed the reasons to change as far outweighing the reasons to stay the same. He was ready and willing to help his wife change, because he was not as ready as his wife to accept the risks of diabetes. However, he was afraid to bring up the issue of her poor diabetic control because he thought she would get upset and they would have an argument.

THINKING ABOUT CHANGE (contemplation)

Spouse setting the agenda and making an assessment: Two weeks after their 50th wedding anniversary, Mr. D. still had not broached the issue about diabetic control with his wife because he did not want to detract from her enjoyment in calling friends and family to thank them for their attendance. During this time, Mrs. D. modified her diet slightly, but she continued to drink two to three glasses of wine a day, which was more than her usual intake. With gentle prompting from her husband, she checked her blood glucose on several occasions. The blood sugar levels were much higher than before the wedding anniversary.

Soon after her last thank-you call, Mr. D. read a newspaper article about a new drug to treat diabetes. This prompted him to tell his wife how concerned he was about her diabetes, and he suggested that they go and see their practitioner together to talk about the possibility of Mrs. D.'s using this drug. Mrs. D. could see that her husband was concerned about her, and she also was moved by the fact that he had deliberately not said anything that he thought might spoil her enjoyment, so she agreed to an appointment.

Commentary: Mr. D. contained his anxiety and concern about his wife without expressing it to her because he knew she would not respond well to his insistence. He decided to mention this new drug only in passing to check whether Mrs. D. was interested in doing something else about her diabetes. Much to his relief, she was willing to make an appointment with her doctor to discuss the issue. Mr. D. had helped his wife move from precontemplation to early contemplation, even though his reasons for wanting her to see a practitioner were quite different from hers. She only saw the pros of using a new drug in terms of lowering blood glucose so that she did not have to be as careful with her diet.

PREPARING TO CHANGE (preparation)

Practitioner enhancing mutual understanding: Mr. and Mrs. D. went to see her practitioner together. Mrs. D. told her practitioner about her anniversary. He congratulated them and then inquired about whether their celebrations had made it difficult for her to stick to her diet. Mrs. D. looked at her husband, smiled at her practitioner and then informed him that she had not kept to the diet and had had a few drinks. She then changed the direction of the discussion by telling the practitioner that the reason they came today was because her husband had read a newspaper article about a new drug to treat diabetes, and she would like to know more about it.

Her practitioner acknowledged her request but also informed her about the need to keep to her diet, reduce her alcohol intake to below low-risk limits and lower her blood glucose levels to the normal range. He advised both Mr. and Mrs. D. that a recent study about type 2 diabetes showed that good blood pressure and glucose control could avoid the complications of diabetes. Mr. D. was impressed with this information, but Mrs. D. appeared unfazed. The practitioner asked her what she thought about this information. Mrs. D. gleefully stated that she enjoyed the food at her anniversary, was not afraid of dying, enjoyed her lifestyle and planned to continue as she was. Mr. D. appeared anxious and concerned.

When the practitioner realized how ineffective the educational approach had been with Mrs. D., he took an alternative approach. He acknowledged her lack of fear about death, but he expressed concern about what might happen to her before she died and the impact this might have on her husband and family. Mr. D. leaned forward and said, "That's what concerns me." Mrs. D. was surprised by her husband's response; she had not thought about her quality of life in this way. The practitioner then asked Mr. D. if he was holding back any concerns about his wife. While Mr. D. explained that he had not said anything for two weeks because he did not want to spoil the anniversary, Mrs. D. looked attentively at him. When Mr. D. leaned back, as if relieved of an emotional burden, he noticed tears in his wife's eyes. The practitioner asked Mrs. D. whether she would be prepared to consider change for the purpose of improving her quality of life and for the benefit of her husband. She took her husband by the hand and told him that she would take better care of her diabetes.

Commentary: During this exchange, Mrs. D. shifted from contemplation to the preparation stage. With the assistance of her practitioner and husband, she began to see that the pros of taking better care of her diabetes outweighed the cons of changing the lifestyle she enjoyed. This shift in the balance occurred because Mrs. D. became aware of her husband's concerns and was thus interested in improving not only her quality of life (integrated motives) but also in relieving her husband's anxiety (external motives). These issues were more important to her than the other change benefits of living longer or avoiding diabetic complications.

DOING IT (action)

Implementing a plan: Mrs. D. and her practitioner negotiated about a treatment plan. After some discussion, Mrs. D. selected a plan of action that included trying the new medication, Metformin. She also agreed to reduce her alcohol intake to less than seven drinks per week, with no more than two drinks on a single occasion. She was interested in whether this medication would also help reduce her blood glucose level. She made a commitment to keep to her diabetic diet, but she did not want to check her blood glucose every day. She was willing, however, to check her blood glucose three times a week before a meal and one hour afterward. She was not interested at this time in reducing her weight.

Commentary: Mrs. D. made several steps toward reducing her blood glucose. Because the negotiated plan represented a significant step in the right direction, the practitioner did not push her to achieve ideal body weight and blood glucose levels. She decided to visit her practitioner every three months to monitor the impact of the new regimen on her hemoglobin A1c.

KEEP DOING IT (maintenance)

Follow through: Mrs. D.'s husband attended all her appointments with her. With the new medications, her blood glucose dropped to near the normal range. She lost four pounds without really trying and reduced her alcohol intake to less than seven drinks per week, only occasionally consuming more than this limit. She also monitored her blood glucose twice a week. At this point, she became interested in losing weight. She thought she would try and lose 10 pounds in six months. After six months, she had lost six pounds and reduced her hemoglobin A1c from 10 to 7.5.

  Commentary: Regular follow-up appointments helped Mrs. D. keep to her diet, lose weight and reduce her hemoglobin A1c without a relapse.

YOUR SUMMARY

Reflect: write a summary about what you have learned that was new for you.

_____
_____
_____
_____
_____
_____
_____
_____
_____
_____
_____
_____
_____
_____
_____
_____
_____
_____
_____
_____
_____
_____
_____
_____
_____

Enhance: write down your ideas about how your new learning could improve your interactions with patients. Add your notes to your learning portfolio.

_____
_____
_____
_____
_____
_____
_____

_____

_____

_____

_____

_____

REFERENCES

1. Botelho RJ. A negotiation model for the doctor-patient relationship. Family Practice 1992;9(2): 210-218

2. Lazare A, Eisenhart S. Outpatient psychiatry. A negotiated approach to the clinic encounter: Conflict and negotiation. Baltimore, MD: Williams & Wilkins; 1979

3. Lazare A. The interview as clinical negotiation. In: Lipkin M, Jr, Putnam SM, Lazare A, eds. The medical interview. New York: Springer-Verlag; 1995: 50-64

4. Fisher R, Ury W. Getting to yes: Negotiating agreement without giving in. Boston: Houghton Mifflin; 1981

5. Hall L. Negotiation: Strategies for mutual gain. Newbury Park, CA: Sage Publications; 1993

6. Putnam LL, Roloff ME. Communication and negotiation. Newbury Park, CA: Sage Publications; 1992

7. Szasz TS, Hollenender MC. A contribution to the philosophy of medicine: The basic models of the doctor-patient relationship. Archives of Internal Medicine 1956;97: 585-592

8. Byrne PS, Long BE. Doctors talking to patients. London: HMSO, Royal College of General Practitioners; 1976

9. Working party of the Royal College of General Practitioners. The future general practitioner: Learning and teaching. London: British Medical Association; 1972

10 Berne E. Games people play. New York; Penguin Books; 1978

11. Scott NCH, Davis RH. The exceptional potential in each primary care consultation. Journal of the Royal College of General Practitioners 1979;29: 201-205

12. Kleinman A. Patients and healers in the context of culture. Berkeley, CA: University of California Press; 1979

13. Rollnick S, Kinnersley P, Stott N. Methods of helping patients with behaviour change. British Medical Journal 1993;307(6897): 188-190

14. Siegler M. Searching for moral certainty in medicine: A proposal for a new model of the doctor-patient encounter. Paul Turner, New York. Academy of Medicine 1981;57(1): 56-69

15. McWhinney IR. Are we on the brink of a major transformation of clinical method? Canadian Medical Association 1986;135: 873-878

16. Pendleton D, Schofield T, Tate P, et al. The consultation: An approach to learning and teaching. 6th ed. Oxford General Practice Series; 1984

17. Levenstein JH, Brown JB, Weston WW, et al. Patient-centered clinical interviewing. In: Stewart M, Roter D, eds. Communicating with medical patients. London: Sage Publications; 1989:107-12

SECTION III

HELPING PATIENTS CHANGE:
A SIX-STEP APPROACH

The six-step micro skill approach is designed to help you negotiate with patients about behavior change in a single encounter or during multiple encounters over time. A chapter is devoted to each step: building a partnership, negotiating an agenda, assessing resistance and motivation, enhancing mutual understanding, implementing a plan for change and following through. By moving back and forth between these steps with patients, you can learn how best to motivate them to change.

CHAPTER 9

STEP 1: BUILDING PARTNERSHIPS

Patients ultimately determine the goal and pace of behavior change. However, your partnership-building skills can significantly accelerate your patients' progress. In this three-part chapter, you will learn about three sets of skills that will enable you to develop effective partnerships with patients.

Part A: Develop empathy to understand patients' perspective

Part B: Relate to patients appropriately and accommodate their preference

Part C: Clarify roles and responsibilities (separate and shared) with patients

Empathic relationships enable you to form effective alliances with patients (see Figure 3.3). Good relationships with your patients have intrinsic worth and value for both parties, but this relational process may not always lead to improved outcomes. What the process *can* do is lay the foundation for developing effective partnerships with your patients so that you can address your differences in perceptions and values about behavior change (discordance) with them before building common ground (concordance). Effective partnerships can help you work through patients' emotional dis-ease, heightened ambivalence, conflicts (intrapersonal and interpersonal) and even enhanced resistance that can be produced by discussing your differences. To weather patients' emotional storms created by the prospect of change, you may need to strain your relationship (or even allow it to temporarily worsen) so that they can improve their health care outcomes. If you successfully help patients navigate through and move beyond these storms, you can strengthen your relational bond with them and work more effectively together on any other health behavior and/or issue.

CHAPTER 9 Part A

DEVELOPING EMPATHY

FOR REFLECTION

How do you empathize with patients who resist changing their risk behaviors?

OVERVIEW

Empathic relationships provide the foundation for promoting behavior change, even though empathic skills alone may not be sufficient to help patients change their behavior. To develop such relationships, you can use a variety of communication skills to understand patients' thoughts and feelings about their risk behavior. Such relationships enable you to work from their perspective and enhance their prospects of change.

An empathic relationship provides the foundation for improving patient outcomes.[1-5] Such relationships may involve[6-9]

- Understanding and/or feeling how your patients feel
- Communicating your understanding of their feelings back to them
- Patients acknowledging that you understand their feelings

With respect to behavior change, patients may be indifferent or have positive, negative or mixed feelings about their risk behaviors. An expanded notion of empathy means that you attempt to understand patients' perspectives (assumptions, expectations, perceptions, values, attitudes, beliefs and culture) about their risk behaviors, that is, why they feel the way they do.

Quite often, patients are not fully aware of all the underlying factors that affect their thoughts and feelings about their risk behavior and behavior change. Some patients may engage in unhealthy behaviors to avoid certain negative feelings (e.g., drinking alcohol to protect themselves against feelings of low esteem) and are unaware of what they are doing. This can make it difficult to empathize with such patients because their "absent" feelings are readily apparent to you, if not to themselves. Patients need courage to admit to these feelings and risk being vulnerable; your empathy helps them become more aware of their feelings about risk behavior and behavior change.

EMPATHIC SKILLS

Good empathic skills are essential for gaining an understanding of patients' perspectives about their risky situations or behaviors. Patients' verbal and nonverbal communications can help you understand the underlying factors that affect their thoughts and feelings about behavior change. Their nonverbal cues can also point to discrepancies between what they say and what they feel. You can help patients use such discrepancies to work toward resolving them; for example, in a case of spousal abuse, you might say, *"You claim that you may leave him in the future if things don't get better, but you looked scared when you said that."*

Because it is usually difficult to understand why patients stay in abusive relationships, particularly when they do not follow our advice to plan for a safe exit, spousal abuse is used throughout this section as an example to highlight the challenge of establishing effective partnerships with patients. To work more effectively with this frustrating situation, we need to examine our own frame of reference (mind-set) in working with patients who stay in such risky relationships. Are we asking questions and making comments from a negative *("She should leave him")*, neutral *("I don't know whether she should leave him")* or positive *("She should stay with him")* mind-set? The following example of a midwife who cared for a patient, Mrs. T., may help you reflect about your mind-set when addressing suspected spousal abuse and how you might approach things differently.

> Mrs. T. was a woman who was emotionally abused by her husband during her 10th week of pregnancy. The midwife's perspective was that Mrs. T. was also being physically abused and that her unborn first baby was at risk for abuse. The midwife felt that Mrs. T. should leave her husband. When Mrs. T. mentioned that her husband argued a lot with her, the midwife inquired directly: "So does your husband ever hit you when you have arguments?"
>
> "No," Mrs. T. responded curtly.
>
> "If your husband ever physically threatened or hurt you or your baby, would you go to a home for battered women?" the midwife continued.
>
> When the midwife persisted in her concerns, Mrs. T. became evasive. She stated that she wanted to work things out with her husband even though the midwife was ready to help her leave the situation. Mrs. T. resented the implication that her husband might do something abusive to their child and resisted any discussion about going to a home for battered women.

Two different perspectives about abused-abuser issues may help you explore your assumptions and mind-set further when addressing suspected abuse. These perspectives may help you work with patients more effectively and understand how they feel, based on what options they may have.

> **A landmark perspective about abused/abuser dynamics**: The cycle of abuse/abused dynamics consists of three phases. The first phase is tension-building. The second phase is acute battering. The third phase is kind and contrite, loving behavior. This cycle repeats itself over and over again.[10]
>
> **A pragmatic perspective about spousal abuse:** Choices for battered women are limited, particularly if they lack self-esteem, self-confidence and adequate job training. Many of them have insufficient financial resources to live independently. Even if they leave, they fear being stalked or killed. Battered women are often at risk whether they stay or leave. Therefore, they face a daunting dilemma. Paradoxically, they may be safer staying in the relationship for the time being, and are more at risk of harm if they choose to leave the relationship without adequate planning or resources.

The following example demonstrates how another midwife, MW, used a variety of communication skills (open-ended questioning, reflective listening, paraphrasing, validating feelings, normalizing behaviors, affirming strengths and asking probing questions) to address Mrs. T.'s suspected spousal-abuse situation.

MW:	*"So how does Jeff help you?"* (**open-ended question**)
Mrs. T.:	*Well, he's okay. He brings in the money, and he's looking forward to having a son. But sometimes, we get into arguments."* (Her tone of voice and nonverbal cues suggested that she disliked the arguments.)

MW: *"So you dislike the arguments?"* (**reflective listening**)

Mrs. T.:   *"Well, sometimes he gets so angry that I want to leave the room, but he won't let me. But things get better after he lets off steam, and he often apologizes afterwards."*

MW: *"Arguments arise and he keeps you in the room against your wishes, but he makes it up to you afterwards. Things get better and then arguments arise again. It seems as though things go in circles.* (**paraphrasing**) *Are things getting better or worse?"*

Mrs. T.:   *"It's worse when I can't tell when he's getting mad."*

MW: *"So sometimes you can sense when Jeff is getting mad, but at other times he gets angry without any reason, and that makes you feel really scared."* (**validating feelings**)

Mrs. T.:   *"With our baby coming, I just want to stay together as a family."*

MW: *"It's normal to want to keep the family together, but that can be very difficult when you feel scared."* (**normalizing behaviors**)

Mrs. T.:   *"We've got to stay together!"*

MW: *"So, you're committed to staying together?"* (**affirming strengths**)

Mrs. T.:   *"Well, I guess that's true."*

MW: *"Suppose things got a lot worse and you became concerned about your own and your child's safety. What would you do?"* (**probing question**)

Mrs. T.:   *"Well, I don't know. I suppose I would go to my mother's house."*

The perspectives about abused-abuser issues and the above discussion helped MW to understand why Mrs. T. chose to stay with her husband, rather than proceeding on the premise that Mrs. T. should leave. At the next prenatal visit, she talked with Mrs. T. without evoking the defensiveness and undue resistance caused by the first midwife, which had prevented Mrs. T. from exploring her feelings and choices. MW posed questions based on the assumption that Mrs. T. was going to stay despite her marital difficulties. Once Mrs. T. realized MW was trying to understand her position, she was more willing to discuss the situation and even move toward some kind of action.

Helping women who you suspect are being abused express their reasons for staying in such a relationship may actually help them talk more freely about their potential options. You may thus benefit by first understanding why they stay in relationships that you suspect are abusive, rather than by jumping ahead to work on helping them leave the relationship when they are not ready.

Although these perspectives about spousal abuse do not address all aspects of this complex issue, they can help you reflect about how your assumptions may facilitate or hinder the process of helping abused patients. This example may help you better understand about the mind-set (negative, neutral and/or positive) upon which you base your assumptions, ask questions, make comments and respond to patients—which will, in turn, affect how well you can empathize with your patients' experiences.

Communication skills (as described in the previous dialogue example) can help you empathize with patients about their risk behaviors or risky situations, and thereby you can establish a good relationship with them. These skills can be used throughout the six steps. Furthermore, many of the micro skills described in subsequent chapters can enable you to better understand patients' perspectives. For example, you can use the decision balance (see Chapters 1 and 13) in ways that enhance your ability to empathize with patients. However, this is just the first step, as you can have effective communication and good relationships with patients without improving health care outcomes. In other words, the process of care can improve without making a difference in the patient's health. The challenge is how to use your communication and relationship skills to change patients' perceptions and values about their risk behaviors so that they decide to take action. Communication and relationship skills are valuable means to that end.

YOUR SUMMARY

Reflect: *write a summary about what you have learned that was new for you.*

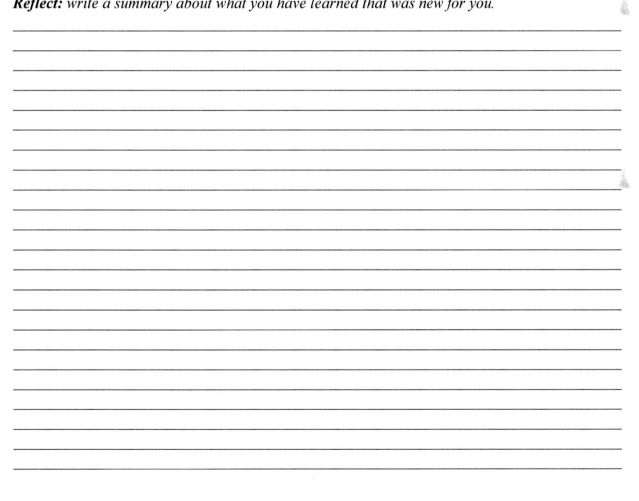

Enhance*: complete a self-assessment of your skills using the worksheet on page 318.* ***Write your goals below for improving specific skills*** *in role plays or patient encounters. After doing these practice sessions, reassess your competence score for these skills and make notes on page 318 to explain why you changed your scores. If possible, keep an audio recording or videotape of your practice sessions.*

_____
_____
_____
_____
_____
_____
_____
_____
_____
_____
_____
_____
_____

REFERENCES

1. Squier RW. A model of empathic understanding and adherence to treatment regimens in practitioner-patient relationships. Social Science & Medicine 1990;30: 325-339

2. More ES, Milligan MA. The empathic practitioner: Empathy, gender, and medicine. New Brunswick, NJ: Rutgers University Press; 1994

3. Spiro H, McCrea M, Perschel E, et al. Empathy and the practice of medicine. New Haven: Yale University Press; 1993

4. Gallop R, Lancee WJ, Garfinkel PE. The empathic process and its mediators: A heuristic model. Journal of Nervous & Mental Disease 1990;178: 649-654

5. Brock CD, Salinsky JV. Empathy: An essential skill for understanding the physician-patient relationship in clinical practice. Family Medicine 1993;25: 245-248

6. Platt FW, Keller VF. Empathic communication: A teachable and learnable skill. Journal of General Internal Medicine 1994;9: 222-226

7. Suchman AL, Markakis K, Beckman HB, et al. A model of empathic communication in the medical interview. Journal of the American Medical Association 1997;277: 678-682

8. Barrett-Lennard GT. The phases and focus of empathy. British Journal of Medical Psychology 1993;66: 3-14

9. Zinn W. The empathic physician. Archives of Internal Medicine 1993;153: 306-312

10. Walker LE. The battered woman. New York: Harper Perennial; 1979

CHAPTER 9 Part B
USING RELATIONAL STRATEGIES

FOR REFLECTION

Which relational strategies can best help patients change?

OVERVIEW

A relational map can help you better understand how to develop effective partnerships with your patients. Understanding this map helps to clarify how your patients can relate to you in three ways:[1]

1. The patient one-up/practitioner one-down position
2. The one-to-one position (egalitarianism)
3. Practitioner one-up/patient one-down position (paternalism or autocracy)

You can select one of three relational strategies to help patients take charge of changing their behavior by

1. Elevating them to take the one-up position
2. Deliberately taking the one-down position
3. Establishing complementary relationships

When you elevate patients to take the one-up position, you assume that patients know what is in their best interest and how to change, if they choose to. When you take the one-down position, you do not assume you know what is best for your patients or how they could best use your expertise, if at all. With complementary relationships, you accept patients at whatever relationship level they are at but also address the underlying factors that could prevent or detract from taking the one-up position. For example, you can boost the patient's confidence by acknowledging strengths and past successes at behavioral change.

A relationship map can help you learn how to develop and maintain effective partnerships with patients. You can also use a variety of relational strategies to enhance patients' responsibility for and active participation in changing their behavior.

RELATIONSHIP MAP

A relationship map can help you track how you and your patients relate to one another in dealing with different health issues.[1] The map (see Figure 9.1) is derived from T. S. Szasz's model of the doctor-patient relationship and includes the one-to-one position (egalitarianism) and the practitioner one-up position (paternalism and autocracy).[2] However, the map adds to that model in four important ways:

1. An additional relationship level, the patient one-up position, describes situations in which patients exert more or total responsibility for their own health care than do their practitioners.
2. The positioning in the practitioner-patient interaction is dynamic; you and your patients may both change positions within a single encounter to address different health care issues.
3. Conversely, these issues can influence the level at which you and your patients interact with each other. You can change the relationship level at any time during your interactions.
4. This map provides a way to track the relational process over time. Such tracking can help you and your patients develop an effective partnership in addressing risk behaviors and their complications. You learn how to make your relationship with patients work toward positive outcomes.

This map helps you guide patients toward the one-up position, in which they assume all or most of the responsibility for taking charge of their health, if appropriate. Such patient empowerment or elevation enhances the prospects of favorable outcomes.[3-7] The challenge is to help patients develop autonomous motives to change. Sometimes, however, patients are too handicapped by illness to assume this position and have genuine dependency needs (temporary or permanent).[4-7]

**Figure 9.1. Relationship Map
for Developing Effective Partnerships**

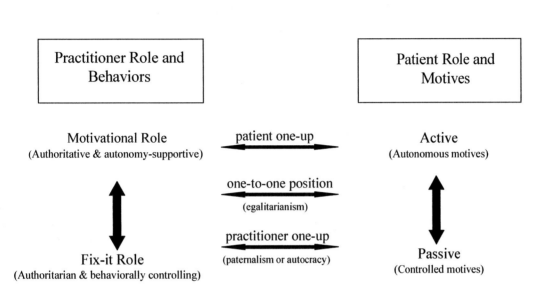

The relationship map can help you assess which is the right relationship level with your patient at a particular time.

THE PATIENT ONE-UP POSITION

The patient one-up position describes a relationship level at which patients assume more or total responsibility than their practitioner for all or most aspects of their health care. In other words, patients take charge of dealing with their health behavior change and the complications of their risk behaviors. They and their families determine how and what health care is to be provided while you defer to their directives and preferences.

However, patients may sometimes take the one-up position inappropriately, perhaps because of emotional reactions (fear, feeling out of control) to disease and illness: for example, a patient who refuses hospitalization for a heart attack or who exercises vigorously too soon after a heart attack. When you understand and address the emotional reasons underlying such behavior, you are in a better position to renegotiate your relationship to the level of egalitarianism so that the patient behaves in a more appropriate way.

Patients may also relate to you inappropriately at the one-up level with respect to addressing risk behaviors. For example, a patient may adamantly state that he does not have a drinking problem, even though there is clear evidence of alcohol dependence. To address this difference in problem definition, you can again try to establish more of an egalitarian relationship. To initiate such a change, you can initially allow the patient to maintain the one-up position but move toward renegotiating the relationship level. Consider the following example:

Renegotiating the relationship level: The practitioner may state, "You don't seem to think that alcohol is having any negative effects on your health." If the patient replies affirmatively or minimizes the consequences of alcohol, the practitioner may reply, "Perhaps you can help me understand your thoughts about that." [Let the patient explain and then respond.] "Let me share my concern about how I think alcohol is affecting your health."

Explain the health consequences: "I think we see things differently. Do you agree?" [Let the patient respond.] "As long as we see things differently, it's going to be difficult for us to work together to help you feel better and improve your health." [Let the patient respond.]

"Help me understand why you are convinced that alcohol is not affecting your health." [Let the patient respond.]

Commentary: The practitioner is attempting to renegotiate the relationship level from a patient one-up to a one-to-one position. Rather than arguing with the patient, the practitioner provides health information that contradicts the patient's understanding and encourages the patient to address the discrepancy between his opinion and the medical facts.

THE ONE-TO-ONE POSITION (EGALITARIANISM)

The practice of egalitarianism has gained prominence in the delivery of health care. Egalitarian practitioners relinquish some control and encourage patients to assume more responsibility for their health care. Such an approach helps to redress the imbalance of power and control in authoritarian practitioner-patient relationships and to reject traditional paternalism in health care.[8]

With health behavior change, you are on an unequal footing with patients at the onset of your interaction, because you have professional expertise about how risk behaviors affect health. However, patients have lay expertise about the patterns and reasons for their unhealthy habits. Together with your patients, you can take advantage of both professional and lay expertise to motivate behavior change. You can educate patients about the risks and harms of a behavior in an authoritative manner that is sensitive and relevant to patients' concerns, feelings and expectations, and they can offer you insight into their behavior. Such a synergistic relationship will help patients decide whether, when, how and what to change.

Illness, however, can diminish patient autonomy to the point where egalitarianism is inappropriate. For example, when patients and/or their families request that you take charge of all medical aspects of care, it would not be appropriate for you to insist that patients share responsibility equitably. Egalitarianism is also questionable when patient autonomy is diminished by conditions such as depression, anxiety, addictions and stress. In such circumstances, patients may suffer when you do not take a leading role in addressing their needs. Patients can feel abandoned if their practitioner assumes an egalitarian relationship when patients need a more paternalistic relationship.

Sometimes you might work better if you relate to your patients at different levels in dealing with behavior change and the complications from their risk behaviors. Patients may want you to take charge in addressing a disease complication; in effect, they expect a paternalistic relationship. In contrast, patients may take charge when it comes to initiating behavior change; in effect, they take the one-up position. The overall relationship may appear as egalitarian, but this label conceals the nuances of sharing responsibility for addressing different issues (e.g., one partner may take more responsibility for one issue, and the converse occurs on another issues).

Paternalism and autocracy are two examples of the practitioner in the one-up position. Practitioners may assume, and patients may expect, this kind of relationship under certain circumstances. Paternalism may be appropriate provided that patients make this choice and that they can opt out of this kind of relationship whenever they want.

PATERNALISM

Paternalism is appropriate in certain situations. For example, you can act in a variety of parental ways with patients: nurturing, advising, controlling and autonomy-supportive. Sometimes a paternalistic manner of giving advice is welcomed. Some patients may implicitly or explicitly expect a paternalistic relationship with you, particularly when dealing with medical issues they do not understand. Some elderly patients and certain ethnic groups expect their doctor to know best. Despite your encouragement to the contrary, some patients prefer that you make decisions about their health care. This can occur in circumstances when the effects of addiction, disease and/or psychological illness impair patients' autonomy. At such times, you may need to adopt a paternalistic relationship. But as patients recover, you need to change your relationship so that patients assume increasing responsibility for their health care. Describing different forms of paternalism—which range between these two extremes, from practitioner-centered to patient-centered—will help clarify when you can appropriately relate to patients in this manner.[9] When used inappropriately, however, such an approach can be interpreted as patronizing.[10]

Practitioner-centered Paternalism

A stereotype of traditional paternalism is a practitioner who always knows what is best for the patient. Such practitioners act in controlling ways and instruct patients to change their behaviors. The advice they give imposes their values on patients, rather than understanding and accommodating patient values. Ethical objections to such paternalism arise from well-justified concerns that it is wrong to impose your values unilaterally without regard to patients' values, preferences and needs. As previously mentioned, some ethnic and socioeconomic groups expect this traditional form of paternalism. Such paternalism (father/mother knows best) is acceptable when patients explicitly state that they trust you to act this way, but you are not obliged to do this just because of patient expectations and dependence. When it is appropriate, you can activate patients to modify their expectations so that they relate to you in a more egalitarian manner and assume more responsibility for their own health care.

Patient-centered Paternalism

As a practitioner, even though you act in authoritative, autonomy-supportive and nurturing ways, you consider the values and needs of patients and their families in working together. With their consent, you act in the best interest of patients, based on your understanding of their values and needs. In effect, you accommodate patients' autonomy and request to act as their parent, rather than imposing your values. This role choice may result from factors as diverse as ethnic values, disease, illness, stress or addictions. As much as possible, you also help patients work toward assuming more responsibility for addressing risk behaviors and their complications. In time, they may relate to you at an egalitarian or even higher level.

AUTOCRACY

When the patient's autonomy is impaired or absent due to a life-threatening event, you must take control to save or to protect life. You take charge in responding to medical, surgical and psychiatric emergencies. When addressing health behavior change, autocracy has limited applications.

In a caring manner, you can deliver poignant, brief and imperative messages about the need to change risk behaviors. Such semiautocratic messages may be effective if patients are in a state of receptive vulnerability. For example, in time-pressured encounters with patients, you can use direct, brief interventions when dealing with the acute complications of risk behaviors. You can also give time-limited directives to the patient (e.g., during pregnancy) not to smoke or drink alcohol.[11] This kind of message might seem autocratic, but the label oversimplifies the complexity of how you can address behavior change as part of your ongoing relationships with patients. Before judging whether these directives are purely autocratic, you need to consider how such directives are embedded in the context of a meaningful and trusting relationship and how patients interpret such messages. With certain patients and under certain circumstances, the autocratic approach may sometimes be effective.

RELATIONAL STRATEGIES

Once you understand the various levels at which you and your patients can relate, you can then help them take charge of change by

- Elevating them to take the one-up position
- Taking the one-down position with them, or
- Forming a complementary relationship with them

You can test which strategy works for individual patients based on what you think will have the greatest impact. When uncertain about a patient's capacity to assume greater responsibility, you can use these strategies tentatively to enhance his or her responsibility and motivation. Alternatively, you can use these strategies more affirmatively when the patient seems capable of assuming greater responsibility.

ELEVATING THE PATIENT TO TAKE THE ONE-UP POSITION
Use this relational strategy when you think the patient can relate to you at a higher level. Elevate your patient to take the one-up position by

- Deferring to the patient's opinion
- Telling the patient he or she has the know-how to change
- Encouraging the patient to make his or her own decisions
- Deferring to the patient about how best to address health behavior change

Examples of questions that elevate the patient to take the one-up position:
- *"Do you think you will always continue this behavior?"*
- *"What would it take for you to decide that you need to change your behavior [stop smoking, reduce alcohol consumption, assume self-care of chronic disease]?"*
- *"What would it take for you to decide to change?"*
- *"At what point in your life do you think it would be sufficiently important for you to change?"*

>   ***Commentary:*** *These questions toss the ball of responsibility to patients, defer to their expertise and encourage them to consider change. The underlying message is that health behavior change is beneficial and possible and that patients have the skills to change. Your tone of voice can convey the message of these questions in a tentative or affirmative manner, depending on how you perceive the patient's level of confidence and competence to change. When patients are competent but lack confidence, ask these questions in an affirmative manner. When you are concerned about patients' competence to change, ask these questions in a tentative manner.*

By elevating patients to take the one-up position, you imply that patients have the ability to change if they want to. Such interventions can further enhance patients' sense of confidence to change. In some situations, patients and their families will need additional advice from you about different methods for changing their behavior. Describe the advantages and disadvantages of various methods but without recommending a particular course of action. This approach enables patients to make their own decisions.

TAKING THE ONE-DOWN POSITION WITH A PATIENT

This approach may be appropriate when patients behave in a dependent manner and expect a paternalistic relationship with you. Take the one-down position by telling patients that you

- Do not know the best option for handling the situation
- Do not know how they can best use their own resources and expertise
- Are uncertain how they should deal with a risk behavior
- Cannot make the decisions for them
- Do not know what are the best decisions for them

This strategy can help patients explore whether they are capable of assuming greater responsibility for dealing with a behavior.

> **Example of a practitioner taking the one-down position:** A practitioner stated to an elderly man who recently developed adult-onset diabetes, "Most patients feel overwhelmed about how to deal with diabetes. We've discussed many recommendations—weight reduction, diabetic diet, taking drugs appropriately, self-monitoring of blood sugar, lowering cholesterol levels, smoking cessation, modification of alcohol use, adjustments in family and work routines, eye checkups with ophthalmologists, foot care and regular appointments with primary care practitioners. But I don't know where you would like to start to address any of these recommendations. What do you think?" Not uncommonly, patients are initially evasive with this approach and may defer to the practitioner by echoing, "Well, what do you think?" The practitioner can then reply, "I'll certainly share with you what I think, but it's important for me to understand where you stand regarding all this information and what you feel you can do at the moment."

> **Commentary:** Discrepancies commonly exist between the ideal recommendations for diabetic care and the real-world practice. You and your patients are apt to have different priorities about how to approach diabetic care. Taking the one-down position helps you understand the patient's priorities. This approach may also elevate some patients to take more responsibility for their diabetic care.

FORMING A COMPLEMENTARY RELATIONSHIP WITH A PATIENT

In this relational strategy, you initially engage patients at the relationship level of the patient's choice but also address the underlying factors that prevent or detract from patients being more active.[3-7] Examples of such interventions include enhancing patients' confidence and competence to change, increasing their family and community support, reducing barriers to change and addressing psychological impediments to change, such as anxiety disorders and depression. In effect, you indirectly empower patients to work toward a complementary or one-up position.

> **Example of working toward a complementary relationship:** Mr. L. seemed despondent, and related at the level of paternalism with his practitioner. He felt that his practitioner was responsible for finding a quick fix to help him change his drinking habit. The practitioner initially interacted with Mr. L. at this level but then boosted his morale by praising him for having cut back on his drinking for three weeks about six years ago. The practitioner reminded Mr. L. that many people who eventually succeed in quitting often make several attempts, persist in trying and regard failures as opportunities to learn how to succeed. This intervention, which focused on strengths and past success, enhanced Mr. L.'s self-esteem and confidence to such a degree that he acknowledged he could change again.
>
> **Commentary:** The practitioner recognized and addressed the patient's despondency in ways that activated the patient to shift the relationship from the level of paternalism to the level of egalitarianism.

USING RELATIONAL STRATEGIES CREATIVELY

You can use relational strategies creatively by sequencing them in ways that have the greatest impact on enhancing patients' responsibility for change. For example, take the one-down position, followed by elevating the patient to take the one-up position. When initially using these strategies and interventions, you may have concerns about manipulating patients. In fact, you are indeed trying to manipulate your patients. But such manipulation is ethical, provided that you have your patients' consent to improve their health and that you act in authentic and genuine ways: for example, recognize what you do not know, rather than presume to know what is best for your patients. Sometimes you know what is best medically but do not know how to use your expertise for their benefit. Relational strategies—such as admitting that you do not always know how best to work with patients about health behavior change—help to bridge your professional world with that of your patients' to help them change.

Although your intentions are to achieve favorable outcomes, you may find yourself using relational strategies inappropriately. For example, you may use the one-down position when patients are unable to exert greater autonomy in dealing with their disease, illness and/or risk behavior. In such circumstances, patients may feel pressured and abandoned. Overall, relational strategies can expand your repertoire of working with patients, but you need to monitor whether you are using them appropriately and effectively.

USING ROLE CHOICES CREATIVELY

You may also find that you need to adopt different roles to address different risk behaviors and their complications when using these relational strategies. For example, a motivational role is appropriate to help a patient modify excessive alcohol intake, while a fix-it role may be suitable for prescribing drugs to treat alcohol-induced hypertension. These roles vary along a continuum between acting as an agent of influence and as an agent of control. As this happens, the patient's role can vary along an active-passive continuum. Your role and that of your patients are complementary, no matter who sets the tone of the relationship. For example, when patients are passive, you are more likely to assume a fix-it role and to take the one-up position with patients and relate to them paternalistically. Conversely, when you adopt this role, patients are more likely to assume a more passive role and adopt the one-down position.

When you adopt a motivational role and activate patients to take responsibility, they are more likely to assume a more active role for change. In such cases, you are more likely to relate to them at the one-to-one level (egalitarianism) or the patient one-up level. When this occurs, they are more likely to experience favorable outcomes.[12]

When your roles do not complement one another, you can run into role conflicts with patients. For example, you may take on a fix-it role and expect a passive patient, but the patient instead actively engages in an unhealthy behavior. Relational strategies and roles therefore have a mutual impact on the way you and your patients interact.

YOUR SUMMARY

Reflect: write a summary about what you have learned that was new for you.

_____
_____
_____
_____
_____
_____
_____
_____
_____
_____
_____
_____
_____
_____
_____

_____
_____
_____
_____
_____
_____
_____
_____
_____

Enhance*: complete a self-assessment of your skills using the worksheet on page 318.* ***Write your goals below for improving specific skills*** *in role plays or patient encounters. After doing these practice sessions, reassess your competence score for these skills and make notes on page 318 to explain why you changed your scores. If possible, keep an audio recording or videotape of your practice sessions.*

_____
_____
_____
_____
_____
_____
_____
_____
_____

REFERENCES

1. Botelho RJ. A negotiation model for the doctor-patient relationship. Family Practice 1992;9(2): 210-218
2. Szasz TS, Hollenender MC. A contribution to the philosophy of medicine: The basic models of the doctor-patient relationship. Archives of Internal Medicine 1956;97: 585-592
3. Wallerstein N. Powerlessness, empowerment, and health: Implications for health promotion programs. American Journal of Health Promotion 1992;6: 197-205
4. Feste C, Anderson RM. Empowerment: From philosophy to practice. Patient Education & Counseling 1995;26: 139-144
5. Rodwell CM. An analysis of the concept of empowerment. Journal of Advanced Nursing 1996;23: 305-313
6. Gilbert T. Nursing: Empowerment and the problem of power. Journal of Advanced Nursing 1995;21: 865-871
7. Skelton R. Nursing and empowerment: Concepts and strategies. Journal of Advanced Nursing 1994;19: 415-423
8. Thomasma DC. Beyond medical paternalism and patient autonomy: A model of physician conscience for the physician-patient relationship. Annals of Internal Medicine 1983;98: 243-248
9. Lomas HD. Paternalism; medical or otherwise. Social Science & Medicine 1981;15: 103-106

10 Brewin TB. Truth, trust and paternalism. Lancet 1985;1: 490-492

11. Cogswell B, Eggert MS. People want doctors to give more preventive care: A qualitative study of health care consumers. Archives of Family Medicine 1993;2: 611-619

12. Kaplan SH, Greenfield S, Ware JE, Jr. Assessing the effects of physician-patient interactions on the outcomes of chronic disease. Medical Care 1989;27: S110-S127

CHAPTER 9 Part C

CLARIFYING ROLES AND RESPONSIBILITIES

FOR REFLECTION

What factors affect your roles and responsibilities in working with patients?
How do you clarify your roles and responsibilities with patients?

OVERVIEW

The following factors can shape and change your and your patients' roles in working together:

- Your patients' perceived confidence and ability to change (self-efficacy)
- Your patients' motives
- Your patients' autonomy
- Your use of authority, influence and control
- The balance of responsibilities between you and your patients

Clarifying your roles and responsibilities can help you enhance the effectiveness of your partnerships with patients over time. The process may activate patients to take charge of their own health care.

As already noted, addressing risk behaviors can be particularly frustrating if you assume responsibility for health care issues that you cannot control. To resolve your frustrations, you can shift your role and redefine responsibilities in order to build an effective partnership with patients.

An example of shifting roles: The practitioner was initially insistent that her patient, Mr. S., lose weight and keep to a strict diabetic diet in order to lower his blood glucose and cholesterol levels. She was convinced that Mr. S. could control his diabetes and hypercholesterolemia by diet and weight reduction. Furthermore, she was adamant that Mr. S. stop smoking in order to protect his heart (fix-it role). Mr. S. told his practitioner that he did not entirely agree with this plan. He was not ready to lose weight or stop smoking, but he was prepared to reduce his alcohol consumption, reduce his fat intake and take hypoglycemic and hypocholesterolemic drugs to reduce his blood glucose and cholesterol levels. Realizing that her patient was not ready to follow what she considered to be the ideal approach, the practitioner switched roles and negotiated with the patient. She asked him whether he might reconsider weight reduction and smoking cessation at a later time. Mr. S. then thought he would try to make only one change at a time, and asked his practitioner what she thought was more important to address first. She advised him that

- Smoking cessation was more important than weight reduction
- He might gain a few pounds after he stopped smoking
- Medications would lower his blood glucose and cholesterol levels
- He might be able to stop taking some medications if he lost 15 pounds.

Commentary: The practitioner initially took the one-up position in relating to the patient, but Mr. S. resented being told what to do. He let his practitioner know that he was not prepared to do everything asked of him. The practitioner then backed down from the one-up position. Instead, she adopted a motivational role that incorporated the input of Mr. S. into the decision-making process to establish a better partnership with him.

Once you have moved away from your initial role, you can further clarify to avoid overstepping the boundaries of defined responsibilities.

Practitioner: "I can prescribe drugs to control your cholesterol [fix-it role], but what concerns me is that half of all people stop taking the drugs regularly after a couple of years. If you decide to use a drug, I can certainly work with you in making this long-term commitment [motivational role]. What do you think about taking a drug for lowering cholesterol?"

Learning Exercise 9.1 Role clarification
    Role clarification can set the stage for you and your patients to define the balance of responsibilities in addressing different issues. Now think about a patient with whom

you became frustrated and confused about roles. Using the ideas presented, how could you have clarified your role and responsibilities with your patient?

Many factors affect the roles that patients and practitioners assume in working together, and role changes may occur without either party being fully aware of the process. Understanding the factors that shape and change these roles can help you to adopt the appropriate one for the situation.

YOUR PATIENTS' CONFIDENCE AND ABILITY (SELF-EFFICACY)

Self-efficacy refers to patients' perceptions about their confidence and ability to change: the "I can do it" attitude.[1-7] Many patients lack confidence even though they are able to change their behavior; consequently, they appear to lack self-efficacy. For example, Mrs. C. related to her practitioner at the level of paternalism because she lacked confidence about asserting herself when practicing safe sex with her boyfriend, despite knowing how to use condoms. Mrs. C. wanted her practitioner to talk to her boyfriend for her. The practitioner changed the relationship level by working with Mrs. C. in ways that boosted her confidence. Eventually, Mrs. C related to the practitioner at the level of egalitarianism and took more responsibility for her health care by talking to her boyfriend herself.

Other patients can project confidence but lack ability. This projection of confidence can deceive how practitioners perceive their patients. For example, Mr. B. took the one-up position in relating to his practitioner. However, he did not quit smoking, in spite of claiming that he could. The practitioner later learned that Mr. B. could not read well; the informational materials the practitioner had given to Mr. B. were beyond his reading abilities. He lacked the ability to quit, and his overconfidence was a way of concealing his embarrassment about his reading deficit. The practitioner had perceived Mr. B. as confident about his ability to change, without realizing the inaccuracy of this perception.

YOUR PATIENTS' MOTIVES

According to the self-determination theory discussed in Chapter 7, patients' motives exist along a continuum: indifference, controlled motives (external and internal) and autonomous motives.[8;9] These motives can influence how patients relate to their practitioner. Patients with freely chosen (autonomous) motives may take the one-up position by telling you what they are going to do. In contrast, patients with controlled motives may relate at the level of paternalism and expect you to tell them what to do. Patients who are indifferent about change may feel helpless, hopeless, fatalistic or resigned about effecting change. Sometimes these patients can make you take responsibility for issues that you cannot control or change—a frustrating experience.

YOUR PATIENTS' AUTONOMY

Patients act autonomously when they determine the extent to which they will take responsibility for dealing with risk behaviors and their complications.[10] In other words, feeling autonomous enables them to share responsibility with and relate to you differently over time, depending on circumstances. Patient autonomy is a dynamic phenomenon.

Personal autonomy refers to the extent to which patients determine whether they will take responsibility for risk behaviors and their psychosocial complications (financial problems, driving while intoxicated, relationship difficulties). Disease-centered autonomy refers to the extent to which patients decide to take responsibility for dealing with medical complications caused by risk behaviors. The extent to which patients exert their autonomy to address these medical and personal issues influences the level at which they relate to you. Patients often change the relationship level. In turn, you can adjust your relationship accordingly.

> **Contrasting "disease-centered" and "personal" autonomy:** When dealing with the medical aspects of hypercholesterolemia and asymptomatic type 2 diabetes, Mr. B. did not want to know the pros and cons of using different drugs for treating high cholesterol and diabetes. He simply wanted his practitioner to tell him what the best drugs were for him.
>
> After he had listened to his practitioner's recommendations, Mr. B. Discussed the impact of his high cholesterol and diabetes on his personal life, and then told his practitioner how he was going to deal with these Health issues. He decided to lose 15 pounds over six months, take the recommended cholesterol-lowering drug, stick to a diabetic diet and recheck the control of his diabetes on a monthly basis. In other words, although he trusted his practitioner's medical expertise and allowed his practitioner to take the one-up position in addressing the medical issues, he took the one-up position in dealing with the personal aspects of health behavior change. The practitioner provided the options; the patient made the decisions.

YOUR USE OF AUTHORITY, INFLUENCE AND CONTROL

Most patients expect you to be an authority on risk behaviors. The use of professional authority may be a state or trait characteristic. A state characteristic is evoked in a particular situation. For example, when dependent patients expect a paternalistic relationship, they may expect and require you to act in an authoritarian or authoritative manner. A trait characteristic relates to a more immutable personal style: the tendency to act in a manner independent of context and circumstances, that is, to habitually behave in this way.

Your style of using authority (authoritarianism vs. authoritativeness) affects whether you will use control or influence when working with patients. Control refers to the extent to which one person attempts to regulate or restrain another person and/or the situation (e.g., disease). Influence refers to how one person helps the other decide whether to change, without any coercion. Authoritarianism is a controlling approach that you use in emergencies, for example, rescuing patients in life-threatening situations. Such control is appropriate in these cases but is not appropriate for motivating change in risk behaviors. In routine health care, such an approach can foster patient dependency to the degree that patients relate to you exclusively at the level of paternalism. They are less likely to challenge your authority, or even ask questions.

When adopting a motivational role, you influence rather than try to control patients' behavior. You use your expertise authoritatively by providing pertinent information to patients. You let them decide how to use this information and whether to change.

Understanding the difference between control and influence is especially important in helping you decide which role will be most effective in addressing particular risk behaviors and their complications.[11] The following examples provides illustrations to help you understand:

- How you can deliver controlling or autonomy-supportive messages to patients
- How patients may interpret these messages
- How you can respond to patients' self-defeating responses to these messages

CONTROLLING VERSUS AUTONOMY-SUPPORTIVE MESSAGES

Health information can be used as a weapon to coerce patients to change (controlling message) or as an aid to influence change (autonomy-supportive message). For example, you could try and scare patients by showing them frightening pictures of smokers' damaged lungs. Such scare tactics work infrequently, because these kinds of controlling messages only help patients develop controlled motives: "I'm going to stop smoking because my doctor told me that it causes lung damage" or "because my family wants me to stop damaging my lungs." With these kinds of motives, patients often do not take full ownership of and responsibility for change. Furthermore, continued reinforcement is typically needed to help patients maintain changes in their behavior.

In contrast, you can deliver autonomy-supportive messages and use your influence, not control, by stating, *"As you probably know, smoking is the cause of your breathing problem. If you quit smoking, your breathing problem will not get worse; it may even improve over time. Could you spend some time just talking and thinking about whether you would like to quit?"* With this example, you emphasized the positive gains or benefits of change rather than using scare tactics. At the same time, patients take some responsibility for change simply by talking or thinking about it.

PATIENT INTERPRETATIONS OF YOUR MESSAGES

Patients may interpret your messages differently from what you intended, even if you deliver them in the same way to every patient. In the following example, a patient in the contemplation stage (Mrs. C.) interpreted a controlling message differently from a patient in the preparation stage (Mrs. P.).

Contrasting interpretations of a controlling message

1. A patient who is ambivalent about change: When the practitioner stated, "You should stop smoking," Mrs. C., who was thinking about change, became irritated by the practitioner's manner, but concealed her irritation by replying, "I know I should give up smoking. My children and husband have been nagging me about it." After their discussion, however, Mrs. C. decided not to think about smoking cessation because she was fed up with people telling her to quit smoking, that is, she became a precontemplator.

Commentary: Mrs. C. interpreted the practitioner's message as controlling and also felt nagged by him. No one seemed to understand her stress, which made her feel more discouraged. She did not tell her practitioner that she had been thinking about using a nicotine patch. Since she perceived her practitioner as nagging her, she changed from feeling that she should stop smoking to feeling disinterested in smoking cessation. Her family and practitioner had inadvertently added to her stress. She used her usual coping style of dealing with added stress by continuing to smoke and becoming less inclined to think about smoking cessation or to seek medical attention for her stress and nicotine addiction. In other words, she changed from having an internally controlled motive toward change ("I ought to quit") to an indifferent one ("I don't care about quitting").

2. A patient who is ready for change: Mrs. P. was ready to change and thus already had an autonomous motive for change. Because she had almost decided to take action herself, she interpreted the same message from her practitioner as autonomy-supportive and replied, "I've been thinking about that for a while, and I'm ready to quit smoking." She felt that she was making the choice for herself rather than for her practitioner, and thus was prepared to set up a quit date with him.

Commentary: The contrasting responses of Mrs. C. and Mrs. P. demonstrate how a controlling message can be interpreted differently, based on the patient's stage of change (contemplation vs. preparation) and their motives to change: "I should/ought/must stop smoking" (internally controlled) vs. "I am going to quit" (autonomous). Because the practitioner did not know each patient's stage of change, he was unable to make a distinction between controlled and autonomous motives toward change. In order to avoid such different interpretations, he needed to clarify both his and each patient's roles in order to define the balance of responsibility.

Conversely, patients who have been victimized in abusive relationships or lived in socially deprived situations may expect others to control them and consequently may interpret your autonomy-supportive messages as controlling ones, that is, try to guess what you want even when offered choices.

RESPONDING TO PATIENTS' SELF-DEFEATING RESPONSES TO THESE MESSAGES

When patients feel as though behavior change is beyond their control, they may feel hopeless and/or helpless about change. They also may feel controlled by others (including their practitioner), by circumstances or by the behavior itself (addiction or habitual routine). As a consequence, patients may deflect taking responsibility for change by making self-defeating statements:

1. *"I don't have the willpower to change."*
2. *"I don't have enough family support to change."*
3. *"I'm addicted to nicotine, and I can't change."*

Controlling messages to these statements (such as judgmental or directive comments) can sometimes make the situation worse. Or you may behave in ways that are subtly controlling without being aware of it. (Reviewing your videotapes or tape recordings of patient encounters can help you identify such behavior.) In contrast, you can counteract patient hopelessness/helplessness with autonomy-supportive messages. For example:

Possible responses to Statement 1: "I don't have the willpower to change"
- *"I'm curious to know what you mean when you say that you don't have the willpower to change." (This probing response helps you to clarify what a patient means to better understand the patient and perhaps lower his or her resistance to change.)*
- *"You have no willpower to change? But you did stop smoking for three months in the past." (Reflective listening and paraphrasing a patient's response statements provide the patient with the opportunity to reflect on his or her response and allow time to explore past successes.)*
- *"What would it take for you to take charge of your health?" (This question reframes "willpower" to "taking charge." This change of words may help the patient avoid blaming himself or herself for a lack of willpower. It also helps the patient to overcome feeling like a victim of circumstance with no choices or control over life. Challenging such assumptions can help the patient realize that there are choices and that he or she can take charge of a behavior.)*

Possible responses to Statement 2: "I don't have enough family support to change"
- *"I'm curious about what you mean when you say you don't have support from your family." (This probing statement helps you clarify what a patient means to better understand the issues faced by the patient. It is especially helpful for a patient who seems unable to get the family support that he or she needs.)*
- *"You don't get enough support? That means you'll have to do it alone." (Again, by using reflective listening and paraphrasing the patient's response, you encourage the patient to explore the issue of support and responsibility for change.)*

- *"How would you get the support from your family that you need? And if you couldn't get the support you need, what else could you do?" (These questions help the patient clarify issues about how to get family support. It also challenges the patient to do what is needed for his or her own health if he or she cannot get family support.)*

Possible responses to Statement 3: "I'm addicted to nicotine, and I can't change"
- *"Tell me what you mean when you say 'addicted to nicotine' or 'can't change.'" (This helps a patient clarify what he or she means and helps you better understand the issues faced by the patient.)*
- *"You're addicted to nicotine, so it's hard for you to think that you can quit alone." (Use reflective listening and paraphrase the patient's response. Then let the patient respond.) "And what do you think about using nicotine patches to help you get over your addiction?"*
- *"How do you think you could overcome your nicotine addiction? Would you like some ideas about how you could do it?" (These questions challenge the patient to consider the possibility of overcoming his or her addiction and let the patient know that help is available if he or she cannot do it alone.)*

Some or all of these responses may help patients overcome their self-defeating behavior and increase their confidence and ability to change.

Learning Exercise 9.2: Addressing hopelessness/helplessness
Think about a patient who made you feel powerless to effect change. On a separate piece of paper, write down a patient statement that you had difficulty responding to, and then think how you could have responded to this patient.

BALANCE OF RESPONSIBILITIES BETWEEN YOU AND YOUR PATIENTS

You and your patients may vary the amount of responsibility each takes for addressing different health issues. As discussed in Part 9B, the balance of responsibility changes with your relationship level, depending on whether it is the one-up (paternalistic and autocracy), the one-down or the one-to-one position (egalitarianism).

Since relational boundaries are flexible, practitioners and patients can change how they share responsibilities in working together over time. Sometimes, an important issue is not addressed: neither you nor your patient take or share responsibility for the issue. Conversely, you and your patient may be in conflict about how to balance responsibility for addressing a particular issue. The following exercise may help you think through such a situation.

Learning Exercise 9.3: Unclear responsibilities
    Think about a patient with whom your respective responsibilities were unclear.
Examples of shared and separate responsibilities for a motivational practitioner are
listed in Tables 9.1 and 9.2. How can the ideas presented in these tables help to clarify
your and your patient's separate and shared responsibilities for health care? Then reflect
about how you could have responded differently to the patient.[12]

Table 9.1. Separate and Shared Responsibilities for Addressing Behavior Change

Practitioner	Shared	Patient
Fosters an empathic and autonomy-supportive relationship	Develop an effective partnership to address behavior change	Is willing to work with the practitioner
Educates patient about risks and harms associated with the risk behavior	Discuss the health implications of the risk behavior for the patient	Provides information about the risk behavior to the practitioner
Attempts to lower patient resistance and enhance patient motivation to change	Explore patient/practitioner differences in perceptions and values about health behavior change	Reflects about and changes perceptions and values about health behavior change
Offers goals for change	Discuss implications of the goals	Selects goals for change
Provides support and encouragement to maintain the goals of change	Develop contingency plans in the event of lapse or relapse	Sustains motivation to maintain the goals of change

Table 9.2. Separate and Shared Responsibilities for Addressing Medical Complications

Practitioner	Shared	Patient
Gathers information about the complications	Develop a mutual understanding about the relationship between risk behaviors and complications	Provides information about the complications
Offers options for addressing the complications	Negotiate about what to do for the complications	Selects options for addressing the complications
Arranges follow-up plans to address any problems if the selected options are not working	Develop contingencies if the plan does not work	Decides whether to adhere to the plan for addressing the complications and for attending follow-up appointments

YOUR SUMMARY

Reflect: write a summary about what you have learned that was new for you.

_____
_____
_____
_____
_____
_____
_____
_____
_____
_____
_____
_____
_____
_____
_____
_____
_____
_____
_____
_____
_____
_____
_____

Enhance: complete a self-assessment of your skills using the worksheet on page 318. **Write your goals below for improving specific skills** in role plays or patient encounters. After doing these practice sessions, reassess your competence score for these skills and make notes on page 318 to explain why you changed your scores. If possible, keep an audio recording or videotape of your practice sessions.

_____
_____
_____
_____
_____
_____
_____
_____
_____

REFERENCES

1. Bandura A. Self-efficacy: Toward a unifying theory of behavior change. Psychological Review 1977;84: 191-215

2. Bandura A, Cervone D. Self-evaluative and self-efficacy mechanisms governing the motivational effects of goal systems. Journal of Personality & Social Psychology 1983;45: 1017-1028

3. Bandura A. Social learning theory. Englewood Cliffs, NJ: Prentice Hall; 1977

4. Bandura A. Self-efficacy mechanism in human agency. American Psychologist 1982;37: 122-147

5. Bandura A. Self-efficacy mechanism in physiological activation and health-promoting behavior. In: Madden J, ed. Neurobiology of learning, emotion, and affect 4th ed. New York: Raven Press; 1991

6. Bandura A. Social foundations of thought and action. Englewood Cliffs, NJ: Prentice Hall; 1986

7. Bandura A. Self-efficacy: The exercise of control. New York: W.H. Freeman; 1997

8. Deci EL, Ryan RM. Intrinsic motivation and self-determination in human behavior. New York: Plenum Press; 1985

9. Deci EL, Ryan RM. A motivational approach to self: Integration in personality. In: Dienstbier R, ed. Nebraska symposium on motivation: Vol 38. Perspectives on motivation. Lincoln, NE: University of Nebraska Press; 1991:

10. Botelho RJ. A negotiation model for the doctor-patient relationship. Family Practice 1992;9(2): 210-218

11. Cumming RW, Barton GE, Fahey PP, et al. Medical practitioners and health promotion: Results from a community survey in Sydney's western suburbs. Community Health Studies 1989;8: 294-300

12. Greenfield S, Kaplan SH, Ware JE, Jr. Expanding patient involvement in care: Effects on patient outcomes. Annals of Internal Medicine 1985;102: 520-528

CHAPTER 10
STEP 2: NEGOTIATING AN AGENDA

FOR REFLECTION

How do you address risk behaviors when patients may not want to talk about them?

OVERVIEW

There are two sets of agendas at the beginning of practitioner-patient encounters, yours and your patient's. The following continua can help you characterize a patient's agenda:

- Single item—multiple items
- Urgent—nonurgent
- Orderly—chaotic
- Explicit—implicit
- Simple—complex

Your agenda for clinical encounters often differs from that of your patients. Many patients are not even thinking about health behavior change when you think they should be. Your task is to acquire the necessary skills to understand the patient's initial agenda and then negotiate toward a shared agenda for addressing behavior change using either a problem-focused or a prevention-focused approach. Such agenda-setting skills serve several important functions: they clarify differences in priorities for the clinical encounter; build common ground about the need to address health behavior change, or at least help you better understand your differences with patients; and use time with patients more efficiently and effectively. In particular, your agenda-setting skills prepare patients to participate actively in assessing how their behavior affects their health.

How do you encourage patients to become more willing to talk about their risk behaviors, particularly when they are not even thinking about change? For example, when patients develop complications such as acute or chronic bronchitis from smoking, many of them want you simply to cure or fix the acute problem and not really address the smoking issue.

Consider gaining patients' permission to discuss their risk behaviors, rather than imposing your agenda. This latter approach can make patients feel like they have no choice but to submit to your authority; consequently, they participate passively in the discussion. By gaining patients' consent, they can become more open to, and active in, discussions about their behaviors.

Alternatively, you can negotiate with patients to develop a shared agenda about addressing their presenting complaints and the relationship of these complaints to their risk behaviors.[1-3] Both gaining patients' consent and negotiation can help you build an effective alliance with patients, activate them to take more responsibility for change, and encourage them to think about their behaviors after leaving the clinical encounter.

CLARIFYING AGENDAS

More often than not, you and your patients have differences in your priorities for any single encounter, so it is important to look at both agendas in order to bring about change. The following learning exercise may prepare you to develop your agenda-setting skills by recognizing such differing priorities.

Learning Exercise 10.1: Review a videotape

Videotape or audiotape a complicated patient encounter involving multiple agenda items. As you listen to the taped encounter, record the different agenda items as they are brought up by you and your patient in sequence, using the table below.

Your Agenda Items	Rank order priority	Your Patient's Agenda Items	Rank order priority
1.		1.	
2.		2.	
3.		3.	
4.		4.	
5.		5.	
6.		6.	
7.		7.	
8.		8.	

After writing down the agenda items for both you and your patient, set priorities by assigning a number (1, 2, 3 and so on) to each agenda item in descending order of importance for you and your patient. Now contrast the priorities on these two agenda lists. This learning exercise can help you discern who controls how the agenda is set up and addressed.

After reading about the agenda-setting skills described in this chapter, replay the tape and stop it to identify where you could have adapted these skills to use with your patient. If time does not permit such close self-examination, just think about how you could use these skills with your patient.

TWO AGENDAS

You and your patients usually have different agendas and priorities that must be recognized and addressed during clinical encounters if you are to successfully arrive at a shared agenda for change.

PATIENTS' AGENDA

When patients come to see you, you can characterize their agenda for the encounter by using the following measurements.

Single Item—Multiple Items

This continuum refers to the number of items that you and your patients come prepared to talk about in a clinical encounter. However, during the interaction, either you or your patient may bring up additional agenda items. When dealing with multiple agenda items, you may need to postpone discussing some items until the next encounter.

Urgent—Nonurgent

You and your patients may have different perspectives about the degree of urgency when addressing different agenda items. When this occurs, it may create difficulties in working together unless you and your patients repeatedly address your differences in perspective and agree on an appropriate timetable to deal with various agenda items.

Orderly—Chaotic

Patients come to you in different states of preparedness. Some patients use the time prior to the clinical encounter to think about or write down what they want from you. Others have chaotic, shifting agendas that may stem from emotional, psychological and personality factors. These patients may cause you frustration unless you structure the interview.

Explicit—Implicit

Patients often come to you with a clear understanding of what they want to talk about, that is, an explicit agenda. Other times, they are embarrassed or ashamed to bring up an agenda item (e.g., risky sexual behavior or excessive drinking) and are likely to be reluctant to do so. Other patients do not even have a clear understanding of what issues need to be addressed. For example, patients may not recognize, or want others to know, that they are depressed, have a somatization disorder or have an unrecognized alcohol problem that is, they have a hidden agenda. These agendas are more difficult to identify and address.

Simple—Complex

Based on the patients' overall agenda, you can evaluate their agenda for a single encounter using the simple-complex scale. The difference between a simple and complex agenda is based on your assessment of the patient's situation. What is complex for one practitioner may be simple for another, and vice versa. Typically, a complex agenda is compounded by multiple medical, psychological and/or social factors that make your task of delivering effective patient care more complicated. The case example of Mrs. C. (described in Part 9C) is an example of a complex agenda. Your experience of dealing with such agendas may range from a straightforward, routine or ritualistic encounter to an overwhelming and dramatic one.[4]

YOUR AGENDA AND TASKS

Your initial task is to identify patients' presenting problems, hidden agendas and/or unrecognized problems. As you may come to the clinical encounter with an agenda that may differ from that of your patients, effective negotiation can help make the encounter less overwhelming and more manageable for both parties. As part of this process to set reasonable goals for what can be accomplished, you may opt to

- Identify the patient's agenda items and priorities
  "What do we need to deal with today? Anything else? And where do you want to begin?"

- Express your agenda items and priorities
  "Let me explain what I would like to address today and why."

- Negotiate which items to address for this and subsequent encounters
  "We will address your concern about x [e.g., chest infection], but I am also concerned about y [e.g., how smoking is making your chest infection worse]. Is it okay for us to talk about y as well as x [seeking permission]?" Even if the patient says no to this question, you can ask in a nonjudgmental manner why he or she does not want to talk about this issue. This follow-up question can provide you with invaluable information as to why a patient resists change. (With multiple agendas, you can negotiate with patients about priorities for any particular clinical encounter.) "Let's decide what we can deal with today and what we may need to leave for the next appointment."

Once you have successfully established your respective priorities, you can both move toward a shared agenda about addressing health behavior change.

TOWARD A SHARED AGENDA

Both problem-focused and prevention-focused approaches can help you negotiate a shared agenda with patients and enhance their willingness to reflect on and address their risk behaviors. The distinction between these approaches depends on whether or not patients have health problems caused by or worsened by a behavior (e.g., the effect of smoking on bronchitis). In this case, you can use a problem-focused approach. If your patient has risk behaviors without complications (e.g., unsafe sex), you can use a prevention-focused approach.

THE PROBLEM-FOCUSED APPROACH

A problem-focused approach involves identifying whether any of the patient's complaints (e.g., cough, elevated blood pressure or hyperglycemia) are associated with specific behaviors (excessive smoking, alcohol and drug use or nonadherence to a recommended diet). If there are possible associations, you can use different kinds of questioning techniques to make the connection clear to patients. When you think that patients are unaware of the connection between their presenting complaint and their risk behavior, prefacing statements may help them understand the rationale and purpose for inquiring about this connection. Exploratory questions help patients understand that there is, or may be, a connection between the complaint and a risk behavior. Leading questions help you work from the patients' perspective, especially to clarify their views about the beneficial effects of risk behaviors.

Using Prefacing Statements

The purpose of using prefacing statements is to provide a rationale to patients for exploring how their risk behaviors may be associated with their health problems. The following examples of simple and elaborate prefacing statements demonstrate how you can use them with patients.

Simple Prefacing Statements. The following example of Mrs. K. demonstrates how you can make simple prefacing statements so that a patient becomes more willing to address a risk behavior.

> Addressing obesity, hypertension and drug treatment. Mrs. K., a midlevel manager, works in a company that has significantly downsized its management staff. She has been under tremendous stress during the past year. She has gained 30 pounds, and the nurse at work referred her to a physician because her blood pressure was 160/100. Mrs. K. eats to relieve her stress at work and is particularly worried about her hypertension. Given a family history of stroke, Mrs. K. wanted to take medication to reduce her blood pressure.

Practitioner: "We need to talk about using medications and losing weight. Let me explain. If you lose weight, you might be able to lower your blood pressure to a point where you won't need to take medication. Perhaps we can talk about weight reduction before talking about taking medication. What do you think?" (Let the patient respond.)

When patients are willing to explore the connection between their health problems and their risk behaviors, you can then proceed to assess the behavior before assessing the health problems. Some patients, however, may not want to talk about risk behaviors, such as lack of self-care for chronic disease. With such cases, you may make better use of your time by asking patients if they are willing to explain why they do not want to discuss these issues. By taking this approach, you are working with, rather than against, patient resistance. Listening to why patients do not want to talk about their behavior can help you better understand their reasons for not wanting to change. Sometimes, patients even open up and discuss how their behavior might affect their health.

When patients are reluctant to accept any connection between their complaints and their behavior (e.g., hypertension and alcohol use), you may ask them in a nonjudgmental manner why they think there is no connection. Afterwards, you can provide specific information about how a particular behavior relates to their complaints in a way that creates discrepancies in their reasoning. You can then ask them what they think about the discrepancies between their reasons and the medical facts you have provided. You support and place the onus on patients to address these discrepancies, rather than arguing with them about facts versus opinions.

Elaborate Prefacing Statements. With complicated situations and complex agendas, you may need to provide more elaborate prefacing statements.

>   **Addressing narcotic use for pain control:** Mrs. C., a 50-year-old woman with chronic pancreatitis and abdominal pain, was admitted to the hospital. She had a past medical history of gross obesity and ileo-jejunal bypass operation for weight reduction. After she had been in the hospital for two weeks, her attending physician went on vacation for one week and asked the physician on call to see this patient.
>   Mrs. C. was being intravenously fed, had no appetite and was receiving 15 mg of morphine intravenously per hour, 125 mg of meperidine every three hours and two narcotic transdermal patches. Given that her pancreatic condition was stable, the covering physician considered whether to wean her off the large doses of narcotics and restart oral feeding, in spite of her poor appetite and nausea. He spoke to Mrs. C. for about five minutes. Before negotiating whether to reduce her use of narcotics, he made a series of prefacing statements about how he viewed her situation.
>   Physician: "I will be looking after you for a week while your doctor is away. I'd like to work with you so that you can make as many decisions about your care as you want. [This approach put the patient in the one-up position.] I

don't know, but I may see the situation differently from your regular doctor and could give you a second opinion. Is that okay? [Mrs. C. nodded in agreement and then stated that she would appreciate that.] Let me explain how I see the situation. You are taking large amounts of narcotic medications, which we use when people are dying of cancer. So you must be in a lot of pain. You are also having complications that we often see when people are dying, for example, of malnutrition due to poor appetite, and deep vein thrombosis from not being physically active. But I don't think you are dying, although you are at risk of developing further complications if we don't help you eat better and become more physically active."

Mrs. C. agreed that these issues were important to her, and she wanted to do something about her appetite and nausea. The physician responded, "Well, I agree with that. But let me explain something else. I suspect that the narcotic medications are taking your appetite away and making you feel more nauseated." Mrs. C. stated that she had not really thought about it in that way. The physician then asked her what she wanted to do.

Mrs. C.'s agenda was to get off the intravenous feeding and eat normally. She also wanted a different drug to treat her nausea and to increase the meperidine dosage from 125 mg to 150 mg every three hours. She did not think the morphine was helping her much, so she wanted to decrease it from 15 mg to 10 mg per hour. Her physician agreed and changed the medications in accordance with her suggestions.

On the following day, Mrs. C. forgot to put her narcotic patches on after a shower. Her abdominal pain and retching worsened. Her physician explained to her that her symptoms were worse probably because of narcotic withdrawal, rather than because of a deterioration of her underlying condition. She reaffirmed her desire to minimize the amount of narcotics because she did not like the withdrawal symptoms. Over the course of the week, she stopped using morphine, changed to oral meperidine, used only one narcotic patch and began eating food.

Commentary: These elaborate prefacing statements helped the physician and Mrs. C. begin to set a common agenda before negotiating whether and how much to reduce narcotic medications. The physician provided a rationale about his perspective and tried to make connections between his perspective and what he thought was important to Mrs. C. She, in turn, was able to make her wishes known and make her agenda part of the shared agenda. In effect, they collaborated in shared decision-making to address a complicated situation and complex agenda.

Learning Exercise 10.2: Unaware patient

Think of a patient who was unaware or not fully convinced of the connection between health problems and risk behaviors. Consider how to use prefacing statements that would help your patient recognize the connection, and write your statements below. If you have difficulty completing this task, reread the examples provided. Completing this task is worthwhile because it may help you clarify whether your perspective differs from that of your patient. If you have difficulty in generating a prefacing statement, talk it over with a colleague or teacher to help form additional ideas of what to say.

Prefacing Statements
Brief statement about the nature of the problem:
Give your own examples of simple and/or elaborate prefacing statements:

Using Exploratory Questions

The purpose of exploratory questions is to help patients explore the relationship between health and behavior. These kinds of questions can take two forms, linear or circular. Linear causality (cause-effect) questions can be either closed-ended or open-ended. Closed-ended linear questions (yes-no answers) are brief, to the point and useful for brief encounters. For example, "Has your behavior [e.g., smoking] affected your health [e.g., breathing problem]?" Open-ended linear questions encourage patients to talk about the relationship between health and behavior in more detail. For example, "In what ways has your behavior [e.g., alcohol use] affected your health?" Circular questions go beyond how patients view the relationship between health and behavior, and incorporate the perspective of a third party. Such questions can prepare patients to explore issues related to family, health and behavior. For example, "What concerns does your spouse [or partner] have about how your behavior [e.g., dietary indiscretion or drug nonadherence] affects your health?"

Learning Exercise 10.3: Minimizing patient

Think of a patient who does not see much of a connection between his or her health problems and behavior. Think of how you could use exploratory questions to help the patient begin to make a connection between his or her health problems and behavior, rather than you trying to make this connection for your patient. Write your statements below.

Exploratory Questions
Write a brief statement about the nature of the problem:
Give your own examples of exploratory questions:

Using Leading Questions

You may have been taught not to use leading questions, particularly when collecting medical information. For example, when you ask a leading closed-ended question ("Did you experience a gripping chest pain?") as opposed to an open-ended question ("What was the chest pain like?"), patients may provide information that does not fully reflect their experience, and may lead to inaccurate diagnoses.

In some cases, patients may be reluctant to provide information about their risk behaviors, such as excessive alcohol use, drug abuse and nonadherence to prescribed medications. In these situations, leading questions may help you better understand your patients' perspective and elicit a more accurate account of their feelings about their risk behavior. For example, a leading open-ended question ("What do you like to drink?") may be more effective than a neutral closed-ended question ("Do you drink alcohol?"). Leading questions can help you think about and work from patients' frames of reference rather than from your own frame of reference.

Learning Exercise 10.4: Nonadherent patient
Think of a patient who engaged in risk behaviors and/or was nonadherent to your recommendations. Imagine yourself working with this patient. Think about using leading questions to help you gain a more accurate picture of what is going on for the patient, and write them down below. Creating your own leading questions can help you learn to work more from the patient's frame of reference.

Leading Questions
Write a brief statement about the nature of the problem:
Give your own examples of leading questions:

THE PREVENTION-FOCUSED APPROACH

When patients have risk behaviors without complications, you can use a prevention-focused approach. The Canadian and U.S. Prevention Task Force recommendations and other evidence-based protocols for chronic disease are useful for determining the appropriateness of this type of intervention.[5-7] The following example illustrates a generic approach to address risk behaviors such as tobacco, alcohol and drug use and dietary issues.

> *Using a prevention-focused approach: A prefacing statement helps you focus on how patients' behavior affects their health. For example: "I would like to check up on whether there is anything you can do to improve your health. Is that all right?" (Let the patient respond.) You can then ask about such behaviors as smoking history, alcohol and drug use, diet and sedentary lifestyle.*

Some risk behaviors are difficult to address because they are potentially embarrassing for both you and your patients. Instead of face-to-face approaches, you can use questionnaires or computer-assisted assessments. Patients often are more willing to acknowledge concerns this way.[8] To address sensitive issues in person, it is essential to have a repertoire of agenda-setting skills, particularly for teenagers who do not yet have any complications from risk behaviors such as STDs and unwanted pregnancies. The following examples show how such issues can be raised in a way that allows patients to respond when they would otherwise have failed to address the behavior.

> **HIV concerns:** "Many people have unanswered questions about how they may get infected with the HIV virus." (This prefacing statement, followed by a pause, may help some patients respond without further questioning. If not, continue.) "Do you have any questions or concerns about HIV?" Or "Do you know all the ways that you can get an HIV infection?" (Let the patient respond, and if the patient is sexually active, continue by asking) "For example, from having sex without a condom, from blood transfusions that have the HIV or from oral or anal intercourse without a condom." (Let the patient respond, proceed to take a sexual history and counsel accordingly.)
>
> **Pregnancy:** Prefacing statements can also help you address this sensitive issue, particularly when counseling teenagers about unwanted pregnancies. "Some teenagers get pregnant by accident and others by choice. Do you know of anyone at school who has had a baby that was not planned?" (If the teenager says no, continue.) "Then what about anyone who got pregnant by choice?" (Let the patient respond.) "Where do you stand on this issue?"

Specific examples of consent-gaining and leading questions for the prevention-focused approach are provided in Chapters 15-16 (Part B) and Chapter 17.

YOUR SUMMARY

Reflect: write a summary about what you have learned that was new for you.

_____
_____
_____
_____
_____
_____
_____
_____
_____
_____
_____
_____
_____
_____
_____
_____
_____
_____
_____
_____
_____
_____
_____
_____
_____
_____
_____

*Enhance: complete a self-assessment of your skills using the worksheet on page 319. **Write your goals below for improving specific skills** in role plays or patient encounters. After doing these practice sessions, reassess your competence score for these skills and make notes on page 319 to explain why you changed your scores. If possible, keep an audio recording or videotape of your practice sessions.*

_____
_____
_____
_____
_____
_____
_____
_____
_____

REFERENCES

1. Butler NM, Campion PD, Cox AD. Exploration of doctor and patient agendas in general practice consultations. Social Science & Medicine 1992;35: 1145-1155

2. Bergh KD. Time use and physicians' exploration of the reason for the office visit. Family Medicine 1996;28: 264-270

3. Beckman HB, Frankel RM. Soliciting the patient's complete agenda: A relationship to the distribution of concerns. Clinical Research 1985;33: 714A

4. Miller WL. Routine, ceremony, or drama: An exploratory field study of the primary care clinical encounter. The Journal of Family Practice 1992;34: 289-296

5. U.S. Preventive Services Task Force. Guide to clinical preventive services: Report of the U.S. Preventive Services Task Force. 2nd ed. Baltimore, MD: Williams & Wilkins; 1996

6. Canadian Task Force on the Periodic Health Examination. The Canadian guide to clinical preventive health care. 1994. Ottawa, Minister of Supply and Services, Canada

7. Ellrodt G, Cook DJ, Lee J, et al. Evidence-based disease management. Journal of the American Medical Association 1997;278: 1687-1692

8. Skinner HA, Allen BA, McIntosh MC, et al. Lifestyle assessment: Just asking makes a difference. British Medical Journal 1985;290: 214-216

CHAPTER 11

STEP 3: ASSESSING RESISTANCE AND MOTIVATION

FOR REFLECTION

How do you assess patient resistance and motivation?

OVERVIEW

This chapter will help you learn how to assess patient resistance and motivation. You will also learn how a disease-centered assessment differs from a motivational assessment.

A motivational assessment can be a disarming and positive experience for patients because you first try to understand how they benefit from their risk behavior. This assessment also prepares patients to confront themselves about whether to change, so that they decide why, what and how much to change. To conduct such an assessment, you can use any of the following options:

- Ask about readiness to change
- Itemize benefits and concerns about the status quo versus change
- Use a decision balance
- Assess resistance and motivation based on how patients think and feel
- Explore motives for change
- Inquire about competing priorities and energy to change
- Assess confidence and ability to change (self-efficacy)
- Ask about supports and barriers to change

Ultimately, behavior change is an individual responsibility, but one that is influenced by many external factors. The first part of this chapter provides an individual perspective on change, while the last part addresses the social, community and cultural factors that can act on individuals in positive and negative ways.

Motivational assessments help patients consider, initiate and maintain behavior change. As discussed in Chapters 6 and 7, resistance (reasons to stay the same) and motivation (reasons for change) are expected parts of the change process. By assessing patients' levels of resistance and motivation, you can more readily assist them in moving toward change. This chapter will help you learn how to conduct motivational assessments from individual and systems perspectives and understand the differences between disease-centered and motivational assessments.

Your style in addressing such health issues may vary along two dimensions: practitioner-centered to patient-centered[1] and controlling to autonomy-supportive.[2] These dimensions were described in Chapters 7 and 9 (Part C). To conduct a motivational assessment effectively, you need to use a patient-centered and autonomy-supportive approach, whereas disease-centered assessments tend to use a practitioner-centered and controlling approach.

DISEASE-CENTERED ASSESSMENT

A disease-centered assessment is used primarily to evaluate patients' risks and harm caused by their unhealthy behaviors. With this approach, assessment and implementation plans are independent, linear activities: first diagnose, then treat. This type of assessment may address patients' presenting complaints, the degree of risk associated with the unhealthy behavior and the severity of harm from risk behaviors. Assessing these risks and consequences defines the need and justification for why patients should change their behavior. For example, a physician assesses a patient's cough and smoking habit, prescribes antibiotics for acute bronchitis and then advises the patient to stop smoking (intervention). Such an assessment is clearly practitioner-centered and controlling.

Disease-centered assessments, however, do not address how we may perceive these risks and harms differently from our patients, nor do they help us appreciate how patients think and feel about the benefits of their risk behaviors. For example, some patients perceive alcohol as "a friend who helps me not only to enjoy life but also to cope with my problems." For such patients, alcohol use has many benefits with minimal risks. In contrast, we may view alcohol as having many risks and harm with only minimal benefits, and even regard alcohol as "a disease promoter who befriends yet deceives patients." In other words, we think predominantly in disease-centered ways (hazardous, harmful or dependent use of alcohol). In contrast to this negative perspective, patients view alcohol use in beneficial ways, disconnected from their health issues.

Unless we try to understand our differences in perceptions, some patients will regard our questions and advice as attacks on a "friend" (alcohol). They will respond evasively, defensively or offensively. In effect, we are asking them to be disloyal to their friend. We need to address our differences in perception by first exploring with patients how their friend is helpful and then how their friend may not always be helpful. This approach helps patients explore their relationship with alcohol in both positive and negative ways. Such a motivational approach is an alternative to the disease-centered approach of confronting or arguing with patients and labeling them as being in denial when they do not change. The next section may help you understand more about the difference between disease-centered and motivational assessments.

MOTIVATIONAL ASSESSMENT

A motivational assessment[a] helps you to

- Clarify how you and your patients have differences in perception and values about health behavior change
- Understand why patients adopt risk behaviors
- Explore whether, when, why, what and how much patients want to change

A motivational approach involves three interrelated activities: (1) conducting an assessment, which will be discussed in this chapter, (2) enhancing mutual understanding (see Chapter 12) and (3) implementing plans (see Chapter 13). This approach is very different from the disease-centered, linear approach (see Figure 11.1). For example, assessments can act as interventions in their own right. You may ask patients about their perceptions regarding the benefits of and concerns about a specific behavior. This inquiry alone may motivate patients to change their behavior, that is, you serve as a catalyst for change when assessing risk behaviors, without giving encouragement to change. In addition, interventions can enhance the quality of the assessment by helping you and your patients improve mutual understanding about risk behaviors. For example, you can intervene by asking patients to change their behavior as an experiment. This intervention helps patients assess the role of that behavior in their lives and may result in their being willing to implement a permanent plan for change.

---

a. This assessment can be used to address other health care decisions, such as death and dying issues, nursing home placement, functional activities of daily living (physical, occupational and speech therapy), use of medications, rehabilitative treatments, psychiatric referral or treatment decisions (e.g., alcohol and drug problems), the use of community services (e.g., Alcoholics Anonymous) and safety issues (when to stop driving due to medical conditions, such as dementia).

Figure 11.1. Disease-centered and Motivational Assessments

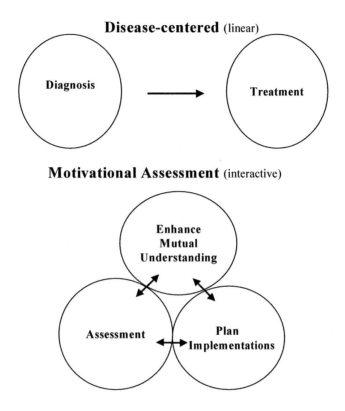

To conduct a motivational assessment, you may use any of the options listed in Table 11.1. For example, by asking patients to itemize the benefits from and concerns about maintaining their risk behaviors versus adopting healthy behaviors, you can begin the process of understanding how you and your patients differ in your perceptions and values about health behavior change. Given the time constraints in most clinical encounters, you can choose the options that are most appropriate to help an individual patient. Thus, it may be more effective to ask about the patient's benefits from drinking alcohol, such as for relaxation, before quantifying the use of alcohol. Your prior knowledge of your patient can help you sequence these options in ways that addresses his or her needs.

Table 11.1.

Motivational Assessment
A. Readiness to change
B. Benefits and concerns—status quo vs. change
C. Decision balance
D. Resistance and motivation
E. Motives for change
F. Competing priorities and energy to change
G. Confidence and ability (self-efficacy)
H. Supports and barriers to change

ASSESS READINESS TO CHANGE

When you ask patients about their readiness to change, they fall somewhere along a continuum:[3-6]

- Not considering change (precontemplation)
- Thinking about change (contemplation)
- Preparing to change (preparation)
- Taking action (action)

Helping patients assess their readiness to change can help you
- Select appropriate assessment options
- Minimize patient resistance
- Work at an appropriate pace of change

Consider when it is appropriate for you to ask patients about their readiness to change. For example, with smoking cessation, many patients are familiar with the risks and harm and some are already thinking about quitting, so you may begin by asking about readiness to change. In contrast, patients who drink above low-risk limits may not consider themselves to be at risk for any health problems. They are not even thinking about change. However, they may be willing to respond to questions about why they like to drink alcohol and their concerns about drinking.

With the "thinking-about-change" and "preparing-to-change" groups, you can use the motivational interventions (described in Chapters 12 and 13) to help patients shift from the contemplation to the preparation and action stages.

ASSESS BENEFITS AND CONCERNS (STATUS QUO VERSUS CHANGE)

You can itemize the patient's benefits from and concerns about staying the same versus changing. This process can prepare you for using a decision balance (see Chapter 11) with your patient.

Itemize the Benefits of Risk Behaviors

Your familiarity with the negative consequences of risk behaviors may prevent you from fully empathizing with patients because you do not understand the benefits that they derive from these behaviors. By asking about these benefits, you can understand better the driving force for your patients' seemingly irrational behavior. A list of such benefits can be organized into an inverted hierarchy of categories based on lifestyle, emotional, interpersonal, coping, social and spiritual reasons (see Figure 11.2). These benefits may also help you understand why patients relapse.

Figure 11.2: An Inverted Hierarchy of Benefits

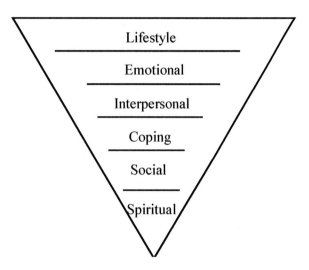

The example of Mr. B. may show how these benefits can create layers of reasons for engaging in risk behaviors.

Mr. B. drank excessive amounts of beer and used alcohol to relax—an emotional reason for drinking. Upon learning this, the practitioner taught Mr. B. relaxation exercises. Mr. B. then reduced his alcohol use, but still drank excessively. The practitioner discovered that Mr. B. was using alcohol to self-medicate panic attacks and social anxiety and referred him to a specialist for dual diagnosis. The specialist advocated abstinence and the use of antidepressants to suppress the panic attacks. Mr. B. initially abstained, but then relapsed because of social pressure from his friends. The specialist addressed these reasons for relapse by helping him develop self-assertive skills to deal with his friends. Again, Mr. B. initially abstained, but then relapsed because he was lacking purpose and meaning in his life without his old friends. The specialist finally persuaded Mr. B. to attend Alcoholics Anonymous to help him find new meaning and purpose in his life.

Commentary: This example, though simplistic, demonstrates the different levels at which practitioners and specialists can work sequentially or concurrently to address the layers of reasons why patients engage in risk

167

behaviors. Practitioners may need to develop more sophisticated interventions to address the complex reasons for patients engaging in such behaviors.

Lifestyle Benefits. Lifestyle benefits for continuing risk behaviors include factors that relate to personal preferences (enjoy the taste of beer) and/or daily activities (see Table 11.2). For example, a patient's limited budget may cause a conflict of needs between paying for medications or paying for food. Another example is the inconvenience of special diets in terms of shopping for and preparing particular foods, and also the extra costs and changes in mealtime arrangements that may be involved.

Table 11.2.

Lifestyle Benefits
• Satisfy basic needs
• Avoid financial cost of medication
• Avoid inconvenience to self
• Avoid inconvenience to family
• Avoid disrupting routines/rituals

Emotional Benefits. Some patients engage in risk behaviors to change their mood. The emotional benefits are deliberately paired because patients may state a mood-enhancing reason that may conceal a mood-diminishing one. Three examples from Table 11.3 are described below the table.

Table 11.3.

Emotional Benefits	
Mood-enhancing	Mood-diminishing
• Feel good or high	• Reduce feeling of depression
• Express anger	• Suppress anger
• Enhance self-esteem	• Suppress self-deprecation
• Enhance confidence	• Reduce feelings of inadequacy
• Give courage	• Reduce fear
• Enhance sexual pleasure	• Reduce sexual anxiety/tension
• Enhance friendly feelings	• Numb feelings of isolation
• Feel powerful	• Reduce sense of victimization
• Unwind or relax	• Reduce anxiety and panic
• Enjoy social activities	• Reduce social anxiety
• Enhance intimacy	• Reduce or avoid intimacy

Feel good or high—reduce feeling of depression

If patients tell you they use alcohol to feel better, you may accept this response at face value or explore whether the patient is depressed. They may drink alcohol to numb the feelings of depression, an ineffective treatment, because alcohol only temporarily depresses the central nervous system. Alcohol may temporarily relieve feelings of depression for a few hours, but over time, it simply makes the depression worse.

Express anger—suppress anger

Some patients use drugs and alcohol to suppress their anger or to express usually suppressed anger. In effect, they use stimulants to help regulate their emotions. Excessive use may have just the opposite effect; these patients may lose their ability to regulate their anger appropriately.

Enhance self-esteem—suppress self-deprecation

Some patients use drugs and alcohol for the purported benefit of feeling better about themselves, but in fact they are only superficially enhancing their self-esteem by suppressing their basic sense of worthlessness and negative feelings about themselves.

Interpersonal Benefits. Patients may engage in risk behaviors to deal with interpersonal issues (see Table 11.4), and these are often related to the emotional reasons listed above. For example, a wife had a relationship problem with her husband that increased her anxiety. She smoked cigarettes not only to cope with her relationship difficulty but also to reduce her anxiety.

Table 11.4.

Interpersonal Benefits
• Overcome difficulties making friends
• Deal with relationship difficulties
• Escape from difficult relationships
• Get back at someone by acting self-destructively

Coping Benefits. Patients may engage in risk behaviors as a way of coping with stressful events, such as an illness in the family, or difficult situations, such as work-related issues (see Table 11.5).

Table 11.5.

Coping Benefits
Coping with stressful events
• Losses (disability, loss of function)
• Illness in the family
• Death of a family member/friend
• Unresolved grief
Coping with work-related issues
• Work overload
• Unemployment
• Job insecurity
• Company downsizing

Social Benefits. Patients may engage in risk behaviors because of social needs and norms, such as developing a sense of belonging and adhering to (or avoiding) certain group expectations. They may adhere to peer influences and norms (see Table 11.6) for many different reasons: for example, to gain a sense of group belonging and identity. Some adolescents may identify with a drug subculture as a way to leave home and differentiate from their family.

Table 11.6.

Social Benefits
Adhering to
• Influence
• Family norms
• Cultural norms
• Work norms

Spiritual Benefits. Spiritual benefits relate to deeper personal needs (see Table 11.7). Patients who are unable to meet their spiritual needs may adopt risk behaviors as a way to address their lack of meaning and purpose in life. For example, a patient stated that he drank alcohol to fill a spiritual void. Other patients may use alcohol/drugs to avoid existential angst, or overeat to fill a sense of emptiness or lack of fulfillment in their lives. Adolescents from poor families who live in aversive environments become involved in drug subcultures as a way of developing a sense of connection, purpose and meaning rather than struggling to overcome poor employment prospects and oppressive social conditions.

Table 11.7.

Spiritual Benefits
Help to deal with a lack of
• Life-fulfilling values
• Sense of community
• Connection to a higher power
• Purpose in life
• Meaning of life

Many other factors (such as family upbringing, beliefs, values, culture, education, and work, school and peer influences) determine the benefits of patients' risk behaviors. While you may not fully understand how patients benefit from their risk behaviors, the learning exercise below may help you gain insight on this issue.

Learning Exercise 11.1: Imagine you are a patient with a risk behavior
Think of a patient, family member or friend who has a risk behavior. Now, imagine that you are this individual. From his or her perspective, list as many benefits of this risk behavior as possible in the table below.

Benefits of a Risk Behavior

For reflection: What was it like for you to think about the benefits of a risk behavior from someone else's perspective?

Commentary: Patients may struggle to identify the benefits of their risk behavior, particularly with a well-ingrained habit. They may not know why they do what they do; their behavior is on autopilot. This exercise helps you gain insight into their perspective. Your knowledge about the benefits of risk behaviors in general can also help them reflect about and rediscover their benefits. They then become more aware of the driving force for their unhealthy habits. To transform an unhealthy habit into a healthy one, you need to help them explore their health choices and provide opportunities for reflection—in effect, assist them to deprogram and reprogram their autopilot.

Key Point
Understanding the benefits that patients derive from an unhealthy behavior can help you understand the driving force
for maintaining the status quo.
Your challenge is to
redirect this force in a healthy direction.

Itemize Concerns about Risk Behaviors

By asking your patients whether a behavior (e.g., smoking, alcohol use, dietary indiscretion or unsafe sex practices) is of concern to them and then itemizing those concerns, you can assess whether they think their risk behavior is negatively affecting their health. After listening to their response, you can then share any key concerns that they did not mention: for example, alcohol-related problems (indigestion, hypertension) or smoking-delayed healing of peptic ulcers. However, it is better not to emphasize your concerns unless patients are willing to accept them. Otherwise, you are imposing your view, and patients are less likely to take ownership of these additional concerns. This two-step strategy of asking patients about their perspective before sharing your perspective can clarify the extent to which you and your patients share similar concerns and perceptions. For example, patients may identify that smoking causes heart disease, but minimize this concern.

> *Learning Exercise 11.2: Compare concerns about staying the same*
> *Use the same patient, family member or friend that you used in the previous exercise. Imagine you are this individual again. From this person's perspective, list as many concerns as possible about his or her risk behavior in the middle column. Then list your concerns as the practitioner in the right-hand column.*

Comparing Concerns

Risk Behavior	His or Her Concerns	Your Concerns

> *For reflection: What was it like for you to compare concerns from the individual's perspective with concerns from yours?*
> *Commentary: This exercise helps you understand how you and your patients can have the same or different concerns. In Step 4 of the six-step approach (enhancing mutual understanding), you will learn to educate patients about the concerns that are not on their list and then ask their permission to make additions to the list if these concerns are relevant to them. This process may also help you learn how you perceive the benefits of and concerns about a risk behavior differently from your patients'.)*

Key Point
Learning about why your patients minimize their concerns about
their unhealthy behaviors can help you better understand
why they lack motivation to change.

Itemize Concerns about Adopting Healthy Behaviors
Patients may not fully anticipate what may make change difficult or what may trigger a relapse. To address these issues, you can ask whether patients have any concerns about adopting a healthy behavior.

Learning Exercise 11.3: Compare concerns about changing
Now think of a goal for change (stop smoking, exercise more, change diet or lose weight) and write it below, using the same person again as your example. From his or her perspective, list as many items as possible about your concerns if you were to change an unhealthy behavior.

Goal for Change	Drawbacks/Concerns about Change

For reflection: *What was it like for you to think about change from this person's perspective? Taking his or her perspective helps you to anticipate issues you may encounter when you attempt to help patients change.*

Another key issue is the selection of the goal for change, based on the patient's readiness to change. This can have a major impact on the patient's commitment in working on such a goal. For example, a problem drinker in precontemplation is more likely to respond favorably to thinking about change than to setting a goal for change by cutting down, keeping to low-risk limits or abstaining from alcohol. Likewise, a problem drinker in the contemplation stage is more likely to consider a trial of low-risk drinking or abstinence for two to four weeks than to keep to low-risk drinking or abstinence indefinitely.

Key Point
Understanding your patients' concerns about changing
an unhealthy behavior can provide opportunities
for reducing their resistance.

Itemize Benefits of Adopting Healthy Behaviors

First, you need to ask patients to itemize the benefits of change before educating them about additional benefits. Even if you and your patients have a similar list of benefits, you may perceive and value these benefits differently.

Learning Exercise 11.4: Compare benefits of changing
Again, imagine you are the same patient. From the patient's perspective, list the benefits of change in the middle column. Then, from your perspective as the practitioner, list the benefits of change in the right column.

Comparing Perceived Benefits

Risk Behavior	Benefits from the Patient's Perspective	Benefits from Your Perspective

For reflection: What was it like for you to compare benefits from the individual's perspective and from yours?

Commentary: This exercise helps you understand how you and your patients can have the same or different benefits. In step 4 of the six-step approach (enhancing mutual understanding), you can educate patients about the benefits that are not on the patients' list, and then ask their permission to make additions to their list, if these benefits are relevant to them. This process may also help you learn how you perceive the benefits of change differently from your patients.

Key Point
Understanding how your patients perceive the benefits of changing
an unhealthy behavior can provide opportunities
for enhancing their motivation.

USE A DECISION BALANCE

The decision balance is an essential component of a motivational assessment because it summarizes the benefits and concerns for patients about staying the same or changing their risk behavior in an easy-to-understand chart (see Table 11.8). This simple tool helps patients organize their thoughts about change by providing a structure for understanding the unique combination of items that influence their behavior.

Each item on their decision balance is like a headline to a story. Your task is to capture the essence of these stories so that you can use this tool in a highly sophisticated manner. This tool can also help you and your patients better understand the emotions, perceptions and values that lie beneath their thought processes. With such an understanding, you are then in a better position to individualize your approach to patients.

It takes practice to use the decision balance effectively. Preprinted decision balances can make this task easier when you first begin to use them with patients. If none are available, you can easily draw one for patients; see the example in Table 11.8. The second row is for the risk behavior: put **Benefits** before **Concerns**—**BC** means "Before Change." The bottom row is for the goal for change: put **Concerns** before **Benefits**—**CB** means "Change Behavior." Patients are more cooperative if you provide a stage-specific rationale and gain their consent to use a decision balance, particularly patients who are not thinking about change.

> ***Precontemplation:*** *"You aren't sure whether alcohol is causing your high blood pressure. Would you mind if we did a decision balance together to help you think about whether to change the amount of alcohol you drink?"*
> ***Contemplation:*** *"You told me that alcohol helps you relieve your stresses, but it could also be causing your high blood pressure. Could we do a decision balance together to help you decide whether to stop drinking for at least two weeks to see if your blood pressure goes down?"*
> ***Preparation:*** *"You are willing to stop drinking for two weeks but are under a lot of stress at the moment. If we did a decision balance together, it could help you set a date to change. Is that okay?"*
> ***Action:*** *"You are ready to set a date to change. If we did a decision balance together, it could help you prevent a relapse once you cut down or stop drinking."*

Table 11.8. Decision Balance

Reasons to Stay the Same	Reasons to Change
Benefits of your risk behavior?	**C**oncerns about your risk behavior?
Concerns about change?	**B**enefits of changing?

Consider using the decision balance in the sequence shown on Table 11.8 as a way to help patients think more seriously about their risk behavior and change options. Some patients become resistant or reluctant to talk about these behaviors if you first focus on concerns. For example, patients may have been told many times before about the negative consequences of their risk behavior. By focusing on the benefits of the risk behavior first, you are more likely to engage your patients in discussion.

Also, rather than suggesting that your patients should change, ask them to consider what it would be like if they were to change: *"Suppose you were to change. What concerns would you have if you did?"* Often, patients are surprised by this question, and you may have to provide some examples. Then you can ask them about the benefits of change. Afterward, you can ask patients if they would like to keep the decision balance to think more about these issues.

ASSESS PATIENTS' RESISTANCE AND MOTIVATION

You can also ask patients to rate their resistance and motivation to change based on a scale of 0–10.

> *"The left column of your decision balance represents your reasons to stay the same. The right column represents your reasons to change. On a scale of 0–10, 0 meaning none and 10 meaning very high, what score would you give for your reasons to*

stay the same? [Let the patient respond.] And what score would you give for your reasons to change?"

Caution is needed, however, when asking precontemplators about their resistance and motivation scores. They may resist working with you if you use the phrase *resistance score*. When patients are highly invested in the status quo and do not want to change, you can use the term *your reasons to stay the same score* instead. You can also use this phrase if patients do not understand the word *resistance*.

In contrast, ambivalent patients in the contemplation stage implicitly understand that resistance and motivation are internal oppositional forces. The words *resistance and motivation scores* provide an explicit way for patients to think and talk about how these two oppositional forces change over time.

Patients' resistance and motivation scores may also differ based on how they think and feel about change. To clarify this, you can ask the question "Are your resistance and motivation scores based on what you think or feel about change?" Some patients can immediately identify one way or the other. Patients with analytical and/or logical dispositions often give their think scores first. Conversely, patients with intuitive and emotional dispositions typically give their feeling scores first. Still other patients will struggle to understand the difference between their thoughts and feelings about change. You may have to give them extra time and support to help them become more aware of the differences.

Dr. O., a middle-aged, overweight physician, gave a resistance and motivation score of 3 when filling out his decision balance. When asked by his doctor whether these scores were based on what he felt or thought, Dr. O. immediately recognized that the numbers he had given represented his think scores for resistance and motivation. He was giving some thought to exercising.

Dr. O.'s Decision Balance

Reasons to Stay Sedentary	Reasons to Exercise
1. Benefits of staying the same Prefer to play music, than exercise, to relax Avoid something that I hate (jogging)	2. Concerns about staying the same Slowly gaining weight More likely to get depressed when not active
3. Concerns about changing Difficulty finding a good time to do it Get injured	4. Benefits about changing Get into shape Feel better
Resistance Score = 3 Think score = 3 Feeling score = 10	**Motivation Score** = 3 Think score = 3 Feeling score = 0

His doctor reflected back to a possible discrepancy between Dr. O.'s verbal and nonverbal cues by saying, "You say that you are giving some thought to exercising, but I also got the impression that you don't like exercising very much. So what scores would you give to your resistance and motivation, based on how you felt about exercise?" Dr. O. gave a resistance score of 10 and a motivation score of 0, based on how he felt. He preferred to play the piano. This process helped him better understand his cognitive-emotional discrepancies about this health behavior.

The important issue is not the scores themselves, but to generate a dialogue that clarifies the implications and meaning of the scores. You can also ask patients to continue to score resistance and motivation over time to discover what helped to increase or decrease their scores, for better or for worse.

EXPLORE MOTIVES FOR CHANGE[2]

According to the self-determination theory discussed in Chapter 7, motivation to change is a dynamic state affected by a blend of motives. Patients may list the same reasons for staying the same and changing, and even have the same resistance and motivation scores, but have very different underlying motives for why they want to change. They have a blend of motives that range along a continuum from autonomous to controlled, unless they are completely indifferent about behavior change. One category of reasons usually predominates at any given time. Furthermore, their motives may change over time.

Autonomous Motives

Patients with autonomous motives act out of a sense of pure volition: "I'll change because it is important to me." They act in accordance with their personally developed and deeply held values about health. They have a proactive attitude toward initiating and maintaining change.

Internally Controlled (Obligatory) Motives

Patients with obligatory motives are afflicted with a sense that they "should, must, or ought to change." They experience internal conflicts and are, in effect, internally controlled. These patients have ambivalent feelings and an obligatory attitude toward change.

Externally Controlled Motives

Patients with externally controlled motives respond to factors outside themselves. They initiate and maintain change provided that others (family, practitioners, primary and secondary prevention programs) reinforce it. Without such external reinforcements, they are likely to revert to their previous patterns of behavior. These patients have a reactive attitude toward change and may experience negative emotions about initiating change. Their behavior often resonates with values generated by external influences (e.g., media advertising about physical appearance, image-making by the tobacco and alcohol industry) rather than from personally developed and deeply held values about health care.

Indifference

Patients who are indifferent about changing their behaviors may not even resist you. They are beyond caring about their health. Many factors may account for this indifference:

- Psychological conditions (depression, stress, anxiety, cognitive impairment)
- Personality traits or disorders (impulsiveness, risk-taking, antisocial behavior)
- Social, cultural and contextual factors (learned helplessness due to psychosocial impoverishment or neglect, poverty, parental neglect and deviant subcultures)
- Spiritual distress (lack of personally developed and deeply held values)

To work meaningfully with patients, you need to move beyond the surface issues of behavior change to understanding their indifference. By stepping back from addressing their behavior, you can identify and address the deeper issues underlying their indifference. For example, depression can impair a patient's ability to change. Because the patient responds with indifference to your motivational approach to behavior change, you may need to treat the depression first. Identifying indifference early can reduce your frustration in working with resistant patients.

Patients may change their motives over time in response to a number of factors, including cultural norms, social situations and family influences, but also how you interview the patient. Whatever the origin of the influence, autonomy-supportive approaches enhance the prospects of patients developing autonomous motives; conversely, controlling approaches decrease the likelihood of patients developing such motivation and may even increase the likelihood of their being either externally motivated or indifferent.

Depending on your impression about the patient, you may select any of the following statements for any unhealthy behavior:

- *"I get the impression that you can't be bothered with change; what do you think?"*
- *"I get the impression that you're only thinking about change because that's what your spouse [or any other family member] wants you to do. So, what do you think?"*
- *"I get the impression that you're only thinking about change because you feel that you ought to change. So, what do you think?"*
- *"I get the impression that you're thinking about change because you really want to change for yourself. What do you think?"*
- *Or, "Tell me what is the driving force for why you want to consider change. Is it because of family and friends? Is it because you feel you ought to change? Are you*

doing it for yourself because it is important to you, or perhaps for a combination of reasons? Which is most important?"

INQUIRE ABOUT PATIENTS' COMPETING PRIORITIES AND ENERGY TO CHANGE

Competing priorities, stresses and time pressures can make it difficult for patients to change, and drain their energy to make changes. You can ask them to rate their energy to change, using a scale of 0–10, and to monitor over time what helps to increase and decrease their score.

"What are your competing priorities that make it difficult for you to change at the moment? [Let patient respond] On a scale of 0–10, what score would you give to your priority to change?"

"On a scale of 0–10, how much energy can you put into changing your behavior?"

ASSESS PATIENTS' CONFIDENCE AND ABILITY (SELF-EFFICACY)[7-9]

While patients often give realistic appraisals of themselves, sometimes they underestimate or overestimate their confidence and abilities. Ask patients

"On a scale of 0–10, how would you rate your confidence to change?" and *"On a scale of 0–10, how would you rate your ability to change?"*

You can reassess the patients' scores later to check whether anything increased or decreased their confidence and ability to change.

ASK ABOUT SUPPORTS AND BARRIERS TO CHANGE

As described in Chapter 5, supports and barriers can make individual behavior change more or less difficult for patients. In particular, family members can help or hinder a patient's prospects for change.

Family Perspective

A family may feel responsible for the health of its individual members, even though health behavior change itself is ultimately an individual responsibility. Although research evidence is not available to justify the routine use of family-oriented assessments and interventions in secondary prevention programs, they may be useful options when individual-focused interventions do not work or when dealing with tertiary prevention.[10] In other words, complex problems may require more comprehensive assessments and interventions. Whenever working solely at an individual level is insufficient to help patients change, you can expand your assessment beyond the individual to include a family, social, community and/or cultural perspective. A systems perspective also helps you take a broader view about health behavior change and identifies the external forces (family, community, society) that support or hinder the change process for individual patients.

Decision Balances for Family Members

Family members frequently accompany patients to health care settings, and patients often want their family members to be involved in their health care.[11] Not uncommonly, family members are more concerned about the risk behavior than the patient is. In fact, family members can fall into the same trap of the fix-it role by being ahead of patients in their readiness to change when the patient is still not ready. Out of frustration and concern, family members may nag patients to change, a tactic that seldom works and may unintentionally enhance patient resistance.

To help patients and family members avoid this unproductive dynamic, you can explain the readiness for change continuum and point out possible discrepancies. For example, a patient may be in the precontemplation stage, while family members want the patient to take action. To help family members understand their differences better, you can ask them to complete a decision balance independently of the patient so that they can compare notes with the patient's decision balance to see how their views differ about issues related to health behavior change. Furthermore, you can ask family members to look at their decision balance and provide a score from 0–10 (0 = not important, 10 = very important) for resistance and motivation. This explanation may help families reflect about a circular dynamic whereby family members approach and nag patients and patients get annoyed and avoid family members.

Following his family doctor's suggestion, Dr. O. asked his wife to fill out a decision balance (see responses below) from her perspective about his weight problem.

Mrs. O.'s Decision Balance

Reasons to stay sedentary	Reasons to exercise
1. Benefits of staying the same Plays music instead of exercise Avoids the effort of exercising when feeling tired	2. Concerns about staying the same Weight gain and high blood pressure Risk of stroke
3. Concerns about changing Will need to buy new clothes if he loses weight	4. Benefits about changing Lose weight Look better
Resistance Score = 1	Motivation Score= 10

After looking at his wife's decision balance, Dr. O. learned how his wife viewed his weight problem differently from the way he did. His wife learned more about how her husband's view of the need to exercise was different from hers. This process of sharing their differences in perceptions about change helped Mrs. O. better understand how her husband struggled with his weight and exercise issues. Dr. O. became more willing to think about change, and Mrs. O. stopped expecting him to start exercising in the near future.

Commentary: The use of the decision balance in this manner can help families break the unproductive dynamic of nagging a person who does not want to change. They can then compare and contrast their items on the decision balances and their perceptions about the change process. This can help them to better understand their different viewpoints and work in a more cooperative, or at least a less antagonistic, manner with one another.

INCORPORATING OTHER METHODS

A motivational approach also provides a framework within which you can integrate other approaches, such as cognitive-behavioral methods. For example, you can suggest to patients that they consider using a diary to monitor the following: cues, triggers, situations associated with risk behaviors; thoughts before, during and after the behavior; feelings before, during and after the behavior; and consequences for self and others. Patients can then decide for themselves whether these methods can help them change. The introduction of these approaches, however, can sometimes be used in controlling ways—telling patients to monitor and record information about their behavior when they are not really motivated to do so.

YOUR SUMMARY

Reflect: write a summary about what you have learned that was new for you.

_____
_____
_____
_____
_____
_____
_____
_____
_____
_____
_____
_____
_____
_____
_____
_____
_____

_____
_____
_____

Enhance*: complete a self-assessment of your skills using the worksheet on page 320. **Write your** **goals below for improving specific skills** in role plays or patient encounters. After doing these practice sessions, reassess your competence score for these skills and make notes on page 320 to explain why you changed your scores. If possible, keep an audio recording or videotape of your practice sessions.*

_____
_____
_____
_____
_____
_____
_____
_____
_____
_____

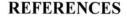

REFERENCES

1. Stewart M, Brown JB, Weston WW, et al. Patient-centered medicine: Transforming the clinical method. Thousand Oaks, CA: Sage Publications; 1995

2. Deci EL, Ryan RM. Intrinsic motivation and self-determination in human behavior. New York: Plenum Press; 1985

3. Prochaska JO, DiClemente CC. Transtheoretical therapy: Toward a more integrative model of change. Psychotherapy Theory, Research and Practice 1982;19(3): 276-288

4. Prochaska JO, DiClemente CC. Toward a comprehensive model of change. In: Miller WR, Heather N, eds. Treating addictive behaviors: Processes of change. New York: Plenum Press; 1986:3-27

5. Miller WR, Rollnick S. Motivational interviewing: Preparing people for change. New York: Guilford Press; 1991

6. Heather N, Rollnick S, Bell A. Predictive validity of the Readiness to Change Questionnaire. Addiction 1993;88: 1667-1677

7. Bandura A. Social foundations of thought and action. Englewood Cliffs, NJ: Prentice Hall; 1986

8. Bandura A. Self-efficacy: The exercise of control. New York: W.H. Freeman; 1997

9. DiClemente CC. Self-efficacy and the addictive behaviors. Journal of Social and Clinical Psychology 1986;4: 302-315

10. Campbell TL, Patterson JM. The effectiveness of family interventions in the treatment of physical illness. Journal of Marriage and Family Therapy 1995;21 (4): 545-583

11. Botelho RJ, Lue B-H, Fiscella K. Family involvement in routine patient care: A survey of patient behaviors and preferences. Journal of Family Practice 1996;42: 572-576

CHAPTER 12

STEP 4: ENHANCING MUTUAL UNDERSTANDING

FOR REFLECTION

How can you address differences in understanding, perceptions and values about health behavior change with your patients?

OVERVIEW

You and your patients will usually have differences in understanding, perceptions and values about health behavior change. You will be more effective in helping your patients to change if you first understand these differences before trying to address them.[1;2] To work toward this goal, you may also need to address your differences in role expectations, agendas and assumptions with your patients. Then you can use these differences to enhance mutual understanding and make a difference.[3] Four essential skills can help you motivate your patients to change their behavior.

1. Educating patients about risk behaviors and the benefits of change can help develop a common understanding with them about the need for change.
2. Using nondirect interventions can clarify how you and your patients perceive and value the benefits and concerns about behavior change differently. These interventions help you explore why patients do not want to change, are ambivalent about it or indifferent to it. This process can lower patient resistance to change.
3. Using direct interventions can help patients change their perceptions and values in ways that motivate them to change their behavior.
4. Addressing perceptions about patients' confidence and ability to change can identify impediments to implementing a plan. After patients have rated their confidence and ability to change, you can consider and act on whether you agree with their self-assessment.

You can use these skills to make a successful transition from conducting an assessment to implementing a plan.

Enhancing mutual understanding (Step 4) with patients is essential for making a successful transition from assessment of resistance and motivation (Step 3) to plan implementation (Step 5). The process can help patients take charge of their health so they decide what to do in the next phase: implementing a plan.

WORKING WITH YOUR DIFFERENCES

To resolve some of your differences in understanding, perceptions and values about health behavior change with patients (see Figure 12.1), you can

- Explore your areas of agreement and disagreement
- Work toward understanding each other's perspectives
- Build agreement and reduce disagreement

Figure 12.1.
Enhancing Mutual Understanding

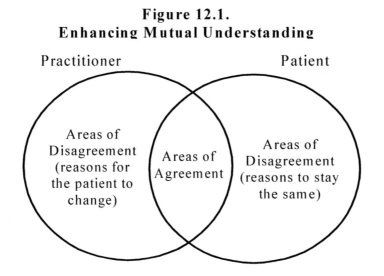

Because misunderstandings can occur at any of the six steps, enhancing mutual understanding is an important option at any step. Before addressing how to work on Step 4, you may need to consider a series of issues that relate to previous steps in order to avoid misunderstandings that prevent you from working effectively with your patients. In other words, you may have to resolve your misunderstandings by returning to an earlier step.

BUILDING PARTNERSHIP ISSUES
One important aspect of the partnership-building process is to address differences in role expectations (described in Chapter 3 and discussed in Chapter 9, Part C) between

you and your patients. Role mismatches occur when you expect patients to assume a particular role but they do not, and vice versa. It is therefore important that you renegotiate your role to develop a more effective relationship, a process that can be done at any point in the six-step approach.

Changing from a fix-it to a motivational role: In frustration, a fix-it practitioner decided to renegotiate his role with his patient, Mrs. S., a diabetic, by stating, "I think that I'm trying too hard to help you stay healthy." The practitioner noticed a perplexed look on the patient's face. "Let me explain. I can't make you change your diet, but I could help you think about whether to improve your health." Mrs. S. was surprised by his approach and complimented him for his concern for her health. She explained that her life was too overwhelming at the moment, but that she would be willing to think about change in about two months.

Changing to a motivational role when the patient expects a fix-it role: Mrs. T., a 79-year-old woman, was a smoker with chronic obstructive pulmonary disease who was on oxygen at home. She expected her doctor to improve her lung condition. While Mrs. T. was in the waiting room, the medical assistant asked her to fill in a decision balance about smoking before seeing her doctor.

Mrs. T.'s Decision Balance

Reasons to smoke	Reasons to quit
1. Benefits of smoking An old friend Helps with depression	2. Concerns about smoking Can't walk far Feels guilty
3. Concerns about quitting Withdrawal symptoms Loneliness	4. Benefits of quitting Feel better Save money

After attending to the presenting complaint, the doctor looked at her decision balance and asked why she wrote down "an old friend" as a benefit of smoking. Since her husband had died three years ago, Mrs. T. explained that she had come to regard smoking as her old friend. The doctor asked what was her most important reason to quit. She told him that she wanted to feel better. He reflected back to Mrs. T., "On the one hand, you like smoking because it's an old friend, but on the other hand, you would feel better if you quit smoking." Mrs. T. then noticed that she had put down "feels guilty" as a concern about smoking, and made the spontaneous remark that an old friend would not make her feel guilty. In effect, she identified her own discrepancy and generated her own ambivalence about change. The doctor encouraged Mrs. T. to think more about slowing the progress of her lung disease as a way to feel and function better so that she could improve her quality of life, regardless of how long she lived.

Commentary: In both examples, the practitioner adopted or was placed in the position of adopting a fix-it role—assuming too much responsibility for issues that he could not fix or control. If you clarify your roles and responsibilities with patients, you are more likely to work more effectively together. Over time, a motivational role can help many of your patients take responsibility for changing their behavior and improving their quality of life.

AGENDA-SETTING ISSUES

Sometimes a patient may appear to be motivated to change but is simply complying with your agenda, even though he or she has not really bought into the discussion about health behavior change. When this occurs, you may need to take a step back to address this issue, because as long as the agenda is perceived as yours, the patient is unlikely to change.

Renegotiating and developing a mutual understanding about the agenda: At the next appointment, Mrs. T. appeared disinterested in talking about smoking. Her doctor said, "Last time, you seemed interested in talking about smoking, but this time, you don't. What's going on?" Mrs. T. stated that the more she thought about quitting, the more she thought about her deceased husband. As she started to feel lonely and depressed, she felt less motivated to think about quitting, and told her doctor to stop the quit-smoking lecture, because she did not care if she lived or died.

ASSESSMENT ISSUES

You often do not have the time to assess patients with regard to their knowledge and understanding about health behavior change; their perceptions about the benefits of and concerns for the status quo and change; their level of resistance and motivation; factors that affect their perceptions about these benefits and concerns; factors that affect their energy, motivational reasons and self-efficacy; and the barriers to and supports for change. Inevitably, you may make inaccurate assumptions about patients. When these assumptions cause misunderstandings, you can reassess the factors contributing to the difficulties in working together.

Reassessing factors that affected Mrs. T.'s resistance: At the next follow-up appointment, Mrs. T.'s doctor asked her if smoking cigarettes helped her to avoid thinking about her husband and to ward off feelings of depression. Mrs. T. acknowledged that this was true. She could not even think about quitting smoking until her depression was treated. Her doctor then reassessed his position in light of this fact, and realized he needed to treat her depression before setting a quit-smoking agenda.

To move on to the next step (enhancing mutual understanding), you can use four skill sets to work on resolving your persisting differences.

FOUR ESSENTIAL SKILLS

Patients may perceive the choice about behavior change differently from you. For example, they perceive the reasons to stay the same (the cons) as being more important than the reasons to change (the pros). In contrast, you perceive the pros as outweighing the cons. Patients can resist working with you as a consequence of these differences in perceptions, but also because of your interviewing approach. Four sets of skills can help you work with patient resistance and redirect this energy in a healthy direction (see also Chapters 15-17).

1. EDUCATING PATIENTS ABOUT HEALTH BEHAVIOR CHANGE

You can educate patients by using approaches that range from practitioner-centered to patient-centered and from controlling to autonomy-supportive (see Table 12.1).

Practitioner-centered Education—A Monologue

In the fix-it role, we educate and give advice in an authoritarian or authoritative manner, without knowing if patients need or want such information. The advantage of this direct approach is its simplicity and brevity. The authoritarian approach is controlling and paternalistic in its delivery style.

> ***Authoritarian monologue:*** *Using a threatening or solemn tone of voice, a practitioner "educated" a patient about the reasons why he must quit smoking: "Smoking is the cause of your heart problems. You must quit smoking; otherwise, you will die from a heart attack." This scare tactic works infrequently, particularly when the patient does not care if he lives or dies because of the physical limitations imposed by his heart problem. Otherwise, health behavior change would be a simple task; you would only have to scare patients to death and they would change.*

Alternatively, with an authoritative approach, we work in an autonomy-supportive way and relate to patients in an egalitarian manner. We educate patients about how their behavior affects their health but do not attempt to control their behavior. However, with this approach, we still tend to provide the same kind of health information to all patients, without knowing what their expectations, needs and preferences are.

> ***Authoritative monologue:*** *Using an autonomy-supportive approach, the practitioner stated in a concerned tone, "You know what my advice would be, but it's up to you to decide whether to quit or not. Can I explain how smoking is damaging your heart and lungs?" This permission-granting approach still uses a practitioner-centered way of educating the patient about his health problem. In other words, it focuses on what the practitioner is concerned about, without understanding the particular concerns of the patient.*

Patient-centered Education—A Dialogue

In the preventive or motivational role, you take into consideration the patients' concerns, feelings, expectations and/or consequences regarding their risk behavior.[4] You try to provide health information tailored to their needs and preferences in an authoritative and personally meaningful way.

> **Patient-centered education:** Dr. P. asked Mr. C. whether anyone in his family had a drinking problem. Mr. C. told Dr. P. that his father had had a drinking problem and had died from cirrhosis when he was only 55. Dr. P. explained to Mr. C. that he was at increased risk of developing a drinking problem and getting cirrhosis like his father. Mr. C. had difficulty accepting this idea because he did not think that he was like his father. He had a strong liver and did not get drunk easily like his father or his friends. Contrary to what Mr. C. thought, Dr. P. told him that this fact put him at increased risk of developing cirrhosis because he could drink much more alcohol than his friends. Over time, his high alcohol intake could gradually damage his liver, so that his tolerance to alcohol would gradually decrease and he would eventually get drunk more easily, like his father. Mr. C. expressed some disbelief and then some concern about this information. He did not like the idea of family history repeating itself. Dr. P. asked him if he would like to have a blood test to see if there were any early signs of liver damage. Even though Dr. P. anticipated that Mr. C.'s liver enzymes would probably be normal, he thought it was worthwhile doing the test to emphasize to Mr. C. the need to keep them normal and to encourage him to reduce his alcohol intake or, better still, abstain from alcohol.

Table 12.1. Approaches to Providing Education and Advice

Practitioner-centered Education: Monologues	Patient-centered Education: Dialogues
Educates about risks and harms in ways that are not based on understanding patients' needs or their life experiences.	Educates about risks and harms based on understanding patients' needs or their life experiences.
Tells patients that they ought to, must or should change their behaviors (controlling advice).	Influences patients to change but lets them decide what to do (autonomy-supportive counsel).

While such tailored information helps you develop a common understanding with patients about the need to change, most patients will still not change their behavior. This is because knowledge alone is generally not enough. You also need to use motivational interventions (nondirect and direct) to help patients change their perceptions and values about their reasons to stay the same (cons) and their reasons to change (pros). This process can tip the balance of the pros and cons in favor of patients adopting healthy behaviors.

2. USING NONDIRECT INTERVENTIONS TO LOWER PATIENT RESISTANCE

Patients may resist working with you if you do not understand their reasons for engaging in a risk behavior. Nondirect interventions can help you better understand why patients do not want to change or are ambivalent and indifferent about it. They also can help patients clarify their perceptions and values about staying the same versus changing their risk behavior.

With nondirect interventions, you take a neutral stance to explore patients' perceptions and values about the benefits and concerns of the status quo versus change, without implying they should change. This does not mean that you abandon your values or opinions. Instead, you put them on the sidelines while attempting to understand your patients more deeply. In effect, you allow patients to confront themselves about these issues in nonthreatening ways. Paradoxically, they can then become more receptive to the possibility of change and thereby lower their resistance and increase their motivation.

A metaphor may help you understand the distinction and relationship between resistance and motivation to change. Resistance (tails) and motivation (heads) are the opposite sides of the same coin. When tails are up (high resistance and low motivation), patients are not even thinking about change. Conversely, when heads are up (low resistance and high motivation), patients are more likely to be in the preparation, action or maintenance stage. When the coin is spinning, resistance and motivation are about equal, and patients are ambivalent about change. Understanding this dynamic can help you work with patients in more deliberate, sensitive and effective ways.

Nondirect interventions can help patients lower their resistance to change by helping them identify their "known" (conscious), "forgotten" (subconscious) and "unknown" (unconscious) benefits (reasons) for continuing their risk behavior. Some patients initially struggle to identify the benefits of their risk behaviors because they rarely think about them. Other patients are at a complete loss to identify any reasons for their long-standing habit because they have completely lost touch with the original benefits for engaging in the risk behavior. You can provide examples of benefits (see Tables 11.2-11.7) to help prompt patients to identify the benefits of their risk behavior. Yet, even if patients identify some benefits, they may resist working with you because of other unrecognized benefits ("unknown" reasons). Thus, it is important to attempt to identify the different levels of reasons.

> **Layers of Reasons:** "I eat to make myself feel good and happy" was a conscious (known) reason for a grossly overweight patient to eat. In working with her practitioner, she discovered that she also ate too much when she felt overwhelmed, anxious and/or depressed (forgotten reasons). When her practitioner referred her to a therapist so that she could address issues related to her emotional abuse as a child, she also discovered an unknown reason for overeating. Her father had used the withdrawal of food as a way to control her "bad" behavior. Consequently, she now felt that eating food was one of the few

things in life that she could control, and she used eating as a way to cope. Despite this new understanding, she still had difficulties stopping herself from overeating when she was particularly stressed. However, she did manage to lose weight when she felt less stressed.

Commentary: The patient gained a deeper understanding about her overeating because her practitioner and therapist worked with her to uncover her forgotten and unknown reasons for overeating. Such a process can help when patients encounter difficulties in changing their behavior.

Key Point
Exploring patients' "known" reasons not to change and uncovering their "forgotten" and/or "unknown" ones can help lower their resistance to change.

Based on the items in the patient's decision balance, you can select any nondirect intervention (see Table 12.2) in any particular order that you think will be most effective in exploring the patient's ambivalence and lowering his or her resistance score.

Table 12.2

Nondirect Interventions
• Use simple reflection to elicit patient's ambivalence
• Probe priorities to explore patient's ambivalence
• Use double-sided reflection to summarize patient's ambivalence
• Acknowledge patient's ambivalence
• Emphasize patient's personal responsibility and choice
• Use explore-the-future questioning

For example, a practitioner (MP) used *simple reflection* to elicit ambivalence from Mr. O., a middle-aged married man with a drinking problem. MP noted, "So, you like drinking with your friends in the bar." Mr. O. replied that he liked his friends' company while drinking in the bar, but didn't have anything in common with them when they were not drinking. MP *probed priorities* to explore ambivalence by asking Mr. O. what was most important, his friends or his drinking alcohol. Mr. O. stated that friendship was important, but then he surprised himself by saying that he didn't know whether his friends would still be his friends if they were not drinking alcohol together.

MP summarized Mr. O.'s ambivalence by using *double-sided reflection*: "So, on the one hand, your friends seem okay when you're drinking, but, on the other hand, you may not count many of them as your friends when you're sober." Though MP paused for a few seconds to allow Mr. O. to reflect, the patient still looked puzzled. MP *acknowledged Mr. O.'s ambivalence* by stating, "You seem to have some mixed feelings about drinking alcohol and making friends."

Using *explore-the-future questioning*, MP continued: "What sort of things did you do with your friends in the past 5 to 10 years that are different from what you do now? And what sort of things do you think you will do with your friends in the future, say five years from now?" Mr. O. described a number of hobbies that he used to do with friends, and thought that he might do something like that again in the future. MP *emphasized personal responsibility and choice* by encouraging Mr. O. to decide how best to spend his time.

Additional examples of nondirect interventions for addressing smoking cessation, alcohol risk and harm reduction and self-care of diabetes are described in Part B of Chapters 15 and 16 and in Chapter 17. In those chapters, you can select concrete examples of nondirect interventions from a menu of options to use in role plays and in your daily work with patients.

The strategy of using nondirect before direct interventions can help decrease the likelihood of patients externalizing their resistance in ways that work against you. It can also help deepen your understanding about why patients engage in risk behaviors. Once you have worked your way through some or all of these nondirect interventions, you can ask patients whether this exploratory process helped to lower their resistance score. Afterward, you can use direct interventions to help patients alter their perceptions and values in ways that help them increase their motivation score.

3. USING DIRECT INTERVENTIONS TO ENHANCE PATIENT MOTIVATION
Direct interventions can help patients explore, think and feel differently about the benefits and concerns of the status quo and change. This process can help them alter their perceptions and values about their reasons to stay the same and their reasons to change. You may need to caution patients, however, that while direct interventions may help them think more deeply about change, such interventions may also make them feel uncomfortable.

> *"I'd like to help you find ways of increasing your motivation score so that you can improve your health, if you like. [Let the patient respond.] It can make you pause to think about changing your habit. If it makes you feel too uncomfortable, just let me know and I'll stop."*

You can thus support patients as they work through their emotional discomfort in productive ways. Now let's look more closely at some powerful interventions to enhance motivation (see Table 12.3). Several examples will illustrate how some direct interventions are more complex to use in practice than nondirect interventions.

191

Table 12.3.

Direct Interventions
• Use benefit substitution
• Use back-to-the-future questioning
• Clarify values
• Use amplified reflection
• Use discrepancies
• Challenge rationalizations
• Reframe items, issues or events
• Use differences in motivational reasons

Questions about ***benefit substitution*** help patients explore whether they can obtain the same benefits derived from their risk behavior without engaging in the actual behavior. Some patients are slow to generate ideas about alternative ways of obtaining the same benefits because they have never thought about this question. You can ask these patients to look at the benefits they listed on their decision balance and then generate an alternative list for each benefit. If patients are willing, you may also offer suggestions after they have struggled and worked on developing their own ideas. If patients resist this exploration, you can pose a value clarification question (see below): "What does this tell you about how important this behavior is to you?"

Back-to-the-future questioning is a nonthreatening and hypothetical way of exploring patients' values with respect to long-term perspectives on their health. For example, you can ask the patient, *"If you had a heart attack now, do you think you'd quit smoking?"* In other words, is the short-term benefit of the risk behavior more important to the patient than the long-term protection of his or her health? If patients think that their risk behaviors are more important than their health, you can ask them why.

Value clarification questions challenge patients to reflect about and change the priorities of their values in relation to their health and other aspects of their life. The process of contrasting values may help generate the motivation necessary to promote change. For example, you can ask them if their risk behavior (smoking, alcohol, drugs) is more important to them than their relationship with their spouse, children and/or grandchildren.

Amplified reflection helps you challenge patients' positions or claims that you disagree with, but without getting into circular arguments that involve claims/ counterclaims. In effect, you exaggerate the claim that patients make so that your comments challenge patients not to remain fixed in their position or claim. These interventions can be helpful when patients repeatedly make statements that help them avoid issues or blame others for their problems.

192

Using amplified reflection, value clarification and back-to-the-future questions: Mr. S. smoked a pack of cigarettes a day, had end-stage emphysema and was able to walk only about 30 yards with oxygen before stopping to regain his breath. During Mr. S.'s hospitalization for emphysema, Dr. M. asked Mr. S. about his smoking. Mr. S. stated how much he enjoyed cigarettes. Dr. M. replied, "I suppose that you enjoy cigarettes so much that you're a diehard smoker [amplified reflection], and nothing would make you change." Mr. S. paused before agreeing, but he was surprised by what his doctor had said. Dr. M. asked Mr. S. whether there was anything in his life that was more important than smoking (a value clarification intervention). Mr. S. replied promptly and adamantly that smoking was the only pleasure left in his life. After pausing for a moment, he stated that he hated paying taxes for cigarettes so much that he would drive to an Indian reservation where he could buy cigarettes tax-free. Dr. M. asked Mr. S. what he would do if he could not drive to the Indian reservation if his breathing problem got worse (back-to-the-future question). Annoyed by the implication of this question, Mr. S. unexpectedly stated that he would cut down to five cigarettes a day if it meant that he would still be able to drive to the reservation for his tax-free cigarettes.

A year later, when Mr. S. was readmitted to the hospital, Dr. M. asked him if he remembered what they talked about at his last hospitalization. Mr. S. stated with pride that he cut down to five cigarettes a day and that this was the longest time that he had been out of a hospital.

You can also generate emotional energy to change by pointing out to patients any *discrepancies* between their self-interest and their behavior. This emotional energy arises from a sense of dissatisfaction or dis-ease with their current situation. Patients may work toward reducing this dis-ease by resolving the discrepancy.

Identify discrepancies between behavior and self-interest: A 20-year-old college student, Ms. A., who smoked one pack of cigarettes a day and drank excessive amounts of alcohol on weekends, appeared for her annual gynecological examination in order to get a refill of birth control pills. Her practitioner asked her, "Could you ever imagine yourself giving up smoking?"

"Not at the moment, but I would give it up if I got pregnant," Ms. A. replied.

The practitioner identified this discrepancy and reflected it back to the patient. "That's very interesting. So you would value the health of your baby more than you do your own."

"Well, I suppose that's right," Ms. A. said hesitantly.

Her practitioner proceeded further: "Is there anything else that might help you give up smoking sooner?"

"Well, I suppose if I had a boyfriend who didn't smoke, then I would give it up," Ms. A. said without hesitation.

The practitioner identified this as another discrepancy and said in a low-key manner, "But if you continue smoking, do you think men who don't smoke will be interested in you if they see you smoking?"

Ms. A. was taken aback by this opened-ended question and remained silent for a few seconds. "Well, I suppose that's an interesting point," she said quietly.

At this point, her practitioner thought that she might be becoming resistant, and explained, "Let me be clear about what I'm doing. I only want to help you improve your health, but that's only if you want me to help you. I'll stop talking about smoking if you want me to."

"No, I understand that you're trying to help me stay healthy," Ms. A. replied.

Not sure about how to proceed, the practitioner noted, "I've said a couple of things that might help you think more about whether to smoke or not. I'd like to say one more thing that might help you think more about this. Is that okay?"

Although Ms. A. was reluctant to hear what the practitioner might say, her curiosity got the better of her: "Okay. Go ahead."

Her practitioner then identified another discrepancy (between an external and an integrated reason toward change). "It seems that you're willing to change provided that it will benefit others, such as your baby or a nonsmoking boyfriend. But what about doing something for yourself?"

"That's really something to think about," Ms. A. replied in a reflective tone.

Among direct interventions, ***challenging rationalizations*** is perhaps the most sophisticated skill to use effectively, because patients will come up with the most intriguing rationalizations for their behaviors that you will sometimes get stuck for a reply. Comments that challenge rationalizations help you disrupt patients' defensive routines so that they pause and reflect about the inconsistency of their rationalization. Patients often make statements such as, "I'm under too much stress at the moment to quit smoking right now" that provide you with opportunities to challenge their rationalizations. You could reply, "Probably you'll always be under some kind of stress. In fact, this may be the best time to think about quitting, because if you quit now, you'll be in a better position to stop yourself from smoking a cigarette when you're under a lot of stress." Patients will give you ample opportunities to generate your own ideas about how to challenge their rationalizations in supportive and nonthreatening ways.

Reframing items, issues or events helps patients decide whether to alter their perceptions about the items on their decision balance. Patients may change their perceptions to increase the importance attached to their concerns about the risk behavior and the benefits of change and/or decrease the importance they attached to the benefits of risk behaviors and the drawbacks of change. For example, patients may cite "nagging family members" as a concern of the risk behavior in a dismissive manner. You may help patients to change their perceptions and enhance the importance of this concern by stating, "The amount that they nag you is a measure of how much they care for you."

Patients often have ***differences in motivational reasons*** for addressing their risk behaviors. As you listen to patients, you can gather information to compare what motivates them to address different behaviors or issues.

Using differences in motivational reasons: Mr. U., a 26-year-old student who had a five-year relationship with his girlfriend, went to see his family physician because he had a urethral discharge. He had gone to a party about four weeks earlier and had had unsafe sex with a woman who was apparently on the birth control pill. As Dr. M. listened carefully to Mr. U.'s account of this sexual encounter, Mr. U. mentioned that in spite of being under the influence of alcohol, he was very careful to make sure that he would not get this woman pregnant (he asked her if she was on the pill) because he did not want to become a father. Dr. M. reflected back to Mr. U. that while he was highly motivated in being responsible about not bringing new life into the world, he was willing to risk contracting an STD or HIV from a woman whose sexual history was unknown to him. Mr. U. at first minimized the risk of contracting HIV. However, when Dr. M. pointed out the discrepancy between his motivation to avoid being a father and his lack of motivation to avoid contracting HIV, Mr. U. gave further thought to the issue of using condoms on a regular basis with casual relationships. The impact of using difference in motivation (between the reasons for avoiding pregnancy and not using safe sex practices) helped him shift from being a precontemplator to a contemplator with regard to using condoms.

After helping Mr. U. think about this casual sexual encounter in a new way, Dr. M. pointed out that there is still a remote possibility that Mr. U. may have contracted the HIV virus, and that the test might not become positive for six months. He advised Mr. U. to use condoms for the next six months with his girlfriend, but Mr. U. thought he would have difficulty doing this because his girlfriend was on the birth control pill. Dr. M. pointed out a dilemma that Mr. U. may have preferred not to address. Either he had the option of not telling his girlfriend about this other relationship, not using condoms and running the risk of passing the HIV virus to her, or he had the option of telling her about this relationship and using condoms to ensure that she would be safe.

The art of using direct interventions is to use the ones that you think will be the most effective in increasing the patient's motivation score and decreasing the resistance score in the decision balance. These interventions can help patients change their perceptions about benefits and concerns in ways that assign greater value to the reasons to change (concerns about maintaining risk behavior and benefits of adopting a healthier one) and less value to the reasons not to change (benefits of maintaining a risk behavior and concerns about adopting a healthier one). Additional examples of direct interventions for addressing smoking and excessive alcohol intake are in Part B of Chapters 15 and 16. Most of the nondirect and direct interventions are derived from the work of Miller and Rollnick.[5] The underlying approach is also influenced by the work of Prochaska and DeClemente and of Deci and Ryan.[6-8]

Monitor Changes in Resistance and Motivation Scores

To assess the impact of these interventions on your patients, you can ask them if they have changed their resistance and motivation scores and why. Their explanations for changing them provide invaluable information about why things are getting better or worse over time. This process also can help to confirm whether your impression about what helped (or not) was accurate. You may be surprised by the inaccuracies of your predictions. Sometimes your best-delivered interventions are less effective than you think they are. Conversely, your poorly delivered interventions can have an impact far beyond your expectations.

Patients may give optimistic scores just to please you. If you feel that this is happening, you can gently question them about whether they really mean what they say. "You gave yourself a 2 for your resistance and a 10 for your motivation score. I would have thought that you would have made an attempt to quit smoking by now. Did you really mean to give yourself those scores?" Such a discussion can help patients reflect more deeply about the discrepancy between their well-meaning intentions and the probability that their intentions will result in a change.

4. ADDRESSING PERCEPTIONS ABOUT PATIENTS' CONFIDENCE AND ABILITY TO CHANGE

Patients vary in how they assess their confidence and ability to change (self-efficacy).[9-11] A simple framework (see Table 12.4) can help you to understand how confidence and ability aren't always evenly matched.

Table 12.4. Perceptions about Self-efficacy

Dimensions of Self-efficacy		Confidence	
		Low	High
Ability	Low	Low confidence/ low ability	High confidence/ low ability
	High	Low confidence/ high ability	High confidence/ high ability

It is also important to distinguish between patients' perceptions and your perceptions about them. To help you address this issue, you can ask patients to score their confidence and ability to change, using a scale of 0–10. You can then use these scores to assess whether you agree with their self-assessment.

Some motivated patients underestimate their ability to change because they lack confidence. Their reasons may be related or unrelated to their risk behavior: for example, drug addiction, depression, low self-esteem and stresses. The following example describes a patient who wanted to change but lacked the confidence.

> Mrs. S., a two-pack-a-day smoker with multiple failed quit attempts, gave herself a score of 1 for her confidence to quit and a score of 0 for her ability to quit. Her practitioner noted: "You keep thinking of quitting, but you seem to underestimate your confidence and ability to change. The nicotine withdrawal symptoms make you relapse, and your sense of failure makes you lose your confidence. You can change if you learn from your quit attempts instead of putting yourself down. Nicotine replacement therapy can also help to increase your confidence to quit."

You can help patients build their confidence, learn from their quit attempts, prolong them and eventually quit for good. The relational strategies described in Chapter 9 (Part B) may also help you enhance patients' perceptions about their confidence. Or you can identify patients' strengths that they can use to address behavior change.

Conversely, some unmotivated patients are confident that they can change and have a perception of high confidence and high ability, but you may disagree with their self-assessment.

> Mr. D. (a heavy drinker dependent on alcohol) gave himself a 10 for both his confidence and ability scores. The practitioner asked, "Then you would have no problem if you quit drinking for two weeks?" Mr. D. nodded in agreement, but stated that he did not want to change. "Suppose you tried to quit for two weeks and discovered that you couldn't stop drinking? What would you think then?" asked the practitioner. Mr. D. was surprised by this idea and stated that he would have to reassess his scores. The practitioner followed up by asking, "Do you think that it would be worth trying to stop drinking alcohol for two weeks to prove that you're not dependent on alcohol?"

You can help these kinds of patients explore whether they have assessed their level of confidence and ability to change appropriately. When patients lack the ability to change, you also may need to help them develop specific skills to achieve their goals for change, so that their confidence and ability are more evenly matched.

YOUR SUMMARY

Reflect: write a summary about what you have learned that was new for you.

_____
_____
_____
_____
_____
_____
_____
_____
_____
_____
_____
_____
_____
_____
_____
_____
_____
_____
_____
_____
_____
_____
_____
_____

Enhance: complete a self-assessment of your skills using the worksheet on page 321. ***Write your goals below for improving specific skills*** *in role plays or patient encounters. After doing these practice sessions, reassess your competence score for these skills and make notes on page 321 to explain why you changed your scores. If possible, keep an audio recording or videotape of your practice sessions.*

_____
_____
_____
_____
_____
_____
_____
_____
_____

REFERENCES

1. Botelho RJ, Skinner HA. Motivating change in health behavior: Implications for health promotion and disease prevention. Primary Care (Saunders) 1995;22: 565-589

2. Brown JB, Weston WW, Stewart MA. Patient centered interviewing: Part II: Finding common ground. Canadian Family Physician 1989;35: 153-157

3. Bateson G. Mind and nature: A necessary unity. New York: E.P. Dutton; 1979

4. Stewart M, Brown JB, Weston WW, et al. Patient-centered medicine: Transforming the clinical method. Thousand Oaks, CA: Sage Publications; 1995

5. Miller WR, Rollnick S. Motivational interviewing: Preparing people for change. New York: Guilford Press; 1991

6. Prochaska JO, DiClemente CC. Transtheoretical therapy: Toward a more integrative model of change. Psychotherapy Theory, Research and Practice 1982;19: 276-288

7. Prochaska JO, DiClemente CC. Toward a comprehensive model of change. In: Miller WR, Heather N, eds. Treating addictive behaviors: Processes of change. New York: Plenum Press; 1986: 3-27

8. Deci EL, Ryan RM. Intrinsic motivation and self-determination in human behavior. New York: Plenum Press; 1985

9. Bandura A. Self-efficacy: Toward a unifying theory of behavior change. Psychological Review 1977;84: 191-215

10. Bandura A. Social foundations of thought and action. Englewood Cliffs, NJ: Prentice Hall; 1986

11. Bandura A. Self-efficacy: The exercise of control. New York: W.H. Freeman; 1997

CHAPTER 13

STEP 5: IMPLEMENTING A PLAN FOR CHANGE

FOR REFLECTION

How can you help patients develop and implement an appropriate plan for change?

OVERVIEW

Many factors affect whether patients develop an appropriate plan for change. This chapter will describe how to

- Evaluate commitment toward a plan of change: Your level of commitment as well as that of your patients may vary when addressing different health behaviors. Furthermore, patients also have different competing priorities, levels of energy and motives that affect their level of commitment to change.

- Decide about goals for change: The range of goals for implementing a plan may exist along the following continua: stages of change (contemplation-preparation-action), short-term to long-term goals and pragmatic to ideal recommendations. Either you or your patient may select the goals for change unilaterally. Alternatively, you may negotiate with patients about the goals for change.

- Work toward solutions: A focus on solutions rather than on problems may help some patients enhance their prospects of implementing a plan for change.

Once you have developed some mutual understanding with your patients about the need for behavior change, you can move toward implementing a plan for change. The level of mutual understanding will obviously influence the extent to which your patients will be willing to implement such a plan. Various other factors will affect the successful outcome of this implementation. These include the need to evaluate commitment toward a plan for change, decide about goals for change, and work toward solutions. Refer to Part B of Chapters 15 and 16 for a more specific discussion of how to implement a plan for excessive alcohol intake and smoking cessation.

EVALUATE COMMITMENT TOWARD A PLAN FOR CHANGE

The level of your and your patients' commitment affects whether you and your patients will successfully work on behavior change together.

YOUR COMMITMENT

Your commitment to helping patients may vary in response to different risk behaviors and chronic diseases. For example, with patients who drink excessive amounts of alcohol, you are more likely to intervene in the late phases, when complications have occurred, than in the early, asymptomatic phases. Early intervention is effective, particularly before patients have become dependent on alcohol. Late-phase interventions, however, are quite understandable, given that most health care settings are not set up either to identify such patients early on or to intervene in a systematic and proactive manner, before complications have occurred.

On the other hand, if you are taking care of patients with diabetes, you respond differently. You help patients in the early phases to achieve normal blood glucose levels so that they can reduce their risk of developing complications. However, your response to some of your patients who do not take good care of their diabetes in the early phases may be similar to your response to patients with excessive alcohol intake. You and your patients may not take effective action in the early phases to avoid complications.

The purpose in pointing out such discrepancies in commitment is to highlight how your level of commitment for addressing different health behaviors may vary. As was noted in Chapter 1, physicians with specific health behaviors (e.g., nonsmoking, low-risk drinking or abstinence, regular exercise) are more likely to counsel patients to pursue such behaviors.

PATIENTS' COMMITMENT

Before deciding about a plan for change, you also need to evaluate the extent to which patients are committed to behavior change in terms of their competing priorities, energy and motives.

Competing Priorities

Competing priorities affect the timing of when patients are likely to initiate change. Even when patients are convinced about the need for health behavior change, competing priorities may reduce the time they can devote to it: for example, overwhelming work and family commitments. If you do not understand their competing priorities, you may find working with your patients frustrating because you will expect change to occur when patients are not yet ready to initiate it. Asking patients about their competing priorities can help you avoid such frustration.

Energy

Even when patients choose health behavior change as their top priority, they may not change because they lack the energy. Life circumstances make it difficult for them to change. Asking patients whether they have the energy to make any changes at this time can again help to avoid frustration for everyone.

Motives

Even when patients are ready and have the energy to change, you should ask them why they want to change, in other words, their motives for change. This is because they may not make a total and personally meaningful commitment to change because of controlled motives: as long as they feel they ought to change, or they are changing because others want them to change, they are less likely to be successful. In such situations, you can work with patients over time to develop autonomous motives so that they freely choose to pursue a goal for change, without any internal or external coercion.

DECIDE ABOUT GOALS FOR CHANGE

You and your patients can discuss and select from a range of goals. When setting a goal, you and your patients may make this decision collaboratively or unilaterally. With the latter option, you either highly recommend a specific goal to patients or you offer them a range of goals and let them make the decision for themselves.

RANGE OF GOALS

The range of goals for implementing a plan may exist along the following continua:
- Stages of change
- Short-term to long-term goals
- Pragmatic to ideal recommendations

Stages of Change

Patients' stages of change shape what they are prepared to do in terms of developing a workable plan. The goal for change may exist anywhere along the contemplation-preparation-action continuum. When patients are not ready for change, you can help them think more about change. Patients may be willing to keep a diary to explore the issue of behavior change, discuss change with family members and/or complete a decision balance alone or with family members. When patients are thinking about change, you can help them prepare to change. At this stage, patients may be willing to attend educational meetings, gather further information about change and read pamphlets and self-help books about behavior change. Once they have reached the action stage, they can decide whether to aim for short-term instead of long-term goals and whether to select a pragmatic over an ideal recommendation.

Short-term to Long-term Goals

The duration of change may range from short-term (from a day to several weeks) to long-term goals (from weeks to months or years). For example, when patients are unsure or ambivalent about the need for change, they may consider a short-term goal; for example, a trial of quitting smoking for two to four weeks. Short-term goals provide patients with learning opportunities that enable them to understand the implications and challenges of the long-term goals they face.

Pragmatic to Ideal Recommendations

The ideal recommendations for behavior change are derived from consensus statements and national advisory bodies. The U.S. Prevention Task Force and Canadian Task Force based their latest recommendations on grades of scientific evidence to support or refute preventive practices.[1-3] Not all recommendations from consensus statements are based on evidence; some recommendations are based on expert testimony from individuals whose professional careers are invested in particular areas or from some professional organizations that have a self-serving interest in making recommendations.

When recommending ideal goals, your challenge is to decipher and differentiate recommendations based on scientific evidence from recommendations based on expert testimony. Some of the latter may not be in the best interest of patients. In addition to this challenge, your task is to help patients achieve goals for change based on the best possible evidence and to make informed decisions that cannot be entirely addressed by the best available evidence.

Finally, the choice of a goal for change can also affect your patients' commitment to working on the related behavior change. You may recommend an ideal goal for change, such as to quit smoking or abstain from alcohol. Some patients are unwilling to accept the ideal recommendations as their short-term goals for change. Such an ideal recommendation can actually prevent some patients from making smaller, incremental changes or even of entertaining the idea of change, because the recommendation is too extreme. For example, a two-pack-a-day smoker may be willing to reduce his or her smoking to one pack a day, but to set a goal to stop smoking completely at this time is unrealistic. A goal of reducing the level of smoking may also help patients to better prepare for the challenge of quitting completely later on. Rather than assuming that the ideal recommendations are the goals for change, you should help work toward reducing the risks and harms associated with unhealthy behaviors in an incremental way. A small step toward the ideal recommendations is better than no change at all.

GOAL-SETTING

When setting a goal and selecting a method for achieving that goal, patients can make decisions either unilaterally or collaboratively with you. For example, a patient may decide to quit smoking without asking you for advice, or a patient may ask you to prescribe something for withdrawal symptoms. Or you may decide what needs to happen without any input from your patients by selecting a diabetic drug without giving them the advantages and disadvantages of other drug options. A limitation of this practitioner-centered approach is that your patients may decide what to do without your input and not get the prescribed drug. Alternatively, you can engage patients in the decision-making process and negotiate about treatment options and goals for change by deciding whether to use diet and/or drugs to control noninsulin-dependent diabetes.

Practitioner-initiated Goal-Setting

Basically, you tell patients what are the ideal goals for change and persuade them to set a date to change. Some patients may want you to behave this way. To avoid giving such advice when patients do not want it, you can ask them whether they would like you to simply give the ideal goals for change or whether they would like to discuss a range of options.

Patient-initiated Goal-setting

You can ask patients about their goals for change without providing any recommendations. Some patients understand what needs to be done, and they tell you what they are prepared to do. Alternatively, you can inform patients about the ideal recommendations and provide a range of options for change, but let them select their goals for change. When patients do this volitionally, they are more likely to follow through with their intentions to change. You can then negotiate a plan for follow-up.

Negotiated Approach to Goal-setting

To implement a plan, you first explore what patients are prepared to do and inquire about their commitment to change. You then make recommendations and negotiate about goals for change.

Combined Approaches

Unfortunately, time does not permit us to negotiate explicitly with patients about all aspects of a complex plan. When addressing a health problem with multiple issues, you may need to use a combination of the above approaches and negotiate with a patient about major issues regarding health behavior change while making some decisions independently of each other. For example, you can negotiate with a patient about whether to use diabetic medications in addition to dietary change, but may not spend any time discussing the different drugs to choose from within a class of medications. Thus, both you and your patients set goals in a variety of ways.

WORK TOWARD SOLUTIONS

Solution-based therapy provides a different orientation to helping patients change, compared to problem-focused approaches.[4-8] Is the glass half full or half empty? The half-full (solution-based) perspective helps you to focus on patients' strengths, competence and confidence. In contrast, the half-empty perspective (problem-focused) focuses your attention exclusively on patients' pathology, weaknesses and inadequacies. Patients may also fall into this trap. An optimistic focus on solutions can counter a pessimistic focus on problems.

Solution-focused interventions can remind you and your patients that they often have much more expertise about the change process than they may realize. The MED-STAT acronym (**m**iracle, **e**xceptions, **d**ifferences, **s**caling, **t**ime-outs, **a**ccolades, **t**asks) provides ways to focus on the positives, the possibility of change and the prospects of success, so patients begin to feel empowered to change.[9] By focusing on what was positive about the patient's change effort or attempt, you may preempt patients' self-defeating responses when they do not fully achieve their goal. Doing something, learning from that and building on small successes is better than going for the gold, failing and then doing nothing.

The MED-STAT acronym provides a way to remind you about some of the options in using a solution-focused approach. Although these options are described in this chapter, you can use them at any step in the six-step model, if it seems appropriate. Any single intervention or combination of interventions may help your patients use their inner resources to change more effectively. (The MED-STAT acronym is also employed in tables in Chapters 15-16 [part B] and Chapter 17.)

MIRACLE QUESTION
The miracle question encourages patients to imagine what life would be like if they achieved their ideal goals for change: "Suppose a miracle happened and you changed tomorrow, what would your life be like then? How do you think your family and friends would respond?" This question helps patients to
- Challenge the status quo and embed the idea that change is possible
- Explore both the positive and negative impacts of change on their lives

- Develop more realistic goals for change, particularly with hard-to-achieve ideal goals, such as weight loss and dietary changes
- Explore how others would react to these changes

EXCEPTIONS

To establish what causes patients to make an exception in a certain behavior, you can either explore with them the extremes of their behavior or ask them how and why they handle similar situations differently. For example, what was going on for patients when they were more adherent to the recommendations for self-care (diets, exercise, drug adherence, low-risk drinking) compared to a time when they were less adherent? You can ask them *"What was going on when you did less [smoking, drinking], and what was going on when you did more [smoking, drinking]?"* Alternatively, you can ask patients how and why they behaved differently in similar situations, for example, ordering a taxi or having a designated driver when drinking too much alcohol, as opposed to drinking and driving: *"What was going on when you handled the same situation differently?"*

DIFFERENCES

The process of identifying differences in how patients reacted in a similar situation can help them to focus on what they did well and then help them to apply those skills to situations that they handled less effectively. For example, you can ask, *"What is different about those two times? What made you handle the two situations differently?"* This approach can encourage patients to use their strengths.

SCALING

Patients can reevaluate any of the following factors: competing priorities, energy, motivation, resistance, confidence, ability and achievability of their goals by using a scale of 0–10. You can say to patients, *"On a scale of 0–10, how would you now rate your [competing priorities, energy, motivation, resistance, confidence and/or ability]? How would you rate whether you can achieve your goal for change? What would help to increase your score? Can you make a list of that? Was there a time when your scores were higher than now? What would it take to tip the balance in favor of a higher score?"*

The art of using scaling questions effectively is to select one or two items that are the most relevant to the patient's needs at that time. Over time, you can choose different items depending on what change the patient needs to address.

Patients often give realistic appraisals in response to any of the features described in the above question, but sometimes they underestimate or overestimate them. Thus an overconfident, dependent drinker in the precontemplation stage may lack the ability to change but still claim, *"I could quit anytime without any problems."* Such patients may lack both the motivation and skills and need specific help to address both issues. In contrast, other patients may have the skills to change but lack the confidence to achieve their goal.

TIME-OUTS

Time-outs help patients reflect about their routine habits and challenge them to consider alternative ways of dealing with situations, particularly when stress is the trigger for the risk behavior. They can help patients disrupt their automatic way of thinking about their behavior and dealing with situations. Again, the emphasis is on helping patients tap into their own internal resources to initiate the process of change. Allow time for silence when using the following suggestions in order to let patients do the work. *"What ideas do you have about how you could have handled those times differently when you did more [smoking, drinking]? What were you doing right when you did less [smoking, drinking]?"*

ACCOLADES

Ask patients to remember what it was that helped them make other successful changes in the past, and ask how those experiences might help them to change now. You can identify patients' strengths and praise them for their past successes to enhance their confidence to change: *"You clearly have the skills to change. But what would it take for you to keep using them?"*

TASK APPRAISALS

Task appraisals can help patients evaluate whether their goals are appropriate for them and what is a suitable timetable for taking steps toward change. For example, you can ask them, *"Is the goal you have chosen [to think about change, prepare for change or make a change] the best one for you at this time?"* or *"When would be a good time to work on your goals?"*

YOUR SUMMARY

Reflect: *write a summary about what you have learned that was new for you.*

_____
_____
_____
_____
_____
_____
_____
_____
_____
_____
_____
_____
_____
_____

_____
_____
_____
_____
_____
_____
_____
_____
_____

Enhance*: complete a self-assessment of your skills using the worksheet on page 322.* ***Write your goals below for improving specific skills*** *in role plays or patient encounters. After doing these practice sessions, reassess your competence score for these skills and make notes on page 322 to explain why you changed your scores. If possible, keep an audio recording or videotape of your practice sessions.*

_____
_____
_____
_____
_____
_____
_____
_____
_____

REFERENCES

1. U.S. Preventive Services Task Force. Guide to clinical preventive services: Report of the U.S. Preventive Services Task Force. 2nd ed. Baltimore, MD: Williams & Wilkins; 1996

2. Canadian Task Force on the Periodic Health Examination. The Canadian guide to clinical preventive health care. 1994. Ottawa, Minister of Supply and Services, Canada

3. Ellrodt G, Cook DJ, Lee J, et al. Evidence-based disease management. Journal of the American Medical Association1997;278: 1687-1692

4. De Shazer S. Keys to solutions in brief therapy. New York: W.W. Norton & Co.; 1985

5. De Shazer S. Clues: Investigating solutions in brief therapy. New York: W.W. Norton & Co.; 1988

6. De Shazer S. Words were originally magic. New York: W.W. Norton & Co.; 1994

7. Chandler M, Mason W. Solution-focused therapy: An alternative approach to addictions nursing. Perspectives in Psychiatric Care 1995; 31: 8-13

8. Berg I, DeJong P. Solution-building conversations: Co-constructing a sense of competence with clients. Families in Society: The Journal of Contemporary Human Services 1996; June: 376-391

9. Giorlando ME, Schilling RJ. On becoming a solution-focused physician: The MED-STAT acronym. Families, Systems & Health 1997;15: 361-373

CHAPTER 14
STEP 6: FOLLOWING THROUGH

FOR REFLECTION

How can you best arrange follow-up for your patients?
How can you help your patients ensure change and prevent relapse?

OVERVIEW

Appropriate follow-up arrangements can help you enhance the prospects of patients initiating and maintaining change and preventing or addressing relapse. You can best arrange such follow-ups by

- Providing a rationale, purpose and reasons for follow-up appointments
- Setting the timing, duration and frequency of follow-up appointments
- Using various methods to ensure change and prevent relapse

Patients who attend follow-up visits are more likely to change their behavior. The process and practice of how follow-up visits are made can affect the attendance or no-show rates. For example, physicians make follow-up visits more frequently when patients present for traditional biomedical problems, compared to health-promotion and disease prevention issues, independent of their patients' level of motivation. When physicians judged patients' motivation low for health-promotion and disease prevention issues, patients were four times more likely to be relegated to self-care.[1] To counteract this trend, you can provide an appropriate rationale for patients to make a follow-up appointment, such as a better understanding of why they lack motivation to change. Methods for negotiating follow-up appointments are described in Chapters 15, 16 and 17 for excessive alcohol intake, tobacco cessation and self-care of diabetes, respectively.

RATIONALE, PURPOSE AND REASONS FOR FOLLOW-UP

Although the rationale that you provide for making a follow-up appointment may not entirely reflect your purpose, the intent of such a rationale is to increase patients' commitment to a follow-up appointment. For example, you may suspect that a patient is dependent on alcohol and is damaging his liver. You decide to do a liver enzyme blood test. You provide the rationale that it is necessary to make a follow-up appointment in the near future to check up on his liver but do not explicitly disclose that you will also address the alcohol issue in more detail at the next appointment. This strategy can help when you suspect that your patient may disengage if you focus on his drinking problem when he does not want to address it.

After giving a rationale, you can check with patients to see whether they understand the need for ongoing care and clarify their understanding of the need for a follow-up. You can also encourage patients to write down any questions they may have and bring them to their next appointment.

TIMING, DURATION AND FREQUENCY OF FOLLOW-UP APPOINTMENTS

Traditionally, practitioners state when the follow-up appointment should occur. An alternative approach is to ask patients when they would like to come back. If you are unfamiliar with this option, you may be reluctant to try it for fear of making patients uncomfortable. However, this is an effective way to encourage patients to give their opinion about follow-up arrangements. Some patients are surprised by this approach and expect you to tell them when to return. You can tell these patients that you will share your opinion with them, but you are also interested in what they think. If patients make reasonable requests, you can simply accept their preference. If you have concerns about their preference, you can always negotiate about when to set a date for the next appointment.

METHODS TO ENSURE CHANGE AND PREVENT RELAPSE

Cognitive-behavioral approaches, relapse prevention and/or motivational reevaluation can help patients maintain their plan for change.

COGNITIVE-BEHAVIORAL APPROACHES

Cognitive-behavioral approaches may require patients to self-monitor their risk behavior with respect to the frequency and duration of the behavior—for example, recording blood glucose levels and/or the number of alcoholic drinks—as well as keeping a diary about their thoughts and feelings about change. Patients may also benefit by self-monitoring their progress toward their goal for change.

LAPSE AND RELAPSE PREVENTION

It is important that practitioners clarify to patients the distinction between a lapse and a relapse. A lapse means that a patient deviated temporarily from a prescribed or agreed-upon regimen and then resumed some degree of adherence. In a relapse, a patient maintained significant deviation from an adherence pattern.

Relapse prevention may involve patients addressing their temptations, urges and cravings about engaging in risk behavior. You can also ask patients to anticipate what they will do in high-risk situations when they are most likely to lapse or relapse by helping them develop plans for dealing with these situations. For example, failing to cope with stress and negative emotional states are common reasons for relapse. You can help patients think of alternative coping strategies and help them develop contingency plans and skills to deal with a possible lapse or relapse by creating a list of ways to cope with such high-risk situations.

You can also help patients identify any supports and/or barriers that may influence their adherence to their goals to change. Social and family support may either enhance maintenance or reduce the prospects of relapse; conversely, barriers may contribute to relapse or nonadherence. Patients can plan how to use these supports and also prepare themselves to overcome the barriers to change.

Patients may also wish to keep a list of the positive reasons for adherence and use those reasons as reinforcing mechanisms to maintain behavior change. They may also set up personally meaningful reward systems to maintain adherence.

If relapse prevention involves the use of drugs for treating withdrawal syndromes, you may need to monitor whether patients are using their medications appropriately to treat nicotine withdrawal symptoms, physical urges to drink and/or the medical complications of risk behaviors.

MOTIVATIONAL REEVALUATION

A significant fact about the relapse prevention approach that focuses on enhancing patient skills is that patients who relapse often have similar skills to those who maintain adherence. It is simply that relapsers do not use their skills at times of vulnerability. In other words, patients relapse not from lack of skills but from a lack of sustaining motivation. With such patients, you can ask them to review their decision balance and discuss how they can reduce their resistance and enhance their motivation to change. (In effect, this means that you have to do more work on Step 3 in Chapter 11).

YOUR SUMMARY

Reflect: write a summary about what you have learned that was new for you.

*Enhance: complete a self-assessment of your skills using the worksheet on page 323. **Write your goals below for improving specific skills** in role plays or patient encounters. After doing these practice sessions, reassess your competence score for these skills and make on page 323 to explain why you changed your scores. If possible, keep an audio recording or videotape of your practice sessions.*

_____

_____

_____

_____

_____

_____

_____

_____

_____

_____

REFERENCES

1. McArtor RE, Iverson DC, Benken DE, et al. Physician assessment of patient motivation: Influence on disposition for follow-up care. American Journal of Preventive Medicine 1992;8: 147-149

SECTION IV

SPECIFIC BEHAVIORS

Chapters 15, 16 and 17 address the subjects of excessive alcohol use, smoking, and self-care of chronic diseases respectively. Chapters 15-16 are broken down into two parts; part A discusses facts and issues specific to the particular behavior, while part B provides options for developing learning skills based on the six-step approach. Each chapter reinforces how you can adapt this approach to address other risk behaviors. Whatever your time limitations and the number of patient contacts, you can individualized these options to help motivate patients to change their risk behaviors.

KEY FINDINGS AND SPECIFIC ISSUES

Chapter 15 describes the notion of a risk continuum, the concept of harm reduction and the use of uncertainty to assess alcohol problems. Any reduction in risk and harm is worthwhile, particularly when patients cannot abstain and achieve the ideal goal. This problem is also relevant to other risk behaviors such as dietary adherence and weight reduction. Chapter 16 addresses the need to integrate behavioral interventions with treating nicotine dependence in order to decrease smoking rates. Combining behavioral counseling with medical treatments is also relevant to helping patients overcome other drug addictions. Chapter 17 addresses self-care of diabetes and the need for patients to juggle multiple agendas. This issue is also applicable to other patients who have multiple risk factors, whether or not they have a chronic disease.

DEVELOPING SKILLS

Chapters 15-17 provides a wealth of ideas and encourage you to use your clinical judgment in selecting interventions that will enhance your patients' readiness to change. If you provide continuity of care to patients, you will have multiple opportunities to intervene over time and to develop your professional skills. Your individualized approach can help patients

- Think more about change
- Reduce their resistance to change
- Enhance their motivation to change
- Prepare for change
- Take action to change

Some options are used more than others. For example, you may use the decision balance more frequently than explicitly clarifying your roles with your patients. The important point is to select and use whatever options seem to work for your individual patient.

CHAPTER 15 Part A

EXCESSIVE ALCOHOL USE

FOR REFLECTION

What is the alcohol risk-and-harm continuum?
How can you use diagnostic uncertainty to assess for alcohol abuse and dependency?

OVERVIEW

Brief interventions have been proven to have a positive effect on excessive alcohol intake. To understand the patterns of alcohol use, an alcohol risk-and-harm continuum lists them in descending order of severity, from alcohol dependence to abstinence. Both alcohol abuse and dependency can be classified from mild to moderate to severe. Definitions for each of these terms are provided in this chapter to assist you and your patients when negotiating about a diagnosis. When you are unable to make such a diagnosis, this chapter discusses how you can use diagnostic uncertainty to help patients assess their excessive use of alcohol.

KEY FACTS ABOUT EXCESSIVE ALCOHOL USE

Excessive alcohol use causes massive negative effects on society in health, social and economic consequences.[1;2] Primary care provides multiple opportunities for intervention,[3-9] and mounting evidence supports educating practitioners about using brief interventions with patients who have excessive alcohol intake.[10-14] The overall effect of brief interventions is estimated to be a 24% reduction in alcohol consumption (95% confidence interval, 18-31%).[10] Yet many practitioners remain unconvinced or skeptical about the benefits of these interventions.[15;16]

The majority of randomized studies have shown that patients receiving brief interventions have better outcomes than those in control groups with respect to reducing alcohol consumption, gamma glutamyl-transferase levels, absenteeism from work, alcohol-related problems, hospitalization days and/or mortality for excessive drinkers in hospital and primary care settings.[17-19;20-32] In a primary care study conducted by Wallace and colleagues, the study group that was given brief advice by general practitioners reported a 17.8% greater reduction in alcohol consumption compared with the control group.[23]

The results of this landmark British study were replicated in a U.S. study.[33] At the time of the 12-month follow-up, significant reductions were achieved in the intervention group, which received brief advice about reducing alcohol consumption, compared to routine care in the control group. The mean number of drinks in the previous weeks decreased from 19.1 to 11.5 for the intervention group versus 18.9 to 15.5 drinks per week for the control group. The control group had about a 20% reduction in their alcohol use, a finding that was similar to the Wallace et al. study.[23] This raises the issue of whether these changes came about because the control group members were encouraged by participating in lifestyle assessments or whether the changes represent a regression to the mean.

Another significant finding is that binge drinking was reduced in the intervention group from 5.7 to 3.1 episodes per month after one year versus 5.3 to 4.2 episodes per month after 12 months for the control group. (Binge drinking for women is defined as having more than four drinks on one occasion, for men, more than five drinks on one occasion.) Overall, physician advice reduced the alcohol consumption of patients by four drinks per week, and binge drinking by 1.5 episodes per month.

Men and women in the experimental group had a 14% and 31% reduction in alcohol consumption, respectively. With respect to health care utilizations, there was no difference in the number of emergency room visits between the experimental and control groups for either men or women. Men in the control group, however, experienced significantly more self-reported days in hospitals than those in the experimental group:

314 days versus 178 days. No difference was reported in the number of self-reported hospital days between the two groups for women. This raises the question of why a lower reduction in overall alcohol consumption resulted in fewer hospitalization days for men but not for women. One possible answer is that in this study, the average age was much higher for men than for women, indicating that age may certainly be a contributing factor.

It is important to note that the British and U.S. studies had different definitions of what is considered to be low-risk drinking. Furthermore, practitioners vary in what they regard as safe, low-risk social drinking.[34] For this reason, national advisory bodies have attempted to define what constitutes low-risk drinking. This issue has been and remains a source of debate. Controversy exists in terms of defining the cutoff for low-risk drinking limits because moderate amounts of alcohol (less than three drinks per day) are also associated with enhanced longevity, reduced cardiovascular mortality and reduced ischemic (but not hemorrhagic) stroke rate.[35-40] It is difficult to determine epidemiologically exactly where a significant increase in risk begins. As a consequence, countries vary in how they define low-risk drinking.[35]

Furthermore, these research studies excluded patients who were dependent on alcohol. Another challenge of applying the results of these studies to practice becomes how to deal with patients who, unknown to you, are dependent on alcohol.

SPECIFIC ISSUES

When addressing the subject of excessive alcohol use, a number of issues need to be examined to better understand patterns of alcohol use, the risks and harms of such use and the challenges you face when trying to make a diagnosis.

ALCOHOL RISK-AND-HARM CONTINUUM

The alcohol risk-and-harm continuum (the patterns of alcohol use) consists of abstinence, low-risk use, hazardous use, harmful (abuse) use of alcohol and alcohol dependence, each of which, excluding abstinence, is discussed below. The percentage of the population that suffers from alcohol abuse and dependence is approximately 15-20% and 5%, respectively. The percentage of the population that uses alcohol hazardously varies from country to country, depending on the definition of low-risk drinking and the abstinence rate. The patient's pattern of alcohol use itself can also change over time.

An important issue to consider is what level of prevention (primary, secondary or tertiary) would have the greatest impact on improving the health of the population. Although the health and economic impact of harmful and hazardous drinking (secondary prevention) greatly exceeds that resulting from alcohol dependency,[41] far greater resources are expended on treating alcohol dependency (tertiary prevention in specialist treatment facilities) than in addressing the harmful and hazardous use of alcohol (secondary prevention in primary care and hospital settings). This is despite the fact that secondary prevention approaches have a far greater potential for improving the health of the population at large than tertiary prevention.[42;43] In the U.S. general population, the implementation of safe drinking limits (secondary prevention) would result in an estimated 14.2% and 47.1% reduction in the prevalence of alcohol abuse and dependency, respectively.[44] To reverse the prevention paradox, health care organizations must systematically introduce secondary prevention programs into mainstream practice.[45;46;47;48] One way to achieve this is through a better understanding of the alcohol risk-and-harm continuum.

Low-risk Use

The U.S. National Institute of Alcohol Abuse and Alcoholism (NIAAA) initially recommended no more than two standard drinks (12 grams of pure alcohol per drink) per day for men and one standard drink per day for women.[49] More recently, they changed these recommendations in a physician's guide.[50] Men are at risk for alcohol-related problems if they drink more than 14 drinks in a week or more than 4 drinks on one occasion. Nonpregnant women are considered at risk if they drink more than seven drinks per week or more than three drinks on any one occasion.[50] Another guide for primary care clinicians also adopted these recommendations.[51]

The Alcohol Risk Assessment and Intervention Project, sponsored by the College of Family Physicians of Canada, also has developed guidelines for low-risk drinking.[52] According to their guidelines, men should not exceed four drinks and nonpregnant women should not exceed three drinks on any single day. No one should exceed 12 unit drinks (10 grams per drink) in a week.[53] In Britain, the Royal Colleges of General Practitioners, Psychiatrists, and Practitioners advised what they termed a "sensible" weekly limit of 21 small drinks (8 grams of pure alcohol per drink) for men and 14 for women.[54] More recently, a government publication from England raised the limits to 21 units for women and 28 units for men, despite objections from the medical profession.

As noted, marked variations exist internationally in terms of the amount of pure alcohol in a standard drink.[55] Furthermore, international differences exist with regard to alcohol use during pregnancy. In the United States, pregnant women are advised not to drink alcohol, whereas in England an occasional drink during pregnancy is not considered a significant risk.[56] Putting these controversial issues aside, the most important issue is for each country to define its own limit for low-risk drinking (see Table 15.1).

Table 15.1. Low-risk Drinking Recommendations

	Canada		United States		Britain/England	
Alcohol	Men	Women	Men	Women	Men	Women
Standard drinks/week	12	12	14	7	28	21
Grams/drink	10	10	12	12	8	8
Total grams per week	120	120	168	84	224	168

Hazardous Use

Hazardous use of alcohol is defined as drinking more than low-risk limits without evidence of harm or dependency. These patients are at increased risk for developing alcohol abuse and dependency, particularly if they increase their consumption over time.

Harmful Use (Abuse)

Harmful use of alcohol includes the diagnosis of alcohol abuse and is defined as drinking that causes any negative medical, psychological and/or social consequences. A NIAAA alcohol alert publication compared the *DSM-IV* and *ICD-10* classifications for alcohol abuse/harmful use (Table 15.2).

Table 15.2.

DSM-IV Alcohol Abuse (Harmful Use)
A. A maladaptive pattern of alcohol use leading to clinically significant impairment or distress, as manifested by one (or more) of the following occurring within a 12-month period: 1. Recurrent drinking resulting in a failure to fulfill major role obligations at work, school or home 2. Recurrent drinking in situations in which it is physically hazardous 3. Recurrent alcohol-related legal problems 4. Continued alcohol use despite having persistent or recurrent social or interpersonal problems caused or exacerbated by the effects of alcohol B. The symptoms have never met the criteria for alcohol dependence.
ICD-10 Harmful Use of Alcohol
A. A pattern of alcohol use that is causing damage to health. The damage may be physical or mental. The diagnosis requires that actual damage should have been caused to the mental or physical health of the user. B. No concurrent diagnosis of the alcohol dependence syndrome.

Dependency

The same NIAAA publication also compared *DSM-IV* and *ICD-10* classifications for alcohol dependency (see Table 15.3). You also can use the 25-item Alcohol Dependence Scale instrument to assess the severity of alcohol dependence quantitatively.[57]

Table 15.3. Definitions of Abuse and Dependence

	DSM-IV	*ICD-10*
Symptoms	A. A maladaptive pattern of alcohol use, leading to clinically significant impairment or distress, as manifested by three or more of the following occurring at any time in the same year:	A. Three or more of the following have been experienced or exhibited at some time during the previous year:
Tolerance	1. Need for markedly increased amounts of alcohol to achieve intoxication or desired effect; or markedly diminished effect with continued use of the same amount of alcohol	1. Evidence of tolerance, such that increased doses are required in order to achieve effects originally produced by lower doses
Withdrawal	2. The characteristic withdrawal syndrome for alcohol; or alcohol (or a closely related substance) is taken to relieve or avoid withdrawal symptoms	2. A physiological withdrawal state when drinking has ceased or been reduced, as evidenced by: the characteristic alcohol withdrawal syndrome, or use of alcohol (or a closely related substance) to relieve or avoid withdrawal symptoms
Impaired Control	3. Persistent desire or one or more unsuccessful efforts to cut down or control drinking 4. Drinking in larger amounts or over a longer period than the person intended	3. Difficulties in controlling drinking in terms of onset, termination, or levels of use
Neglect of Activities	5. Important social, occupational or recreational activities given up or reduced because of drinking	4. Progressive neglect of alternative pleasures or interests in favor of drinking; or
Time Spent Drinking	6. A great deal of time spent in activities necessary to obtain alcohol, to drink, or to recover from its effects	5. A great deal of time spent in activities necessary to obtain alcohol, to drink, or to recover from its effects
Drinking Despite Problems	7. Continued drinking despite knowledge of having a persistent or recurrent physical or physiological problem that is likely to be caused or exacerbated by alcohol use	6. Continued drinking despite clear evidence of overtly harmful physical or psychological consequences
Compulsive Use	None	7. A strong desire or sense of compulsion to drink
Duration Criterion	B. No duration criterion separately specified. However, three or more dependence criteria must be met within the same year and must occur repeatedly, as specified by duration qualifiers associated with criteria (e.g., "often," "persistent," "continued")	B. No duration criterion separately specified. However, three or more dependence criteria must be met during the previous year.
Criterion for Subtyping Dependence	With physiological dependence: Evidence of tolerance or withdrawal, i.e., any of items A(1) or A(2) above are present Without physiological dependence: No evidence of tolerance or withdrawal, i.e., none of items A(1) or A(2) above are present	None

RISK AND HARM REDUCTION

Risk and harm reduction refers to lowering the severity of excessive alcohol use for individuals and populations at large with any of the following goals: reduced alcohol intake, low-risk drinking or abstinence. This concept, which aims to reduce the overall percentage of patients who drink above low-risk limits, whatever their severity of excessive alcohol use, can be used to address many other risk behaviors. When it is not possible to achieve the ideal goal for change, you can use this concept to make an incremental reduction in risk and harm associated with any risk behavior.

THE CHALLENGE OF MAKING A DEFINITIVE DIAGNOSIS

In primary care and hospital settings, it is often difficult to conduct comprehensive assessments to make a definite diagnosis of alcohol abuse and/or dependence with confidence. One way is to make a diagnosis unilaterally, using a likelihood of at-risk and problem drinking scale ranging from unlikely to possible to probably to definitely (see Table 15.4).[58] Such a scale can help you track how your and your patient's perceptions of risk differ. The following example is of a patient, Mr. A.

Making Tentative and Definitive Diagnoses. Mr. A. attended his routine physical exam, where MP (motivational practitioner) took an alcohol and drug history. Mr. A. stated that he smoked about 15 cigarettes a day and drank 20 beers on weekends. His only complaint was heartburn and indigestion on the weekend. Although Mr. A. did not view his drinking behavior as a problem, MP was concerned about the probability of alcohol abuse and possible alcohol dependency. To get a better understanding of how he and Mr. A. differed in their perceptions of risk and problem drinking, MP filled out Table 15.4.

Commentary. Based on this partial assessment, MP established that the patient was definitely drinking above low-risk limits, even though Mr. A. did not view his drinking behavior as a health issue. This helped MP realize that his opinion differed from Mr. A's perspective.

Table 15.4. Differences in Perspective about At-risk and Problem Drinking

Likelihood of a Problem	At-risk Drinker (Hazardous use)	Problem Drinker	
		Abuse	Dependency
Definitely	Pr		
Probably		Pr	
Possibly			Pr
Unlikely	Pt	Pt	Pt

Pr = Practitioner's opinion   Pt = Practitioner's opinion of Mr. A's perspective

Even if you are certain of a diagnosis, it is often challenging to inform patients in ways they will accept. Rather than taking full responsibility for making the diagnosis, you can share this responsibility with patients in ways that enable them to take an active role in the process.

Using Uncertainty to Make the Diagnosis

Because of time constraints and diagnostic uncertainty, you may not always feel confident about diagnosing hazardous, harmful and/or dependent use of alcohol. You can, however, educate patients by using a likelihood scale (possibly, probably, definitely) about their possible alcohol use (see Table 15.5). This approach gives you the option of educating patients in a confident manner (using the word *definitely*) or in a tentative manner (using the word *possibly*) for a variety of diagnoses. This approach is an alternative strategy to making the diagnosis unilaterally *and* telling patients about it.

Table 15.5

Using the Likelihood Scale to Educate Patients about Their Alcohol Use
For hazardous drinking: *"I'm concerned that you are [possibly, probably, definitely] drinking above what are considered to be low-risk limits. What do you think?"* [Let the patient respond.]
For harmful drinking: *"I'm concerned that your health [possibly, probably, definitely] may be caused or made worse by alcohol. What do you think?"* [Let the patient respond.]
For alcohol dependence: *"I'm concerned that you are [possibly, probably, definitely] dependent upon alcohol [or have built up a tolerance to the effects of alcohol because . . .]. What do you think?"* [Let the patient respond.]

Using the likelihood scale, you can educate patients about the severity of at-risk (hazardous use) or problem drinking in a nonthreatening way. For example, "The amount you are drinking is definitely above low-risk limits. What I'm concerned about is that your alcohol is probably causing your high blood pressure, and you could possibly be dependent on alcohol without knowing it." It is often easier to reach a consensus with patients about at-risk drinking than it is to gain agreement about alcohol abuse and dependence. Some patients are truly surprised that they drink more than most of the population. They may doubt, resist and resent even a tentative diagnosis of alcohol abuse or dependence. Rather than arguing about the diagnosis, you can educate and help patients better understand how their drinking habit is affecting their health. Alternatively, you can show patients and their families the diagnostic criteria of abuse and dependency and let them deal with the discrepancy between their opinion and professional opinion.

Dealing with diagnostic uncertainty: After doing a partial assessment, MP thought that Mr. A. definitely drank above low-risk limits, probably was abusing alcohol and possibly was dependent on alcohol; he also felt that Mr. A. would deny any of these diagnostic possibilities. MP first educated Mr. A. about low-risk drinking limits, shared his definitive diagnosis (hazardous use of alcohol) with Mr. A., and then asked Mr. A. what he thought about it. Mr. A. was surprised by this information because many of his friends drank even more than he did. MP explained that both Mr. A.'s and his friends' drinking habits were well above average. Mr. A. listened to his practitioner's reasons for raising the issue of low-risk drinking and agreed that he probably drank too much, given the definition of low-risk drinking (i.e., 14 standard drinks per week and no more than 4 drinks on any one occasion). Mr. A. was also willing to accept that alcohol was possibly making his indigestion and heartburn worse. Since MP did not yet have sufficient information to justify his concerns about the possibility of alcohol dependency, he did not raise this issue at this appointment. However, MP did establish more of a common understanding with Mr. A. about hazardous and harmful use of alcohol.

Commentary: By using the likelihood scale to discuss Mr. A.'s excessive drinking, MP was able to track how Mr. A. shifted in his understanding about the severity of at-risk and problem drinking (see Table 15.6). You can use this table as well to track the extent to which you and your patients share similar perceptions about the likelihood for at-risk and problem drinking.

**Table 15.6. Enhancing Mutual Understanding about
At-risk and Problem Drinking**

Likelihood of a Problem	At-risk Drinker Hazardous Use	Problem Drinker	
		Abuse	Dependency
Definitely			
Probably	C		
Possibly		C	*Pr*
Unlikely			*Pt*

C = Common agreement between practitioner and patient
Pr = Practitioner's opinion
Pt = Patient's opinion

If you work too quickly, however, or are too forceful, some patients will resist accepting your educational message. To avoid such resistance, you can use an indirect approach that involves patients in a process of negotiating a common understanding about the diagnosis before moving on to the issue of alcohol dependency. For example, "Your drinking is above low-risk limits, and there is a possibility that it could be causing your high blood pressure." You can then invite the patient to do a trial of abstinence to see if blood pressure goes down, and assess for any withdrawal symptoms before addressing the topic of alcohol dependence. As is described in Part 15B, you can even show patients the criteria for the diagnosis and invite them to give their opinion about how these criteria relate to them.

YOUR SUMMARY

Reflect: write a summary about what you have learned that was new for you.

_____
_____
_____
_____
_____
_____
_____
_____
_____
_____
_____

_____
_____
_____
_____
_____
_____
_____
_____
_____
_____
_____

Enhance*: write down your ideas about how your new learning could improve your interactions with patients. Add your notes to your learning portfolio.*

_____
_____
_____
_____
_____
_____
_____
_____
_____
_____
_____
_____

REFERENCES

1. Pirmohamed M, Gilmore IT. Alcohol abuse and the burden on the NHS: Time for action. Journal of the Royal College of Physicians 2000;34: 161-162
2. Secretary of Health and Human Services. Eighth Special Report to the U.S. Congress on Alcohol and Health. 1993. Arlington, VA, Dept. of Health and Human Services.
3. Buchsbaum DG, Buchanan RG, Lawton MJ, et al. Alcohol consumption patterns in a primary care population. Alcohol and Alcoholism 1991;26: 215-220
4. Magruder-Habib K, Durand AM, Frey KA. Alcohol abuse and alcoholism in primary health care settings. Journal of Family Practice 1991;32: 406-413
5. Leckman AL, Umland BE, Blay M. Prevalence of alcoholism in a family practice center. Journal of Family Practice 1984;18: 867-870
6. Hill A, Rumpf HJ, Hapke U, et al. Prevalence of alcohol dependence and abuse in general practice. Alcoholism, Clinical and Experimental Research. 1998;22: 935-940 ****
7. Burge SK, Schneider FD. Alcohol-related problems: Recognition and intervention. American Family Physician 1999;59: 361-70, 372

8. Buchsbaum DG, Buchanan RG, Poses RM, et al. Physician detection of drinking problems in patients attending a general medicine practice. Journal of General Internal Medicine 1992;7: 517-521

9. Cleary PD, Miller M, Bush BT, et al. Prevalence and recognition of alcohol abuse in a primary care population. American Journal of Medicine 1988;85: 466-471

10. Nuffield Institute for Health, University of Leeds, Centre for Health Economics, University of York, Research Unit, and Royal College of Physicians. Effective health care: Brief interventions and alcohol use. The Department of Health 7; 1993

11. Bien TH, Miller WR, Tonigan JS. Brief interventions for alcohol problems: A review. Addiction 1993;88(3): 315-335

12. Kahan M, Wilson L, Becker L. Effectiveness of physician-based interventions with problem drinkers: A review. Canadian Medical Association Journal 1995;152(6): 851-859

13. McAvoy BR. Alcohol education for general practitioners in the United Kingdom. Alcohol and Alcoholism 2000;35: 225-229

14. Wallace P. Patients with alcohol problems: Simple questioning is the key to effective identification and management (Editorial). British Journal of General Practice 2001;51: 172-173

15. Lawlor DA, Keen S, Neal RD. Can general practitioners influence the nation's health through a population approach to provision of lifestyle advice? British Journal of General Practice 2000;50: 455-459

16. Deehan A, Marshall EJ, Strang J. Tackling alcohol misuse: Opportunities and obstacles in primary care. British Journal of General Practice 1998;48: 1779-1782

17. Kristenson H, Ohlin H, Hultën-Nosslin MB, et al. Identification and intervention of heavy drinking in middle-aged men: Results and follow-up of 24-60 months of long-term study with randomized controls. Alcoholism: Clinical and Experimental Research 1983;7: 203-209

18. Anderson P. Effectiveness of general practice interventions for patients with harmful alcohol consumption. British Journal of General Practice 1993;43: 386-389

19. Anderson P, Scott E. The effect of general practitioners' advice to heavy drinking men. British Journal of Addiction 1992;87: 891-900

20. Walsh DC, Hingson RW, Merrigan DM, et al. A randomized trial of treatment options for alcohol-abusing workers. New England Journal of Medicine 1991;325: 775-782

21. Persson J, Magnusson PH. Prevalence of excessive or problem drinkers among patients attending somatic outpatient clinics: A study of alcohol related medical care. British Medical Journal—Clinical Research 1987;295: 467-472

22. Persson J, Magnusson PH. Sickness, absenteeism and mortality in patients with excessive drinking in somatic out-patient care. Scandinavian Journal of Primary Health Care 1989;7: 211-217

23. Wallace P, Cutler S, Haines A. Randomized controlled trial of general practitioner intervention in patients with excessive alcohol consumption. British Medical Journal 1988;297: 663-668

24. Babor TF, Grant M. WHO Collaborating Investigators Project on identification and management of alcohol-related problems. Combined analyses of outcome data: The cross-national generalizability of brief interventions. Report on phase II: A randomized clinical trial of brief interventions in primary health care. Copenhagen: WHO; 1992

25. Magruder-Habib K, Durand AM, Frey KA. Alcohol abuse and alcoholism in primary health care settings. Journal of Family Practice 1991;32: 406-413

26. Heather N, Rollnick S, Bell A, et al. Effects of brief counselling among male heavy drinkers identified on general hospital wards. Drug and Alcohol Review 1996;15: 29-38

27. Anderson P, Scott E. The effect of general practitioners' advice to heavy drinking men. British Journal of Addiction 1992;87: 891-900

28. Romelsjo A, Andersson L, Barrner H, et al. A randomized study of secondary prevention of early stage problem drinkers in primary health care. British Journal of Addiction 1989;84: 1319-1327

29. Cowan PF. An intervention to improve the assessment of alcoholism by practicing physicians. Family Practice Research Journal 1994;14: 41-49

30. Chick J, Lloyd G, Crombie E. Counselling problem drinkers in medical wards: A controlled study. British Medical Journal—Clinical Research 1985;290: 965-967

31. Maheswaran R, Beevers M, Beevers DG. Effectiveness of advice to reduce alcohol consumption in hypertensive patients. Hypertension 1992;19(1): 79-84

32. WHO Brief Intervention Study Group. A cross-national trial of brief interventions with heavy drinkers. American Journal of Public Health 1996;86: 948-955

33. Fleming MF, Barry KL, Manwell LB, et al. Brief physician advice for problem alcohol drinkers: A randomized controlled trial in community-based primary care practices. Journal of the American Medical Association 1997;277: 1039-1045

34. Wallace P, Cremona A, Anderson P. Safe limits of drinking: General practitioners' views. British Medical Journal—Clinical Research 1985;290(6485): 1875-1876

35. Klatsky AL. Annotation: Alcohol and longevity. American Journal of Public Health 1995;85: 16-18

36. Pearson TA, Terry P. What to advise patients about drinking alcohol. Journal of the American Medical Association 1994;272: 957-958

37. Donahue RP, Abbott RD. Alcohol and haemorrhagic stroke [letter]. Lancet 1986;2: 515-516

38. Stampfer MJ, Colditz GA, Willett WC, et al. A prospective study of moderate alcohol consumption and the risk of coronary disease and stroke in women. New England Journal of Medicine 1988;319: 267-273

39. Klatsky AL, Armstrong MA, Friedman GD. Alcohol and stroke. Journal of the American College of Cardiology 1987;9: 78A

40. Tanaka H, Ueda Y, Hayashi M, et al. Risk factors for cerebral hemorrhage and cerebral infarction in a Japanese rural community. Stroke 1982;13: 62-73

41. Institute of Medicine. Broadening the base of treatment for alcohol problems. Washington, DC: National Academy Press; 1990

42. Skinner HA. Spectrum of drinkers and intervention opportunities. Canadian Medical Association Journal 1990;143: 1054-1059

43. Cahalan D. Problem drinkers: A national survey. San Francisco: Jossey-Bass; 1970

44. Archer L, Grant BF, Dawson DA. What if Americans drank less? The potential effect on the prevalence of alcohol abuse and dependence. American Journal of Public Health 1995;85: 61-66

45. Kreitman N. Alcohol consumption and the preventive paradox. British Journal of Addiction 1986;81: 353-363

46. Rose G. Sick individuals and sick populations. International Journal of Epidemiology 1985;14(1): 32-38

47. Kendell RE. The physician's role. Canadian Medical Association Journal 1990;143: 1042-1047

48. Anderson P. Management of alcohol problems: The role of the general practitioner. Alcohol & Alcoholism 1993;28(3): 263-272

49. U.S. Department of Health & Human Services. Moderate drinking. Alcohol Alert: National Institute on Alcohol Abuse and Alcoholism 1992;16(PH315): 1-4

50. National Institute on Alcohol Abuse and Alcoholism. Fourth Special Report to the U.S. Congress on Alcohol and Health. U.S. Department of Health and Human Services. 1981.

51. Center for Substance Abuse Treatment. A guide to substance abuse services for primary care clinicians. No. 24. Treatment Improvement Protocol (TIP) Series. 1997. Substance Abuse and Mental Health Services Administration.

52. Peters C, Wilson D, Bruneau A, et al. Alcohol risk assessment and intervention for family physicians. Canadian Family Physician 1996;42: 681-689

53. Sanchez-Craig M, Wilkinson DA, Davila R. How much is too much? Further evaluation of empirically-based guidelines for moderate drinking: One-year results of three studies with male and female problem drinkers. Toronto: Addiction Research Foundation; 1994

54. Lord President's report on action against alcohol misuse. London, England: Her Majesty's Stationery Office; 1991

55. Miller WR, Heather N, Hall W. Calculating standard drink units: International comparisons. British Journal of Addiction 1991;86(1): 43-47

56. Knupfer G. Abstaining for foetal health: The fiction that even light drinking is dangerous. British Journal of Addiction 1991;86: 1063-1073

57. Ross HE, Gavin DR, Skinner HA. Diagnostic validity of the MAST and the alcohol dependence scale in the assessment of DSM-III alcohol disorders. Journal of Studies on Alcohol 1990;51: 506-513

58. Botelho RJ, Novak S. Dealing with substance misuse, abuse and dependency. Primary Care 1993;20: 51-70

CHAPTER 15 Part B

REDUCING ALCOHOL RISK AND HARM

FOR REFLECTION

How do you deal with patients who do not respond to your advice to keep below the low-risk drinking limit or to abstain from alcohol use?

OVERVIEW

About 20% of patients who drink excessive amounts of alcohol will respond to health education and advice to reduce alcohol consumption to below low-risk limits. Even when patients have alcohol-related complications, however, they will not respond to your advice to change. Furthermore, many patients are dependent on alcohol without your knowing about it. This section helps you learn how to deal with the full spectrum of resistant patients who have a hazardous, harmful and dependent use of alcohol; it can also help you work with patients who drink and drive, request sedative drugs and/or provide rationalizations to avoid dealing with their excessive alcohol use.

To learn new skills, first work with patients who drink above low-risk limits or have alcohol-related problems. After you have developed some skills, you can learn how to deal with patients with alcohol dependence.

STEP 1: BUILDING PARTNERSHIPS

You can build your partnership with patients throughout the problem-solving process. For example, you can use the decision balance in ways that strengthen your partnership with patients and thereby enhance the prospects of facilitating change.

DEVELOP EMPATHY

You can use a variety of communication skills to develop empathy with patients. Practitioners who develop higher levels of empathy with patients, even at the first encounter, are more successful in helping patients reduce their alcohol intake. [1-4]

Communication Skills for Developing Empathy	
Use open-ended questions	*"So, what is your favorite drink?"*
Use reflective listening	*"So, alcohol helps you relax and deal with your fears."*
Paraphrase	*"You have difficulty understanding where those fears come from."*
Validate feelings	*"These fears are overwhelming and make life difficult for you."*
Normalize behaviors	*"It's normal to have fears and want them to go away."*
Affirm strengths	*"It takes courage to understand and come to terms with those fears."*
Use probing questions	*"When do those fears occur? What do you fear from your past? What fears do you have now and for the future?"*

USE RELATIONAL SKILLS EFFECTIVELY

At any problem-solving step, you can take the one-down position with the patient or put the patient in a one-up position. For example, you can use these relational skills during Step 4 (enhancing mutual understanding) when patients resist the notion that they drink excessively.

Putting the Patient in the One-up Position
"What convinces you that you do not have an alcohol problem?"
"How would you know if you had an alcohol problem?"
"What would convince you about the need to keep to low-risk drinking?"
Taking the One-down Position with a Patient
"I'm not sure what it would take for you to think that you may have an alcohol problem?"
"What would convince you to keep to below low-risk drinking limits?"

CLARIFY ROLES AND RESPONSIBILITIES

More often than not, you and your patients assume roles and responsibilities without any explicit negotiation. The option of explicitly clarifying your roles and responsibilities with your patients is appropriate before the agenda-setting step, but you can use this option at any time, particularly when patient resistance occurs.

Clarifying Your Roles
Clarify your prevention role: *"Alcohol can damage your health before you get any symptoms. Can we do some blood tests to check if alcohol is damaging your liver?"*   Motivational role (treating alcohol abuse): *"I can treat your [alcohol-related problem], but you're not sure if you should stop drinking. Can we take some time to talk about this?"*
Clarifying Responsibility
"I'll tell you about how alcohol affects your health, but I suspect that we see the benefits and harms of your alcohol use differently. Let's talk about this before you decide whether to change or not."

STEP 2: NEGOTIATING AN AGENDA

You can either use a prevention-focused or problem-focused approach to negotiate an agenda with patients about assessing their pattern of alcohol use. After gathering sufficient information to suspect hazardous, harmful or dependent use of alcohol, you can proceed to conduct an assessment.

PREVENTION-FOCUSED APPROACH

The following options can help you identify at-risk patients or hazardous drinkers who do not have any alcohol-related problems.

Use Direct Questions about Alcohol and Drug Use

Direct questions (closed-ended or open-ended) represent the traditional way of obtaining a history of substance abuse (see examples below) When asked direct questions, some patients show signs of resistance. This cue may increase your suspicion of an underlying drinking problem. Sometimes attempts to quantify alcohol consumption make patients less likely to cooperate. In such circumstances, you may choose not to pursue an accurate alcohol history but instead opt for leading or screening questions and/or conducting an assessment.

Consent-gaining Direct Questions
About health: *"What kinds of alcohol do you drink? Beer, wine, hard liquor?" "How many drinks do you have in a week?" "What size drinks do you usually have?" "How much beer, wine or hard liquor do you buy in a week?"*

Use Leading Questions

As some drinkers are vague in quantifying their alcohol use, leading questions may help you obtain a more accurate history. These questions assume that people enjoy drinking alcohol.

Using leading questions to detect excessive alcohol use: Mr. A., age 85, was admitted to the emergency room with chest pains. He disclosed to the emergency room physician that he smoked three packs of cigarettes a day and drank one beer a day. He was diagnosed as having unstable angina with electrocardiogram changes suggestive of an evolving myocardial infarction. After Mr. A. was given thrombolytic therapy, his attending physician visited him in the emergency room to assess his risk for alcohol withdrawal syndrome because his family stated that he drank a lot. He asked Mr. A., "What is your favorite beer?" Mr. A. smiled and mentioned the brand name of an inexpensive beer. The attending physician continued, "How many beers a day do you like to drink?" "Oh, maybe five or six beers a day," replied the patient.

Leading Open-ended Questions
"So, what kinds of alcohol do you like to drink?"
"What are your favorite drinks?"
"What do you like to drink when you go out to a party?"

Administer Screening Questionnaires

The CAGE questionnaire (see Table 15.7) is the briefest instrument for detecting past and present alcohol abuse and/or dependence but is not appropriate for detecting hazardous use of alcohol.[5;6] If you have not used the CAGE questionnaire before, you may feel awkward using it with patients. Prefacing statements can help to reduce your feeling of awkwardness and prepare patients for these questions: for example, "I would like to ask you a few questions about how alcohol is affecting your health. Is that okay?" Alternatively, you can intersperse these questions during your conversations with patients rather than ask them in a sequential manner.

The sensitivity of the CAGE questionnaire ranges from 49-89% and specificity from 79-95%.[7-11] Therefore, a negative response on this questionnaire will still miss many patients who have a problem of harmful use of alcohol, as well as the majority of patients who have a hazardous use of alcohol. Patients with a negative screen on the CAGE questionnaire may still require an assessment if they present with complaints that may be associated with alcohol use or if they drink more than the low-risk drinking limit.

Table 15.7.

CAGE Questionnaire	
C	*"Have you ever felt you should **C**ut down on your drinking?"*
A	*"Has anyone **A**nnoyed you by criticizing your drinking?"*
G	*"Have you ever felt bad or **G**uilty about your drinking?"*
E	*"Have you ever had a drink (an **E**ye-opener) first thing in the morning to steady your nerves or to get rid of a hangover?"*

Decision rule: Two or more positive responses indicates alcohol abuse or dependence. One positive response warrants further assessment.

Another screening instrument is the 10-item AUDIT questionnaire (see Table 15.8) developed by the World Health Organization Early Intervention Project for use in primary care.[12-16] This instrument has an advantage over the CAGE questionnaire in that you can identify both hazardous and problem drinkers (alcohol abuse and dependence).

Table 15.8. AUDIT Questionnaire

Please check the answer to each question that is correct for you:				
1. How often do you have a drink containing alcohol?				
❏ Never	❏ Monthly or less	❏ Two to four times a month	❏ Two to three times a week	❏ Four or more times a week
2. How many drinks containing alcohol do you have on a typical day when you are drinking?				
❏ 1 or 2	❏ 3 or 4	❏ 5 or 6	❏ 7 to 9	❏ 10 or more
3. How often do you have six or more drinks on one occasion?				
❏ Never	❏ Less than monthly	❏ Monthly	❏ Weekly	❏ Daily or almost daily
4. How often during the last year have you found that you were not able to stop drinking once you had started?				
❏ Never	❏ Less than monthly	❏ Monthly	❏ Weekly	❏ Daily or almost daily
5. How often during the last year have you failed to do what was normally expected from you because of drinking?				
❏ Never	❏ Less than monthly	❏ Monthly	❏ Weekly	❏ Daily or almost daily
6. How often during the last year have you needed a first drink in the morning to get yourself going after a heavy drinking session?				
❏ Never	❏ Less than monthly	❏ Monthly	❏ Weekly	❏ Daily or almost daily
7. How often during the last year have you had a feeling of guilt or remorse after drinking?				
❏ Never	❏ Less than monthly	❏ Monthly	❏ Weekly	❏ Daily or almost daily
8. How often during the last year have you been unable to remember what happened the night before because you had been drinking?				
❏ Never	❏ Less than monthly	❏ Monthly	❏ Weekly	❏ Daily or almost daily
9. Have you or someone else been injured as a result of your drinking?				
❏ No	❏ Yes, but not in the last year		❏ Yes, during the last year	
10.Has a relative, friend, doctor or other health worker been concerned about your drinking or suggested you cut down?				
❏ No	❏ Yes, but not in the last year		❏ Yes, during the last year	

Questions 1-8 are scored 0-4 points, and questions 9-10 are scored 0, 2 or 4 points, giving a possible range of 0-40 points.

Patients can complete the AUDIT instrument themselves; given its length, it is unlikely to be used commonly during routine patient encounters. The AUDIT-C (consumption) instrument has been developed. This shortened version consists of the first three questions listed above, giving a possible range score of 0-12.[15] Another instrument, the Five-shot Questionnaire (see Table 15.9), has been developed to meet the need for brevity.[17]

Table 15.9. Five-shot Questionnaire

Please check the answer to each question that is correct for you:				
1. How often do you have a drink containing alcohol?				
❏ Never	❏ Monthly or less	❏ Two to four times a month	❏ Two to three times a week	❏ Four or more times a week
2. How many drinks containing alcohol do you have on a typical day when you are drinking?				
❏ 1 or 2	❏ 3 or 4	❏ 5 or 6	❏ 7 to 9	❏ 10 or more
3. Have people annoyed you by criticizing your drinking?			❏ No	❏ Yes
4. Have you ever felt bad or guilty about your drinking?			❏ No	❏ Yes
5. Have you ever had a drink first thing in the morning to steady your nerves or to get rid of a hangover?			❏ No	❏ Yes

Questions 1 and 2 are scored 0-0.5-1.0-1.5-2.0 points, and questions 3-5 are scored 0-1, giving a possible range of 0-7 points.

A study compared the screening properties of these instruments for detecting alcohol abuse or dependence in general practice (see Table 15.10).[18] The AUDIT-C and Five-shot questionnaires both performed well in terms of sensitivity and specificity for men. In women, the Five-shot Questionnaire has superior sensitivity rates over the AUDIT-C, but the reverse was true for specificity.

Table 15.10. Performance of Screening Tests in General Practice

Screening Test	Males		Females	
	Sensitivity	Specificity	Sensitivity	Specificity
CAGE 2 or >	47.7	92.3	37	96.8
AUDIT 5 or >	82.6	72.9	65.2	91.9
6 or >	74.2	81.4	58.7	95.9
8 or >	60.6	90.3	50.0	98.7
AUDIT-C 5 or >	78.0	74.9	50.0	93.2
6 or >	66.7	84.3	39.1	97.3
8 or >	48.5	94.3	21.7	99.6
Five-shot 2 or >	86.4	63.6	67.4	87.4
2.5 or >	74.2	80.9	63.0	94.7
3.0 or >	62.1	88.3	37.0	97.3

Other attempts have also been made to identify one or two screening questions instead of using questionnaires.[19-21] Based on the National Health Interview Survey, self-report of five or more drinks on one occasion over the past year had a sensitivity and specificity of 0.90/0.53 in men and 0.77/0.77 in women for alcohol abuse and dependence.[22;23] This question (modified to five or more drinks in the last three months) had a sensitivity of 62% and a specificity of 93% in primary care.[21] A positive result tripled the probability of problem drinking from 25% prevalence to a post-test probability of 74%, while a negative test reduced this probability from 25-12%.

Take a Family History

The purpose of taking a family history for alcohol and drug problems is to identify and help high-risk patients as well as family members. Patients who come from families with a history of substance abuse are at increased risk of developing alcohol and drug problems. Family, twin, half-sibling and adoption studies of alcoholic subjects suggest that the risk of inheritance of alcoholism is at least 50%.[24] The questions below can identify other family members who have drug or alcohol problems. For those patients whose family members have current alcohol or drug problems, you can encourage their relatives to seek professional help as well.

Screening for Alcohol and Drug Problems in the Family
"Has anyone in your family had alcohol or drug problems in the past?"   *"Do you think anyone in your family has an alcohol or drug problem now?"*   *"Can they drink more alcohol than most people and not get drunk?"*

PROBLEM-FOCUSED APPROACH

Even if the outcome of the CAGE screening is negative, the following complaints are cues to possible alcohol related-problems:

- *Medical:* Injuries, gastrointestinal symptoms (dyspepsia, peptic ulcer, diarrhea), high blood pressure, minor and major accidents, chronic fatigue, headaches, back pain/chronic pain
- *Psychological:* Sleep problems, anxiety, depression, relationship difficulties, sexual problems
- *Social:* Poor work performance, poor school performance, missing work, loss of jobs, family problems, financial problems
- *Legal:* Driving while impaired or intoxicated; debts

Prefacing statements and exploratory questions help you to explore how patients view the association between their presenting problems and alcohol use.

Prefacing Statements

Prefacing statements link the use of alcohol to patients' presenting complaints in ways that provide a rationale for taking an alcohol history, administering the CAGE questionnaire or conducting an assessment.

Prefacing Statements
Normalizing and validating comments: *"Many people find that drinking alcohol helps them get to sleep. Is that how it is for you? Let me explain how alcohol causes poor sleep even though it helps you to get off to sleep."*
Comments that focus on concerns about the consequences: *"Some people find that drinking alcohol makes their stomach pain worse. Has that happened to you?" "Did you know that alcohol can cause high blood pressure?"*

Use Exploratory Questions

Exploratory questions help you engage patients in assessing how their health problems relate to their alcohol use. They include closed-ended linear questions, open-ended linear questions, rephrasing prefacing statements as questions and circular questions.

Exploratory Questions
Closed-ended linear questions: *Has your stomach problem affected how much you drink?"* *"Has drinking alcohol made your depression (or stomach) feel better or worse?"* Open-ended linear questions: *"How has your drinking affected your health?* *"In what ways has your drinking affected your depression?"* Rephrase prefacing statements as questions: *"How does drinking alcohol affect your sleep?"* *"How is your sleeping problem affected by your use of alcohol?"* Circular questions: *"What concerns your family (spouse or children) about how your drinking affects your health?"*

STEP 3: ASSESSING RESISTANCE AND MOTIVATION

Depending on your patient's responses to negotiating an agenda, you can choose from an array of options to conduct motivational and disease-centered assessments. The distinctions between these assessments highlight some of the ways in which specialists and generalists deal with alcohol-related problems (see Table 15.11). Patients who have a high probability of severe alcohol problems are often referred to specialists, who then conduct lengthy assessments and work with patients intensively for a limited period of time. Specialists diagnose a variety of medical, psychological and social problems, and develop an appropriate management plan. In contrast, generalists encounter patients who may be anywhere along the risk-and-harm continuum. They are often uncertain about the underlying severity of a patient's alcohol problem. A definitive diagnosis may take time.

Table 15.11. Comparing Specialist and Generalist Assessments

Addiction Specialists	Practitioners
Referred patients	Case-finding
Standardized questionnaires and structured interviews	Individualized interviews using brief assessments
Organized, intensive program provided episodically in times of greatest need	Continuity of care provided in context of comprehensive, coordinated care
Linear, medical, or psychiatric assessments	Circular, behavioral assessments
Time-limited (hours)	Brief and recurrent (minutes)
Make a diagnosis & educate patients about it	Negotiate about a diagnosis

MOTIVATIONAL ASSESSMENT

To conduct a motivational assessment, you may use any of the following options: decision balance, readiness to initiate change, motivational reasons for change, energy to change, self-efficacy and supports and barriers. As part of this process, you may also uncover psychiatric and psychological problems (anxiety disorders, depression, emotional disorders, suicidal ideation and intentions and relationship problems), social problems (financial and work issues), legal problems (drinking while intoxicated) and medical problems (indigestion caused by alcohol).

Ask about Readiness to Change

Before using a decision balance, ask about the patient's readiness to change. The patient's response will help you decide whether to provide a stage-specific rationale. Furthermore, you can repeat questions about readiness to change to monitor a patient's progress over time.

Readiness to Change—Direct Questions
"Where are you in terms of dealing with cutting down to low-risk drinking [or quitting]?" (Select one of the following questions according to your impression of the patient.) *"Aren't you interested in changing your drinking habit?"* *"Are you thinking about low-risk drinking or quitting?"* *"Are you willing to keep to low-risk drinking or stop drinking?"*
Readiness to Change—Indirect Questions
Consider any of the following: *"What concerns would you have if you were to cut down below the low-risk drinking limit?" "Do you think that you will ever cut down or quit drinking?"*

Use a Decision Balance with the Patient

A stage-specific rationale helps patients understand why you are using the decision balance, particularly for those patients who are in precontemplation and in contemplation; first provide an appropriate rationale, and then show the patient what a decision balance looks like.

Providing Stage-specific Rationale and Gain Consent to Use the Decision Balance
Precontemplation: *"Alcohol may be making your stomach problem feel worse. Can we use a decision balance so I could understand more about why you like to drink?"*
Contemplation: *"You told me that you are thinking about reducing how much you drink. Can we use a decision balance to help you think more about whether to reduce your alcohol intake to below low-risk drinking limits [or abstain]?"*
Preparation: *"You think you will change soon. Can we use a decision balance to help you set a date to change?"*
Action: *"You are ready to set a date to change. Can we use a decision balance to help you prevent a relapse once you cut down or stop drinking?"*

Showing the Decision Balance to the Patient
"Let me show you what a decision balance looks like. As we use the decision balance, it can help you understand better your reasons to stay the same and your reasons to consider change. But first [pointing to the right column], what you do you like about drinking alcohol? I would like to make a note of what you say. Is that okay? You can keep this decision balance to use when you go home, if you like."

After gaining the patient's cooperation in doing this task, you can ask one or more questions from each quadrant, preferably in the sequence suggested in the table below, or alter it to adapt to the patient's needs.

	Decision Balance	
Risk behavior	*1. Benefits* *"What do you like about drinking alcohol?"*	*2. Concerns* *"Do you have any concerns about how alcohol affects your life?"* *"What concerns do you have about how alcohol affects your family or work?"*
Reducing risk/harm	*3. Concerns* *"What concerns would you have if you were to keep to low-risk drinking limits (or abstain)?"* *"In what way would your life be different if you were to quit for two weeks or longer?"*	*4. Benefits* *"In what ways would your health be better if you were to stop drinking or cut down?"* *"In what ways would other aspects of your life be better if you were to stop drinking or cut down?"*

After completing the decision balance (see below), give a copy with the responses to the patient and keep a copy of it in the patient's records. Alternatively, you can ask patients to complete this task in the waiting room or as a homework assignment for the next visit, perhaps with the input of a family member. At follow-up appointments, you can refer to the decision balance with the patient.

Exploring change	Reasons to drink (Cons)	Reasons to change (Pros)
Excess Alcohol Use	*1. Benefits* *Enjoy drinking with my buddies* *Makes me feel relaxed* *Relieves stress* *Helps relieve back pain*	*2. Concerns* *Hangovers* *Spouse nags me* *High blood pressure* *Occasional stomachache*
Low-Risk Drinking or Abstinence	*3. Concerns* *Miss my friends* *No fun* *Back-pain aggravation*	*4. Benefits* *Reduced risk of hypertension* *Spouse will be happy* *Less stomach upset*
Force of change	*Resistance score =* *Think score = 5 Feel score = 8*	*Motivation score =* *Think score = 5 Feel score = 2*

The reason for inquiring about the benefits and concerns is to help patients think about factors that affect their resistance and motivation to change: in other words, their force of change toward disease or health. By working from the patients' perspective, you can enhance their cooperation to explore how alcohol is affecting their health, family, work and other aspects of their life.

Once you have completed the decision balance, you can ask patients to score how important their reasons are to stay the same (resistance score) and to change (motivation score), using the questions below. Then patients can monitor how their resistance and motivation scores change over time.

Explaining and Obtaining Resistance and Motivation Scores
"The left column represents your reasons to drink (resistance). The right column represents your reasons to cut down or quit drinking (motivation). On a scale of 0–10, 0 meaning none and 10 meaning very high, what score would you give for your reasons to stay the same? [pointing to the left column] *And what score would you give for your reasons to change? Are your resistance and motivation scores based on what you think or feel about change? Now how would you score your resistance and motivation based on what you feel* [if a think score was given] *or think* [if a feeling score was given]*?"*

Decision balances can help patients think more about the possibility of change and clarify their ambivalence about change. The initial intent of using the decision balance is to itemize the benefits and concerns about drinking as usual versus low-risk drinking (or abstinence), without implying that patients should change. This approach can give you an insight into the reasons patients drink alcohol in spite of the associated risks and harms. The process itself is usually insufficient to initiate actual change in patients; it is only a first step in motivating them.

Use a Decision Balance with Family Members

If family members accompany the patient, you can ask them to do a decision balance separately from the patient. Afterwards, they can compare their perspectives. A family member's decision balance can help you and them understand why the patient and family members are at different stages of change. When a family member is at the action stage and the patient is at the contemplation stage about the patient's drinking habit, the family member may nag the patient to change (or be perceived as nagging) and evoke patient resistance. Thus, you can use the decision balance to help the patient and family members understand how they differ in their views about the benefits and concerns about change. This process can help family members understand the patient's resistance and ambivalence, but, more important, it can help them to stop nagging the patient.

At the end of the encounter, you can give the decision balances back to the patient and family members. Patients and family members can continue to work on this task by adding more items to their decision balance and comparing the similarities and differences in their items. If they are willing, they can combine the items from both decision balances onto a new sheet of paper as part of an assignment for the next appointment.

Assess Motivational Reasons, Competing Priorities, Energy and Self-Efficacy

Ask patients why they want to change. This inquiry can help you better understand whether patients are intrinsically or extrinsically motivated to change. You can also inquire about their energy and self-efficacy to change.

Assessing Motives
"Tell me what is driving you to consider changing your drinking habit." (Let the patient respond, and then continue with prompting.) *"Is it because of family and friends? Is it because you feel you ought to change? Are you doing it for yourself because it is important to you or perhaps for a combination of reasons? Which is most important?"*

Assessing Competing Priorities and Energy
"What competing priorities make it difficult for you to change your drinking habit?"
"On a scale of 0–10, how much energy can you put into changing your drinking habit?"

Assessing Confidence and Ability (self-efficacy)
"On a scale of 0–10, how would you rate your confidence to abstain from alcohol (for 2–4 weeks or for life)?"
"On a scale of 0–10, how would you rate your ability to abstain from alcohol (for 2–4 weeks or for life)?"

Assess Supports and Barriers

Supports and barriers may facilitate or hinder patients' changing their drinking habits.

Assessing Supports
"Who is around to support you after you have quit drinking or kept to low-risk drinking? Do you feel that you want help from others to help you quit drinking or keep to low-risk drinking? Have you thought about attending AA meetings or getting an AA sponsor?"

Assessing Barriers
"Is there anyone who makes it more difficult for you to change your drinking habit? Are there any situations that make it difficult for you to cut down to low-risk limits or quit altogether for a while?"

DISEASE-CENTERED ASSESSMENTS

The options for a disease-centered assessment are listed in a sequence that ranges from less threatening to more threatening for the patient:

1. Discuss presenting complaints without addressing the patient's use of alcohol.
2. Link alcohol use to the presenting complaint.
3. Clarify the severity of hazardous, harmful or dependent use of alcohol.

A disease-centered assessment also helps you define the severity of the alcohol problem. If patients are drinking above low-risk limits, then they are hazardous users of alcohol. Part 15A defined harmful and dependent use of alcohol and provided you with guidelines about using diagnostic uncertainty for negotiating with patients about making a specific diagnosis of excessive alcohol use. The language of these criteria has been modified into a questionnaire (Tables 15.12 and 15.13) that you can use with patients as a way to engage them in self-evaluation. You can use this questionnaire with patients during the encounter or by patients alone after the encounter for future discussion. The information that patients provide can be used to educate them about their alcohol use. These questionnaires may also assist you in negotiating with patients about diagnosis. Patients can circle their responses (Y= Yes, Ns = Not sure, N = No).

Table 15.12.

Self-evaluation for Alcohol Problems	Circle One		
During the past year, have you had any problems caused by Or made worse by alcohol use?			
Difficulties in fulfilling your responsibilities at work, school or home	Y	Ns	N
Physical or mental health problems	Y	Ns	N
Repeated alcohol-related legal problems	Y	Ns	N
Social or relationship problems	Y	Ns	N

Table 15.13.

Self-evaluation for Alcohol Dependence	Circle One		
Are you doing fewer other activities (social, occupational, or recreational) because you are more involved in drinking-related activities?	Y	Ns	N
Do you spend a fair amount of time in obtaining alcohol for your pleasure?	Y	Ns	N
Do you spend a fair amount of time recovering from the effects of alcohol?	Y	Ns	N
Do you have difficulty deciding when to stop drinking alcohol?	Y	Ns	N
Do you drink larger amounts of alcohol than you intended?	Y	Ns	N
Do you have urges or cravings for alcohol?	Y	Ns	N
Do you drink even though you know it causes you problems?	Y	Ns	N
Do you need more alcohol than you used to in order to have the same effect?	Y	Ns	N
Can you drink much more alcohol than you used to before you get drunk?	Y	Ns	N
Do you need much less alcohol to have the same effect or to get drunk?	Y	Ns	N
Have you had any withdrawal effects when you stop drinking alcohol?	Y	Ns	N
Does drinking alcohol help relieve your withdrawal symptoms?	Y	Ns	N

A response of "yes" to a question from three or more sections probably indicates physical or psychological dependence on alcohol.

STEP 4: ENHANCING MUTUAL UNDERSTANDING

Educate patients about your assessment and/or discuss further their self-evaluation about their alcohol use. This process may involve negotiating about the diagnosis (refer to Part 15A). After reaching some agreement about the problem, use nondirect and direct interventions, respectively, to lower resistance and enhance motivation to change. Also, consider whether to discuss how you and your patients view their self-efficacy, the same or differently.

EDUCATE PATIENTS ABOUT EXCESSIVE ALCOHOL USE

You can inform patients nonjudgmentally about the outcome of their assessment, so that they think more about the relationship of their alcohol use to their health concerns and the likelihood of hazardous, harmful or dependent use of alcohol. Such education also encourages patients to think more about the risks and harms and, if relevant, the physical and psychological aspects, of addiction.

- **Alcohol use related to presenting complaint or health concerns:** Address patients' presenting complaints but also educate them about how alcohol relates to their complaint.

- **Hazardous use:** Inform patients that they are drinking beyond the low-risk limit[25] and then evaluate what they think about this information. Inform them about how their intake compares with that of the general population and how excessive use increases the risk of developing health care problems, particularly if they have a family history of alcoholism.

- **Harmful use:** Educate patients about how alcohol is causing or contributing to medical, legal, social, sexual, psychological and/or financial problems. Inform them about the need to assess further whether their alcohol use is causing any other health problems. Provide objective data about the medical consequences of drinking alcohol, such as the results of blood tests.

- **Alcohol dependence:** Provide patients with assessment feedback about the level of dependence (e.g., tolerance, loss of control and continued drinking despite negative consequences) and educate them about alcohol dependence.[26]

In the time-pressured environment of primary care and hospital settings, practitioners are often unable to make a comprehensive assessment of alcohol use in a single patient encounter, and consequently cannot make a definitive diagnosis. If necessary, in such situations you can present your assessment to patients in a tentative way (as described in Part 15A) and/or educate patients in personally meaningful ways that enable them to make their own diagnosis.

Counter Patient Resistance to Diagnostic Labeling
Even if you educate patients about their alcohol risk in nonjudgmental ways, some patients may respond defensively by stating that they are not an alcoholic or do not have a drinking problem.

Patient Defensiveness about Alcohol Dependence: *"You're not saying that I'm an alcoholic, are you?"*
Practitioner's Response: *"What do you mean by 'an alcoholic'?"* (Reflective questioning)
"That's a good question, but I don't know the answer. Together we can work out whether you are at risk of becoming one." (Validation with concern)

Patient: *"But I'm not a skid-row alcoholic."*
Practitioner's Response: *"Most alcoholics are not on skid row. Most have a job and an intact family. We no longer use the term* alcoholic *for that reason. Instead, we use the term* alcohol dependency. *Let me explain what this means."* (Reframing patient's definition)

Patient Defensiveness about Alcohol Abuse: *"Are you telling me that I have a drinking problem?"*
Practitioner's Response: *"I don't know about that, but it is important to find out whether alcohol is causing your health problems."* (Reframing the label)
"Let me share with you the medical definition of a drinking problem—alcohol abuse—so that you can decide for yourself." (Clarifying differences)

Patient Defensiveness about Hazardous Use: *"I don't drink any more than my friends."*
Practitioner's Response: *"But you and your friends are in the minority. Most people don't drink as much as your friends do."* (Reeducating patient)

USE NONDIRECT INTERVENTIONS TO LOWER PATIENT RESISTANCE
It is equally important to know not only what to say but also how to say it when dealing with patients. A neutral stance helps you use nondirect interventions more effectively. In other words, you deliberately avoid trying to make patients change. At this stage, you do not state what is best for individual patients or about whether, when, how or why they should change. This nondirect exploration helps patients lower their resistance to change so that they become more inclined to consider it. Even if this does not occur, this approach is less likely to provoke patients to externalize their resistance so that they work against you. It is difficult, however, to maintain a stance of neutrality—not recommending what is best for individual patients—when you feel strongly that patients *should* change.

The different types of nondirect interventions are listed below, with specific examples that you can use or adapt for your own patients. These interventions are also discussed individually in the following sections.

Nondirect Interventions to Lower Resistance
Use simple reflection to elicit ambivalence: *"So you like drinking when you go out?" "So drinking helps you to relax?" "So sometimes you get hangovers?"*
Probe priorities to explore ambivalence: *"What is the most important reason for you to drink? And what is the most important reason for you to change your drinking habit?"*
Use double-sided reflection to summarize ambivalence: *"On the one hand, drinking alcohol is fun, but, on the other hand, you get hangovers the following morning."*
Acknowledge ambivalence: *"So, it seems that you have mixed feelings about drinking alcohol."*
Emphasize personal responsibility and choice: *"What you decide to do about drinking is entirely up to you." "It's up to you to decide whether to change. I'm here only to see if you are interested in improving your health. That's what I see as my role. Only you can decide what is in your best interest."*
Use explore-the-future questioning: *"So, what do you think your health will be like in 5–10 years if you carry on drinking alcohol at the same or higher levels?"*

Use Simple Reflection to Elicit Ambivalence

By further exploring the benefits and concerns about drinking alcohol from patients' perspective, you may elicit some ambivalence from them about their alcohol use. Reflective statements ("So you like drinking with your buddies") encourage patients to elaborate on the statements made during the assessment when drawing up a decision balance.

Probe Priorities to Explore Ambivalence

The purpose of exploring ambivalence is to clarify the key issues that patients are working on, and then to clarify the relative importance of these issues, as marked in each quadrant of the decision balance.

Use Double-Sided Reflection to Summarize Ambivalence

Double-sided reflections can challenge patients to work through their ambivalence about change. Statements such as "On the one hand, you like to drink and party, but on the other hand, you are then less likely to practice safe sex" can clearly summarize a patient's ambivalence toward change. Patients need time, however, to reflect about such statements. Remaining silent after making such statements disrupts patients' automatic defensiveness and gives them a time-out to reflect about inconsistencies in their rationalizations for engaging in risk behaviors.

Acknowledge Ambivalence

Sometimes it is worthwhile to acknowledge explicitly patients' ambivalence to change. This can help patients feel understood in ways that may keep them from feeling discouraged. You can help them to understand that this is part of the normal process when considering change.

Emphasize Personal Responsibility and Choice

Emphasizing personal responsibility can serve several important functions for both you and your patients. For example, when you use nondirect interventions, some patients may interpret your intentions as implying that they should change. When this occurs, you can use variations of the examples described below to minimize patient resistance and help them feel they have a choice. This approach is also useful when you get stuck or when patients resist working with you for other reasons.

Use Explore-the-future Questioning

These types of questions help patients to examine their past and present to explore the future in order to see the impact of their drinking habit. These questions can be modified to help patients explore their family history of drug and alcohol problems.

USE DIRECT INTERVENTIONS TO MOTIVATE PATIENT CHANGE

After patients become more receptive (less resistant) to the possibility of change, you can use direct interventions to enhance their motivation to change. In effect, you act as an advocate for behavior change but without telling patients what they should do. Direct interventions help patients alter their perceptions about the benefits and concerns about behavior change so that they diminish the value they give to reasons to stay the same and increase the value they give to reasons to change. These interventions can help patients do most of the work, but resistance can occur particularly when they feel that you are trying to "make them change" their perceptions and values.

Use Benefit Substitution

You can ask patients how they could obtain the benefits of drinking in alternative ways. This task can be part of the patient encounter, or patients can complete this task for the next encounter or on their own time. After they have worked on developing their own ideas, you may add your suggestions. Again, let the patient do the work first before providing assistance.

Benefit Substitution
"What are other ways of having fun with your friends that don't involve drinking alcohol?"   Or *"You say that you enjoy drinking beer with your friends, but can you still enjoy your friends and drink nonalcoholic beer at lunchtime?"*

Use Back-to-the-future Questions

Back-to-the-future questions help patients anticipate the possibility of future complications or events (negative or positive) occurring in the present. These questions help patients consider what they would do if such a complication or event did occur.

Back-to-the-future
"If you were to develop a health problem from your drinking now, would you stop drinking?" (Provided that the patient shows some interest in prevention, continue.) *"At the moment, you are drinking over the low-risk drink limit and are at risk for developing complications. Do you want to wait and see if you develop a complication before deciding to change?"* (If the patient remains interested in prevention, continue.) *"What would it take for you to decide to drink alcohol below the low-risk limit?"* (If the patient is ambivalent, or not interested in prevention, continue.) *"Would you mind sharing with me why you don't want to avoid complications?"* Or *"Let's suppose that alcohol is damaging your health in a way you are unaware of. Do you think this is a possibility?"* (With a negative response, offer an example such as abnormal liver function enzymes. With an affirmative answer, continue by saying:) *"If we discover that alcohol is damaging your health, what do you think you will do?"*

Clarify Values

Interventions that probe and contrast patients' values may help them think about their life priorities in ways that go beyond what they itemized on their decision balance: for example, how alcohol use stands in relation to other aspects of their life. A probing question involves asking patients to reflect about what is more important in their life than alcohol use. A contrasting question asks patients to compare whether alcohol (or drug) use is more important to them than something or somebody else, such as their relationship to their spouse, children and/or grandchildren. Value clarification questions can be effective in focusing patients who are evasive, avoid responsibility for themselves and/or blame others.

Clarifying Values
Questions that probe values: *"What is more important in your life than drinking alcohol?"* *"What is more important in your life than your health?"* *"What would have to change to make your health more important than drinking alcohol?"*
Questions that contrast values: *"So, having a hangover is worth it to have a good time at the party?"* *"So, what is more important to you: drinking alcohol or having a good relationship with your spouse and being a good parent?"* *"You say that your wife is worried about your having a drinking problem, but you don't think you do. So, what is more important to you: drinking alcohol, or having a wife who is less worried?"*
Questions that contrast values and behavior: *"If you say that your relationship with your wife is more important than drinking alcohol, you're saying one thing and doing another. What would convince you to do what you say?"*

Probing and contrasting values: Mrs. C. used cocaine once a month or so for several years when meeting with a group of friends to drink rum. MP asked, "Do you know of any people who have run into serious trouble with their use of cocaine?" (MP was indirectly attempting to ascertain whether Mrs. C. had any concerns about cocaine use and whether she valued keeping out of trouble.)

He then asked, "Do you think there's any possibility that this might happen to you?" (MP used a back-to-the-future question.) "Are there other things in your life that are more important to you than drinking alcohol and using cocaine?" (MP directly challenged the patient to think about how important cocaine use was compared to other things in her life. MP then asked Mrs. C. about any concerns about cocaine use. Mrs. C. said, "I'm concerned about avoiding sex with HIV-infected cocaine users, preserving my health and avoiding addiction and financial bankruptcy."

Commentary: This approach placed the responsibility on Mrs. C. to reflect and clarify what was more important in her life than using alcohol and cocaine.

Challenge Rationalizations

Patients often provide intriguing rationalizations for their excessive use of alcohol. From the patients' frame of reference, their rationalizations make reasonable or even indisputable sense, but to you, their rationalizations are irrational and flawed. Nondirect interventions help you understand patients' frames of reference. Direct interventions help you challenge patients' frames of reference in ways that may modify or change their rationalizations.

Challenging Rationalizations
"Do you mind if I say a few things that might help you think about your drinking differently?" (With an affirmative response from the patient, continue.) *"It may make you pause and think. You don't have to say anything if you don't feel like it, and if you want me to stop talking about alcohol, just tell me."* (Choose one of the following statements.) *"Many drinkers with family histories of alcoholism don't remember how many years it took for their father [or other family member] to become an alcoholic, so they believe that it is impossible for them to become an alcoholic like their father [or other family member]." "Sensible drinkers can even become alcoholics without knowing it: for example, they don't recognize how much they have developed a tolerance for alcohol."*

Examples of responding to rationalizations: *Mr. D. (age 50) held two jobs to earn enough money to support his family. His second job was as a barman; he regarded this job as recreational, a release from work and family responsibilities. Mr. D. drank well over the low-risk drinking limit. During his encounter with his practitioner, he made a number of comments rationalizing his drinking habit. Dr. M. did not agree with Mr. D., and challenged him.*

Patient: *"I never lose control when I drink alcohol and drive."*

Practitioner (challenging the patient's frame of reference): *"That is what most people think, but alcohol impairs people's judgment so that they think they're still in control. Alcohol affects your ability to drive without your being aware of it."*

Patient: *"I got a DWI but I wasn't drinking out of control."*

Practitioner: *"You may not feel out of control, but that's not the problem. Research shows that you may be able to do routine driving when you drink, but your reaction time and skills in emergency situations are impaired."*[27]

Patient: *"I'm a sensible drinker."*

Practitioner: *"But you can still damage your health even if you're a sensible drinker."*

Patient: *"I hold down two jobs without any difficulty."*

Practitioner: *"You hold down two jobs very well, but that doesn't have much to do with how alcohol is affecting your health."*

Use Discrepancies

During the process of understanding patients' reasons for drinking alcohol, you may identify discrepancies between their behaviors and some aspect of their self-interest, or help them discover these discrepancies for themselves.

Discrepancies between a Behavior and Self-interest
"You enjoy drinking alcohol at parties, but you get a hangover the morning after." "You say that alcohol makes you feel better. But if you felt better, would you still need to drink?"
"I'm not sure if I'm hearing you correctly, but what I think I hear is that your relationship with alcohol is becoming more important than your relationship with your spouse and kids."
"You started drinking at home since your DWI, but now you're trapped at home with a wife who nags you about your drinking."
"You say that alcohol helps you with your depression. At best, alcohol gives you short-term relief by numbing your feeling of depression, but afterwards you'll feel worse because alcohol makes you more depressed. So you drink more. It becomes a vicious cycle. If alcohol really helped depression, you could stop using it after a while because your depression would go away. What do you think is the best way for you to treat your depression?"
"So, now that your kids are getting into alcohol and drugs, you're beginning to take another look at your own use of alcohol. How does their use of alcohol and drugs affect you and your thinking about your alcohol use?"
"You say that alcohol helps you sleep better, but the effects of this drug are complex. Let me explain. Alcohol certainly does help you get to sleep, but it also causes wakefulness during the night. This reduces the amount of deep sleep that your body needs to give you more energy. When asleep, you don't realize that your sleep is poor quality. So, in the evening, when you feel tired and have difficulty getting to sleep, you understandably have a few drinks to help you sleep. Do you understand what I'm saying? (Let the patient respond.) It's a kind of vicious cycle. What makes this worse is that when your body has become accustomed to the alcohol, you experience worse sleep problems when you stop drinking because of the rebound effect. It may take a week or so, sometimes longer, for your body to get over the effects of alcohol. It's quite complicated to understand how alcohol affects sleep. What do you think is the best way for you to improve your quality of sleep and regain your energy, so that you feel better?"

Learning Exercise 15.1: Drug substitute request

In response to practitioners pointing out such discrepancies, patients may request a drug substitute instead of alcohol. Take a minute to reflect about how you would respond to these requests, and fill in your responses below.

Request for a Drug	Your Response
"I can't possibly stop drinking alcohol unless I have something to help me sleep. Can you give me some Valium to take at night?"	
"You just don't understand my difficulties—the sleeping problem and the stresses that I'm under. I really need something at night to help me sleep."	
"There must be some safe pill you could give me to help me sleep."	

Reframe Items, Issues and Events

Reframing techniques help patients to change their views about items, issues or events related to their decision balance. In other words, you help patients turn a reason to drink into a reason not to drink, enhance a reason to stop/reduce drinking alcohol and/or diminish a reason to drink.

Reframing Items, Issues or Events
Change a reason to drink into a reason not to drink: *"You can certainly hold your liquor, but drinking so much alcohol puts you at an increased risk for developing cirrhosis and becoming an alcoholic."*
Enhance a reason to stop/reduce drinking alcohol: *"You say that your spouse nags you about your drinking, but this shows how much your spouse is really concerned about your health. Are you willing to reduce your drinking to stop the nagging?"*
Diminish a reason to drink: *"You say that alcohol helps you get to sleep, but drinking alcohol decreases the quality of your sleep, which then makes you feel tired all the time."*

Use Amplified Reflection

You may identify issues, feelings, concerns or lack of concern and then reflect them back to the patient in an amplified form. For example, a patient mentioned that his father had cirrhosis of the liver, which was probably the cause of his death. He mentioned this without expressing any concern about the fact that his practitioner had just told him that he drank above low-risk limits and had elevated liver enzymes.

Challenging Claims or Positions Using Amplified Reflection
"So, alcohol makes you feel really happy." "So, alcohol makes your pain completely go away." "So, drinking alcohol is the best way for you to have fun with your friends." "So, your [wife/husband] is completely unjustified in [her/his] concerns about your drinking." "Your drinking is increasing your liver enzymes and increasing your risk of developing cirrhosis. Yet when you mentioned that your father died of cirrhosis . . ." (Pause. Let the patient respond and, assuming an indifferent, nonverbal response, then continue.) *"Yet you don't seem at all concerned about what I've just told you."* (Amplified reflection of the patient's nonverbal response)

Use Differences in Motivational Reasons

Identify something other than alcohol use that patients are highly motivated to do (be a good parent or spouse, do well at work, fish for relaxation). Ask them if they could put the same amount of effort and care into changing their alcohol intake as they are putting into these other activities. Or identify a past successful change (e.g., quitting smoking) and ask them to use that experience to help them change their alcohol use.

Using Differences in Motivational Reasons
"You decided to quit smoking by yourself, but what would it take for you to do the same thing in terms of reducing your alcohol intake to below low-risk limits?"

Monitor Changes in Resistance and Motivation Scores

Patients are ready for change when they, not you, perceive the reasons to change (motivation) as outweighing the reasons not to change (resistance).[28] To monitor change over time, you can ask patients if they have changed their resistance and motivation scores and why. Their explanations for changing their scores provide invaluable information about why things are getting better or worse over time.

Monitoring Changes in Resistance and Motivation Scores
"What scores would you now give for your resistance and motivation to change, on a scale of 0–10? Why did you change your resistance score? And why did you change your motivation score? You can learn a lot about yourself even if your scores got worse and went in the wrong direction. Sometimes it helps if your resistance score goes up and your motivation score goes down, as it can show you what it would take to change for good."

CLARIFY DIFFERENCES IN PERCEPTIONS ABOUT PATIENT SELF-EFFICACY

Patients may overestimate or underestimate their self-efficacy (ability and confidence) to change. Some patients who are unknowingly dependent on alcohol may even boast about their ability to quit drinking and also refute any need to change because their drinking is not causing any problems. In contrast, you may know that a particular patient is dependent on alcohol and that alcohol is causing problems for the patient. To address this discrepancy in perception about self-efficacy, you can pose hypothetical statements:

> *"Suppose you were to accept a challenge—say, quit drinking for two weeks—to prove that you could do it without difficulty. What would you think if you discovered that you could not stop drinking and that you were dependent on alcohol without knowing it?"*

On the other hand, some patients underestimate their self-efficacy to change their behavior. You can clearly state how you perceive their abilities to change differently, as a way to boost their confidence and help them realistically reevaluate their strengths.

"On a scale of 0–10, you stated that your ability to stop drinking was a 1, but I see you as a 5 to 6 on that scale. What do you think about the fact that we see things differently?"

(See Chapter 9B for other ways to help patients deal with their sense of hopelessness about change.)

STEP 5: IMPLEMENTING A PLAN FOR CHANGE

The extent to which you and your patients share similar and different perceptions about the benefits, risks and harms of alcohol use influence how you develop an appropriate plan together. If you underestimate the differences in these perceptions, you are likely to experience more difficulties in implementing a plan with your patients.

Clarifying Persistent Differences in Perceptions
"I think it is important for us to be clear about how we each see the benefits, risks and harm of drinking alcohol—the same or differently—because this will affect how we work together. I think I understand what you like about drinking alcohol, but I am more concerned about the risk and harm caused by your drinking than you are. What do you think?"

EVALUATE PATIENT COMMITMENT TOWARD A PLAN

Before selecting goals for change and implementing a plan, consider assessing the extent to which patients are committed to changing their use of alcohol with respect to competing priorities, energy and motivational reasons.

Competing Priorities
"What's going on in your life that makes it difficult for you to reduce your alcohol intake to low-risk levels [or to abstain] now? Is there anything else?" "What would it take for you to put low-risk drinking [or abstinence] at the top of your list of things to do?" "What is stopping you from putting low-risk drinking [or abstinence] at the top of your list of things to do?"

Energy
"What's going on that makes it difficult for you to devote your energy to quit drinking or cut down on your drinking? What would it take for you to put your energy into changing your drinking habit? If you don't have any energy to change, what would it take for you to get your energy back?"

Motives
"What will make you commit yourself to the goal of low-risk drinking [or abstinence]? And what else?" "You say that you are here because your family wanted you to come. But what would it take for you to come for your own reasons?"

DECIDE ABOUT GOALS FOR CHANGE

You need to decide for yourself what you think are the best goals for change based on your understanding of your patients, their readiness to change and the severity of their alcohol risk. The range of goals for implementing a plan may exist along the following continua: stages of change (contemplation-preparation-action), short-term/long-term goals and pragmatic/ideal recommendations.

Range of Goals

Table 15.14 outlines a range of goals for helping hazardous, harmful and dependent drinkers. These options are

- Contemplate further low-risk drinking or abstinence
- Prepare for low-risk drinking or abstinence
- Take action toward change (low-risk drinking or abstinence)

With regard to abstaining, drinking below low-risk limits or reducing their alcohol intake and the duration for these goals, patients may opt for goals that are short-term (2-4 weeks) or long-term (greater than a year). When patients are unsure about the need for change or are ambivalent about it, they may opt for short-term, incremental steps toward change, such as reducing alcohol intake. If patients are reluctant to change, you can suggest that they conduct an experiment and try to abstain for two weeks.

Before selecting goals, decide what your recommendations are going to be for the patient: either to abstain from alcohol or to drink below the low-risk limits. Your opinion and recommendations will influence whether you think you can work with this patient or whether you will need to make a referral to an addiction specialist or a community program such as Alcoholics Anonymous.

Table 15.14.

Goals for Change: Hazardous and Harmful Use of Alcohol

• Think more about:
    Reduced alcohol intake, low-risk drinking, and abstinence
    Use a decision balance to consider these goals
• Prepare for change:
    Plan how to deal with change
    Learn about what constitutes alcohol abuse and dependence
    Inform family and friends about plans to change
• Set a date to change (abstinence, low-risk, or reduced use):
    Short-term (2-4 weeks) vs. long-term goal
    Address alcohol-related problems

Table 15.14. (continued)

Treatment Options for Alcohol Dependence
• Referral to a counselor for an in-depth assessment
• Detoxification (outpatient vs. inpatient)
• Referral to an alcohol program (outpatient vs. inpatient)

• Attend Alcoholics Anonymous meetings
    Attend open meetings
    Get a sponsor
    Attend 12-step, closed meetings

• Use of Naltrexone to prevent relapse [29]

Setting Goals

You can influence the goal-setting process by providing advice in either a disease-centered or patient-centered way or by using a negotiated approach.

Practitioner-centered goal-setting:

Authoritarian (controlling) monologue: *"I think you should stop drinking alcohol altogether so that you don't get cirrhosis."*

Authoritative and autonomy-supportive monologue: *"If you continue to drink, you are at increased risk of developing cirrhosis. If you decide to stop drinking, you won't get cirrhosis."*

Patient-initiated goal-setting:

Advice-giving monologue: *"You seemed concerned when we talked about your father developing cirrhosis. Let me just mention something that you may have already thought about. Given the fact that your liver function tests are abnormal, you are also at risk of developing cirrhosis. Fortunately, the condition is reversible if you do something about it. Now, let me explain. If you were to stop drinking for six weeks, we could check your liver enzymes after that time to see whether they returned to normal."*

If an advice-giving approach does not work, negotiate with patients about whether to change.

Negotiated Approach—An Engaging Dialogue

MP: *"I am concerned because your father developed cirrhosis and your blood test is now showing that your liver enzymes are high."*

Mr. W.:   *"What does that mean?"*

MP :   *"Let me explain. I think the amount of alcohol that you drink is causing some liver damage and putting you at increased risk of developing cirrhosis."* (MP spoke in a low-key way and caring tone of voice. He showed the patient the written report of the test and explained what the results meant.)

Mr. W.:   *"I can't believe what you are telling me. I know that I don't drink as much as my father did."* (Mr. W. paused, as if expecting the practitioner to reply. MP deliberately remained silent to let Mr. W reflect about this information.) *"Is there something that I can do to stop this?"*

MP: *"Before we talk about that, let me explain a little something about your dad. Your father probably did not know that his liver tests were abnormal before he started drinking heavily. Had someone told him, he may have changed his drinking habits before developing cirrhosis."* (MP again used silence to allow the patient to reflect about what he had said.)

Mr. W: *"What are you telling me—to stop drinking?"* (Mr. W. asked in an incredulous tone of voice.)

MP: *"I think you need to decide what is in the best interest of your health. Only you can decide whether you are prepared to do something about the abnormal liver tests and reduce your risk of developing cirrhosis."* (MP respected Mr. W.'s autonomy to decide what to do about his health.)

Mr. W: *"How do you know whether things will get better if I stop drinking? I mean, will I have to stop drinking for life?"*

MP: *"Fortunately, the liver enzyme levels can go back to normal. Let me share with you what I think you can do to check out if this will happen. If you were to stop drinking for six weeks, we could recheck the liver enzymes then to find out whether they've returned to normal. I don't know the answer yet to your second question. Let's first check out whether the liver damage is reversible or not. Time will help us work out whether it's necessary for you to stop drinking completely to avoid developing cirrhosis over time."* (MP noticed that he was overwhelming the patient emotionally and deferred giving any further information.) *"What do you think about what I'm telling you?"*

Mr. W: *"I think I should give up drinking for a while,"* (Mr. W. said, but not as if he were convinced:) *"Do you agree?"*

MP: (deliberately avoided answering that question) *"I am quite willing to tell you what I think you should do. But it is important for me to know what you can do to improve your own health. I am willing to help you in whatever you want."*

Mr. W.: *"I'm still interested in what you think I should do."* (Mr. W. now demonstrated a genuine interest in his practitioner's recommendations.)

MP: *"Are you willing to stop drinking over the next six weeks to see whether your liver enzymes go back to normal?"* (MP carefully posed his recommendation as a question rather than a statement.)

Mr. W.: *"I'm willing to try, but I think that I'll need a sleeping pill because alcohol helps me sleep."*

Requests for Drugs

In response to motivational interventions, patients may reply in ways that challenge you to deal with requests for drugs. With a trial of abstinence, patients may feel that they need to substitute a drug for alcohol to help them deal with depression, anxiety and/or difficulties in sleeping. A learning exercise will help you think about how to respond to such requests.

Learning Exercise 15.2: Responding to the patient's request for sleeping tablets
Imagine that you are the practitioner. After reading the following dialogue, how would you respond to this patient?

Patient:	*"I need a sleeping pill. Why don't you give me some diazepam?"*
Practitioner:	*"So your sleeping problem is so bad that you're willing to substitute one drug for another. Do you see any alternative to using drugs?"*
Patient:	*"Maybe later. Right now, if you don't give me something to sleep, I can't possibly stop drinking alcohol. I have too much stress going on. I need something now!"*
Practitioner:	*"Do you have so much stress that you're willing to risk using another drug, even though it's not dealing with the cause of the problem?"*
Patient:	(after a period of silence) *"Well, I suppose that's right."*
Practitioner:	*"Can I tell you about how diazepam and alcohol affect your sleep?"*
Patient:	*"Well, okay."*
Practitioner:	*"Diazepam and alcohol may help in the short run, but not in the long run."* (This is agreement with a twist: contrasting short-term benefits with long-term concerns.) *"The effects of diazepam wear off in the short run, and then you need to increase the dose to help you sleep. When this happens, you can become addicted to it."* (The educational message focuses on concerns about use.) *"Do you understand why I'm concerned about using drugs to deal with sleep problems?"*
Patient:	*"Well, I guess so. But I really need something for a few weeks to help me sleep. Is there anything else I could use that isn't addictive?"*
Practitioner:	*"You just told me something that's really important."* (Again, the practitioner intervenes to help the patient identify a discrepancy and uses silence to foster self-reflection.)
Patient:	(after a moment of silence) *"You just don't understand my sleeping problem and the stresses that I'm under. If you had my stresses, you would understand my sleeping problem better. There must be a safe pill you can give me. Can't you think of anything else?"*
Practitioner:	(The practitioner noticed that the patient had shifted the agenda, but refocused on exploring whether the intervention had had any impact.) *"A moment ago, I noticed that you were silent. Do you mind if I ask you what was going through your mind?"* (This intervention invites the patient to put aside his defensive routines against considering change.)
Patient:	*"I was thinking that I had better not become like my father."*

Think about whether you would use a drug with this patient before reading on.

Dealing with a Request for Sedative Drugs

Patient: *"You just don't understand my sleeping problem and the stresses that I'm under. If you had my stresses, you would understand my sleeping problem better. There must be a safe pill that you can give me. Can't you think of anything else?"*

Practitioner: *"Well, there are other drugs, such as amitriptyline, that aren't addictive. You use this drug for a few weeks until your sleep problem settles down. But you can't take this drug with alcohol. Would you be prepared to stop drinking if you use this drug?"*

Patient: *"I need something to help me sleep."*

Practitioner: *"Amitriptyline often causes a dry mouth in the morning, but it wears off over time."*

Patient: *"What happens if the drug doesn't work?"*

Practitioner: *"We can talk over the phone about increasing the dose. But are you prepared to stop drinking?"*

Patient: *"Yes, I will."*

Practitioner: *"I'll start you off with a prescription for 25 mg a day and increase it by one tablet every two to three days, up to three tablets a day. If you develop any other side effects besides dry mouth, call me and I'll call you back. How soon can you come back to see me?"*

Patient: *"I could make it next Thursday afternoon."*

Some practitioners would never prescribe amitriptyline for several reasons—substituting one drug for another, for example, or concerns about drug interactions. In contrast, other practitioners may selectively use this drug in certain circumstances. To consider this issue, you can use a decision balance to explore the advantages and disadvantages of prescribing this drug versus never using it.

Set a Date for Change

You can help patients set a date to change based on whatever their goals are: thinking about change, preparing for change, attempting a trial of abstinence or low-risk drinking for two to four weeks or aiming for the long-term goal of abstinence or low-risk drinking.

WORK TOWARD SOLUTIONS

You can use the MED-STAT solution-based approach to help patients evaluate the feasibility of achieving their goals for change.[30]

Interventions	Solution-based Approach
Miracle question (explore change)	*"Suppose a miracle happened tomorrow and you stopped drinking [or kept to low-risk drinking]. What would your life be like then? How do you think your family and friends would respond?"*
Exceptions (identify strengths)	*"What was going on at times when you drank less alcohol compared to times when you drank more alcohol?* (Patient responds that he drinks when he gets angry.) *"What happens on those occasions when you get angry and don't drink alcohol?"*
Difference (use strengths)	*"What can you learn from those occasions when you were angry and didn't drink alcohol?"* (Let the patient respond.) *"How can that help you deal with your anger when you're tempted to drink?"*
Scaling (assess motivation, self-efficacy and outcome expectancy)	*"On a scale of 0–10, how would you rate your [motivation, ability and confidence] not to drink when you get angry? How would you rate whether you can achieve your goal for change [outcome expectancy]? What would increase or decrease your scores? Can you make a list of these reasons? Was there a time when your scores were higher than now? What would it take to tip the balance in favor of higher scores?"*
Time-outs (consider alternatives)	*"What other ideas do you have about how you could handle your anger differently instead of drinking alcohol?"* (Probe silences.) *"A moment ago, I asked you a question and you were silently thinking. What was going on?"*
Accolades (enhance efficacy)	*"You have the skills to keep to low-risk drinking [or abstain], but what would it take for you keep using your skills all the time?"*
Task appraisals (encourage action)	*"How do you know whether low-risk drinking or abstinence is the best goal for you?"*

STEP 6: FOLLOWING THROUGH

RATIONALE, PURPOSE AND REASONS FOR FOLLOW-UP

The rationale for recommending follow-up appointments has to be grounded in your experience with a patient, after you have worked through the problem-solving phases of enhancing mutual understanding and implementing a plan. At one extreme, you may develop a rationale for focusing on a particular alcohol-related problem (e.g., indigestion) without making it explicit that you will explore how alcohol affects indigestion at the next appointment. The rationale given to the patient may not entirely reflect your purpose for the next appointment. This go-slow approach may seem deceptive, but it is helpful when you anticipate that you are dealing with resistant patients who do not think that they have a drinking problem. At the other extreme, alcohol-dependent patients who accept their diagnosis may only need an explanation about the need for detoxification and immediate referral. After providing your rationale for a follow-up appointment, clarify with the patient about his or her reasons for making a follow-up appointment. This may help you understand the extent to which you have a common agreement about the reason for a follow-up.

Rationale for Follow-up Appointment
"I think it's important for you to come back and work out . . ." (choose one or more of the following): *"What's causing your indigestion [or any other alcohol-related harm]."* *"Whether there's a relationship between your alcohol use and your indigestion."* *"Whether to decrease your alcohol intake so it doesn't bother your indigestion as much."* *"Whether you might be developing a drinking problem."* *"Whether you're becoming dependent on alcohol."* (Then arrange a follow-up appointment.)
Clarifying Patients' Reasons to Attend a Follow-up Appointment
"Why is it important for you to attend a follow-up appointment?" *"What do you think is the most important reason for you to attend a follow-up appointment?"* *"What health concerns do you want to address at your next appointment? When do you think will be a good time for you to come back and address your health concerns? You can always call me if you have any concerns about how the medication is working, or if you have any concern about side effects."*

TIMING, DURATION AND FREQUENCY OF A FOLLOW-UP APPOINTMENT

Once you have established the rationale for a follow-up appointment, you can ask patients when they would like to come back and see you and how often. You may not always have the time to negotiate about arranging a follow-up appointment, but an example is provided next.

> *MP asked Mrs. D. when she thought she needed to come back for a follow-up appointment. Mrs. D was taken aback and asked, "When do you think?" MP explained that he was very interested in hearing first about what she thought before saying what he thought. She was surprised by this request. She paused and said, "I don't know." MP remained silent to allow her to reflect. Mrs. D. then asked, "What about four weeks?" MP then had two options: to accept Mrs. D.'s offer or to negotiate about a different time for the follow-up appointment if there was a large discrepancy between his opinion and Mrs. D.'s suggestion.*

Timing, Duration and Frequency of Follow-up Appointment
"When do you think you should come back to see me?" *"When do you think it would be a good time for you to come back to check up on your health concerns?"* *"I think it's important for you to decide how often you should come back for a follow-up appointment. I will certainly share what I think about this, but I'm more interested in what you think."*

METHODS TO ENSURE CHANGE AND PREVENT RELAPSE
A Diary to Track Change

When patients are contemplating changing their drinking habits, you can suggest that they keep a drinking diary as a way to help prepare them for change. Over a one-week period, you can ask patients to keep a record of the times and circumstances under which they drank alcohol and to monitor their urges and what triggered their desire to drink. You can also use drinking diaries as a way to monitor progress toward the goal of low-risk drinking or abstinence.

A Diary for Tracking Change
"Are you willing to keep a drinking diary and write down your thoughts and feelings about your successes and difficulties in working toward your goal?"

Relapse Prevention

As part of relapse prevention, ask patients to monitor their temptations, urges and cravings to drink alcohol. In addition, you can warn patients that positive or negative emotions (feeling happy, bad, guilty, anxious, depressed) are common triggers for relapse, and ask them how they will handle these emotions in alternative ways. You can also help coach them on strategies to anticipate high-risk situations.

Relapse Prevention
Management of risk situations: *"What kind of situations will make it difficult for you to keep to your goal of low-risk drinking or abstinence? In what ways can you deal with those situations?"*
Pharmacologic management: *"Have you encountered any difficulties in taking your Naltrexone on a regular basis? Do you have any concerns about taking the medication?"*
Emotional management: *"When you feel that way [any negative emotions], how do you think you can deal with those feelings instead of drinking alcohol?"*
Reevaluation of supports: *"Would it help to have someone who will help you work toward your goal for abstinence [or low-risk drinking]?"*
Reevaluation of barriers: *"What do you think is making it difficult for you to abstain or keep to low-risk drinking limits? How do you think you're going to handle those situations?"*
Use of positive reinforcement: *"Would it be helpful for you to set up a reward for abstaining or keeping to low-risk drinking limits? What would that be?"*

Motivational Reevaluation

Ask patients to use their decision balance to reevaluate and/or reinforce the need for preventing lapses or relapses.

Motivational Reevaluation
"Let's look again at your decision balance and talk about whether you still think that your reasons to change are really more important than your reasons to stay the same. This may help you stick to low-risk drinking or abstinence when you feel that you could lapse or relapse."

YOUR SUMMARY

Reflect: write a summary about what you have learned that was new for you.

_____
_____
_____
_____
_____
_____
_____
_____
_____
_____
_____
_____
_____
_____
_____
_____
_____
_____
_____
_____
_____
_____
_____
_____
_____

Enhance: write down your ideas about how your new learning could improve your interactions with patients. Add your notes to your learning portfolio.

_____
_____
_____
_____
_____
_____
_____
_____
_____
_____
_____
_____
_____

REFERENCES

1. Miller WR, Baca LM. Two-year follow-up of bibliotherapy and therapist-directed controlled drinking training for problem drinkers. Behavior Therapy 1983;14: 441-448

2. Miller WR, Sovereign RG. The check-up: A model for early intervention in addictive behaviors. In: Loberg T, Miller WR, Nathan PE, et al., eds. Addictive behaviors: Prevention and early intervention. Amsterdam: Swets & Zeitlinger; 1989: 219-231

3. Valle SK. Interpersonal functioning of alcoholism counselors and treatment outcome. Journal of Studies on Alcohol 1981;42: 783-790

4. Luborsky L, McLellan AT, Woody GE, et al. Therapist success and its determinants. Archives of General Psychology 1985;42: 602-611

5. Bradley KA, Bush KR, McDonell MB, et al. Screening for problem drinking: Comparison of CAGE and AUDIT. Ambulatory Care Quality Improvement Project (ACQUIP). Alcohol Use Disorders Identification Test. Journal of General Internal Medicine 1998;13: 379-388

6. Wallace PG, Brennan PJ, Haines AP. Drinking patterns in general practice patients. Journal of the Royal College of General Practitioners 1987;37: 354-357

7. Rydon P, Redman S, Sanson-Fisher RW, et al. Detection of alcohol-related problems in general practice. Journal of Studies on Alcohol 1992;53(3): 197-202

8. Lawner K, Doot M, Gausas J, et al. Implementation of CAGE alcohol screening in a primary care practice. Family Medicine 1997;29: 332-335

9. Lairson DR, Harrist R, Martin DW, et al. Screening for patients with alcohol problems: severity of patients identified by the CAGE. Journal of Drug Education 1992;22: 337-352

10. Ewing JA. Detecting alcoholism. The CAGE questionnaire. Journal of the American Medical Association 1984;252: 1905-1907

11. Buchsbaum DG, Buchanan RG, Centor RM, et al. Screening for alcohol abuse using CAGE scores and likelihood ratios. Annals of Internal Medicine 1991;115: 774-777

12. Saunders JB, Aasland OG, Babor TF, et al. Development of the Alcohol Use Disorders Identification Test (AUDIT): WHO Collaborative Project on Early Detection of Persons with Harmful Alcohol Consumption—II. Addiction 1993;88(6): 791-804

13. Allen JP, Litten RZ, Fertig JB, et al. A review of research on the Alcohol Use Disorders Identification Test (AUDIT). Alcoholism, Clinical and Experimental Research 1997;21: 613-619

14. Piccinelli M, Tessari E, Bortolomasi M, et al. Efficacy of the alcohol use disorders identification test as a screening tool for hazardous alcohol intake and related disorders in primary care: a validity study. British Medical Journal 1997;314: 420-424

15. Bush K, Kivlahan DR, McDonell MB, et al. The AUDIT alcohol consumption questions (AUDIT-C): An effective brief screening test for problem drinking. Ambulatory Care Quality Improvement Project (ACQUIP). Alcohol Use Disorders Identification Test. Archives of Internal Medicine 1998;158: 1789-1795

16. Piccinelli M, Tessari E, Bortolomasi M, et al. Efficacy of the alcohol use disorders identification test as a screening tool for hazardous alcohol intake and related disorders in primary care: A validity study. British Medical Journal 1997;314: 420-424

17. Seppa K, Lepisto J, Sillanaukee P. Five-shot questionnaire on heavy drinking. Alcoholism, Clinical and Experimental Research 1998;22: 1788-1791

18. Aertgerts B, Buntinx F, Ansoms S, et al. Screening properties of questionnaires and laboratory tests for the detection of alcohol abuse or dependence in a general practice population. British Journal of General Practice 2001;51: 206-217
19. Brown RL, Leonard T, Saunders LA, et al. A two-item screen test for alcohol and other drug problems. The Journal of Family Practice 1997;44: 151-160
20. Schorling JB, Willems JP, Klas PT. Identifying problem drinkers: Lack of sensitivity of the two-question drinking test. American Journal of Medicine 1995;98: 232-236
21. Taj N, Devera-Sales A, Vinson DC. Screening for problem drinking: Does a single question work? The Journal of Family Practice 1998;46: 328-335
22. Dawson DA, Archer LD. Relative frequency of heavy drinking and the risk of alcohol dependence. Addiction 1993;88: 1509-1518
23. Dawson DA. Consumption indicators of alcohol dependence. Addiction 1994;89: 345-350
24. Ferguson RA, Goldberg DM. Genetic markers of alcohol abuse. Clinica Chimica Acta 1997;257: 199-250
25. Klatsky AL. Annotation: Alcohol and longevity. American Journal of Public Health 1995;85: 16-18
26. National Institute on Alcohol Abuse and Alcoholism. Alcohol and tolerance. Alcohol Alert 1995;28: 1-4
27. National Institute on Alcohol Abuse and Alcoholism. Drinking and driving. Alcohol Alert 1996;31
28. Prochaska JO, DiClemente CC, Norcross JC. In search of how people change: Applications to addictive behaviors. American Psychologist 1992;47(9): 1102-1114
29. Weinrieb RM, O'Brien CP. Naltrexone in the treatment of alcoholism. Annual Review of Medicine 1997;48: 477-487
30. Giorlando ME, Schilling RJ. On becoming a solution-focused physician: The MED-STAT acronym. Families, Systems & Health 1997;15: 361-373

CHAPTER 16 Part A

TOBACCO USE

FOR REFLECTION

How can you combine behavioral interventions with drug treatment of nicotine dependence to help your patients quit their tobacco use?

OVERVIEW

Traditional approaches to tobacco cessation involve practitioners providing education and advice to patients.[1-5] These approaches, however, help only a small percentage of tobacco users (2-10%) to quit each year.[6;7] Factors that enhance quit rates include the intensity and duration of smoking cessation programs and approaches that use multiple methods rather than single methods. For example, drug treatments for nicotine dependence can complement behavioral treatments and thus enhance quit rates among nicotine-dependent smokers. The key issue is how best to combine behavioral interventions with treatments for nicotine dependence to help smokers quit.

KEY FACTS ABOUT TOBACCO USE

...cco is the single greatest preventable contributor to disease and premature death ...ternationally, causing 4 million deaths a year. Adolescent and adult smoking is ...easing in most parts of the world. Within 20 to 30 years, tobacco use will cause 10 ...llion deaths per year, accounting for one in eight deaths overall; 70% of all these deaths will occur in developing countries.[8] The report *Trust Us: We're the Tobacco Industry* helps us understand how the tobacco industry contributed toward creating this pandemic plague.[g] The World Health Organization launched a Tobacco-free Initiative and the Framework convention on Tobacco Control (www.who.int/toh) to counteract these disease-promoting practices.

Internationally, a number of evidence-based reviews, guidelines and reports have been published about the need to address tobacco use and to treat tobacco dependence.[9-19] A summary of the recent Agency for Healthcare Research and Quality (AHRQ) Guideline on Treating Tobacco Use and Dependence highlights key issues and findings[20] (the full report is downloadable from www.ahcpr.gov/clinic/cpgsix.htm).

1. Tobacco dependence is a chronic condition that often requires repeated interventions to enhance quit rates and permanent abstinence.
2. Effective tobacco dependence treatments are available for patients who are willing to quit.

   - Treatments involving person-to-person contact (or by individual, group or proactive telephone counseling) are consistently effective, and their effectiveness increases with treatment intensity (e.g., minutes of contact).
   - Three types of counseling and behavioral therapies (problem-solving/skills training, intra-treatment social support and extra-treatment social support) were found to be especially effective and should be used for all patients attempting tobacco cessation.
   - In the absence of contraindications, all tobacco users should be offered drug treatments for their quit attempts. First-line options include nicotine replacement therapies (gum, inhaler, nasal spray or patch) and bupropion SR. Second-line options include clonidine and nortriptyline. For patients not ready to quit,

---

a. You can download the full report (html) from www.ash.org.uk/html/conduct/html/trustus.html, or the pdf format from tobaccofreekids.org/campaign/global/framework/docs/TrustUs.pdf.

motivational interventions can help them think about quitting and work toward a quit attempt in the future.

3. Tobacco dependence treatments are both clinically effective and cost effective. Health care systems should reimburse practitioners for tobacco counseling and pharmacological treatment of nicotine dependence.
4. Health care systems must develop the organizational infrastructure support in health care settings so that they can systematically identify all tobacco users and monitor the impact of treatment on patients over time.

Booklets for consumers, clinicians, health care administrators, insurers and purchasers accompany this guideline:

- *You Can Quit Smoking; Helping Smokers Quit* (consumer guide)
- *A Guide for Primary Care Clinicians. Smoking Cessation: Information for Specialists. Quick Reference Guide*
- *Smoking Cessation: A Systems Approach*
- *A Guide for Health Care Administrators, Insurance, Managed Care Organizations and Purchasers*

The economic implications of tobacco use on health are enormous.[21;22] Furthermore, the treatment of nicotine dependence is cost effective: $3,539 per life-year saved.[23;24] In contrast, the cost of three-vessel coronary bypass graft surgery (vs. medical management) is $12,000 per life-year saved, and the cost of the same surgery for mild and severe angina (vs. percutaneous coronary angioplasty) is $23,000 and $100,000 per life-year saved, respectively.[25] In spite of the far superior cost effectiveness of prevention, greater emphasis is still placed on treating tobacco-related diseases.

The data about cessation interventions generate conflicting interpretations. These commentaries range from pessimistic and realistic to optimistic. Pessimistic commentaries make the following conclusions:

- One behavioral intervention for smoking cessation is no better than another in the clinical context.[26;27]
- Behavioral interventions are of limited effectiveness.[28-30]
- A meta-analysis concluded that behavioral interventions are not cost effective.[31]
- Multimodal behavioral therapy actually averaged 2% greater reductions in smoking cessation, compared to the control groups. Little progress has been made in enhancing the smoking cessation rates over the past 40 years.[32]

Optimistic commentaries highlight studies on brief counseling that show higher quit rates (25%) than those for advice (5-10%).[33] Intensive treatments for outpatients and hospital inpatients have achieved long-term success rates ranging from 15-25%.[5;34]

Smokers with cardiorespiratory complications may have higher quit rates when they receive personalized interventions.[35-40]

AHRQ INTERVENTION DATA

Meta-analyses from the AHRQ guideline provide the most comprehensive and up-to-date information about interventions for tobacco cessation. This data is summarized in Tables 16.1-16.5. The percentage of attributable benefit is the impact that the intervention had over no treatment or a control group. The number needed to treat (NNT) is the number of patients that need to be treated to produce one favorable outcome. For more details about confidence intervals and references, consult the full publication.

Table 16.1. Impact of Screening System for Tobacco Users in Health Care Settings on Clinical Intervention and Abstinence Rates

Assessing Impact of No Screening versus Screening System on	Comparing % rates	% Attributable Benefit (95% CI)	Number Need to Treat
A. Clinical intervention rate	38.5 vs. 65.6	27.1 (19.8, 34.1)	4
B. Abstinence rate	3.1 vs 6.4	3.3 (-1.8, 8.5)	30

Clearly, screening systems for tobacco users are essential organizational supports for maintaining higher rates of interventions and for achieving higher abstinence rates.

Table 16.2. Impact of Clinical Interventions on Tobacco Abstinence Rates

Assessing Impact of	Comparing % rates	% Attributable Benefit (95% CI)	Number Need to Treat
No advice vs. physician advice	7.9 vs. 10.2	2.3 (0.4, 4.1)	43
No contact vs. < 3-minute session	10.9 vs. 13.4	2.5 (0.0, 5.2)	40
vs. 3- to 10-minute session	vs. 16.0	5.1 (1.9, 8.3)	20
vs. >10-minute session	vs. 22.1	11.2 (8.5, 13.8)	9
0-1 session vs. 2-3 sessions	12.4 vs. 16.3	3.9 (1.3, 6.6)	26
vs. 4-8 sessions	vs. 20.9	8.5 (5.7, 11.2)	12
vs. > 8 sessions	vs. 24.7	12.3 (8.6, 16.0)	8
No clinician vs. self-help	10.2 vs. 10.9	0.7 (-1.1, 2.5)	143
vs. nonphysician	vs. 15.8	5.6 (2.6, 8.6)	18
vs. physician	vs. 19.9	9.7 (3.5, 16.0)	10
No clinician vs. 1 clinician	10.8 vs. 18.3	7.5 (4.6, 10.3)	13
vs. 2 clinicians	vs. 23.6	12.8 (12.8, 17.9)	8
vs. > 3 clinicians	vs. 23.0	12.2 (9.2, 15.1)	8

Table 16.3. Impact of Different Methods on Tobacco Abstinence Rates

Assessing Impact of No Format vs.	Comparing % rates	% Attributable Benefit (95% CI)	Number Need to Treat
Self-help	10.8 vs. 12.3	1.5 (0.1, 2.8)	67
Proactive telephone counseling	vs. 13.1	2.3 (0.6, 4.0)	43
Group counseling	vs. 13.9	3.1 (0.8, 5.3)	32
Individual counseling	vs. 16.8	6.0 (3.9, 8.3)	17
One format	10.8 vs. 15.1	4.3 (2.0, 6.6)	23
Two format	vs. 18.5	7.7 (5.0, 10.3)	13
Three format	vs. 23.2	12.4 (9.1, 15.8)	8
One type of self-help	14.3 vs. 14.4	0.1 (-1.4, 1.6)	1000
Two or more types of self-help	vs. 15.7	1.4 (-2.0, 4.9)	71

Overall, a multimodal, multimethod and interdisciplinary approach is clearly more effective than relying on one single intervention or discipline.

Table 16.4. Impact of Behavioral Methods on Tobacco Abstinence Rates

Assessing Impact of No Counseling vs.	Comparing % rates	% Attributable Benefit (95% CI)	Number Need to Treat
Intratreatment social support	11.2 vs. 14.4	3.2 (1.1, 5.3)	31
Extra-treatment support	vs. 16.2	5.0 (0.6, 9.4)	20
General problem solving	vs. 16.2	5.0 (2.8, 7.3)	20
Other aversive smoking	vs. 17.7	6.5 (0.0, 13.7)	15
Rapid smoking	vs. 19.9	8.7 (0.0, 17.8)	11

The treatment labels for these behavioral methods are nonspecific and include a variety of interventions. The AHRQ guideline does not address the interactive effects of using different behavioral methods. As a complement to these behavioral methods, vigorous exercise was found to boost quit rates in women.[41]

SPECIFIC ISSUES

A number of factors increase and decrease the prospects of long-term abstinence of tobacco use. Tobacco users who are motivated to quit, ready to quit within a month period, confident in their ability to quit and/or have a social supportive network are more likely to achieve long-term abstinence. Conversely, tobacco users with high nicotine dependence, a history of psychiatric comorbidity and high stress levels are less likely to achieve long-term abstinence.

Behavioral interventions are an integral part of tobacco cessation programs. In addition, most patients need some assistance in overcoming their nicotine dependence. The five A's model, as outlined in the AHRQ guideline, can be summarized as follows:

1. Ask about tobacco use
2. Advise to quit
3. Assess willingness to quit
4. Assist in quit attempt
5. Arrange follow-up

This basic, practical model is a good initial step, but the guideline does not provide practitioners with adequate guidance in how to help patients at follow-up visits or how to engage patients in the change process who are not ready to quit. Part 16B presents how practitioners can learn ways of addressing these clinical challenges.

DRUG TREATMENT OF NICOTINE DEPENDENCE

High levels of nicotine dependence enhance the difficulty of quitting.[42;43] Heavy smokers are half as likely to quit smoking with self-help interventions than are lighter smokers.[44] Withdrawal symptoms may cause a relapse rate of 25-60%; patients relapse most frequently within the first six months (particularly within the first few days or weeks) after quitting.[45] You can use the Fagerström Tolerance Questionnaire (see Table 16.5) to estimate the degree of nicotine dependence of your patients.[44;46]

Table 16.5. Fagerström Test[46]

Questions	Answers	Points
A. How soon after you wake do you smoke your first cigarette?	Within 5 minutes	3
	6-30 minutes	2
	31-60 minutes	1
	After 60 minutes	0
B. Do you find it difficult to refrain from smoking in places where it is forbidden, e.g., at the library, in church, at the theater?	Yes	1
	No	0
C. Which cigarette would you hate to give up most?	First in A.M.	1
	All others	0
D. How many cigarettes a day do you smoke?	10 or less	0
	11-20	1
	21-30	2
	31 or more	3
E. Do you smoke more frequently during the first hours after waking than during the rest of the day?	Yes	1
	No	0
F. Do you smoke if you are so ill that you are in bed most of the day?	Yes	1
	No	0

Reproduced with permission.

Clinically, you can estimate an increased risk for relapse if patients:

- Have had marked withdrawal symptoms on previous quit attempts
- Smoke more than 25 cigarettes a day
- Have difficulty refraining from smoking in restricted areas
- Smoke more in the morning
- Smoke their first cigarette soon after waking (within 30 minutes)
- Smoke when bedridden with illness
- Inhale more deeply[47-49]

If you score four points or more on this test, you may very well be addicted to nicotine. Scores of more than six generally are interpreted as indicating a high degree of dependence, with a more severe withdrawal syndrome, greater difficulty in quitting, and possibly the need for higher doses of medication. The option of using nicotine replacement therapy (gum and/or patch and/or inhaler) to treat the withdrawal syndrome can complement and enhance the outcome of using behavioral approaches.

The typical smoker absorbs about 1-3 mg of nicotine per cigarette, totaling 20-40 mg for each pack per day. To avert significant withdrawal symptoms, patients need at least 50% of their usual amount of nicotine. Nicotine replacement therapy (NRT) improved treatment outcome.[32;44;46;49-57] A meta-analysis of the benefits of nicotine replacement therapy concluded that the patch and chewing gum increased smoking cessation rates 9% and 6%, respectively, compared to controls.[58] NRT has uncertain efficacy in primary care, however, when only minimal behavioral support is provided.[59]

Drug treatment of nicotine dependency helps to ease the withdrawal symptoms and to enhance tobacco cessation rates.[60] A comparison of the impact of different drug treatments for nicotine treatment is summarized in Table 16.6.

Table 16.6. Impact of Pharmacotherapy on Tobacco Abstinence Rates

Assessing Impact Placebo vs.	Comparing % rates	% Attributable Benefit (95% CI)	Number Need to Treat
Nicotine gum	17.1 vs. 23.7	6.6 (3.5, 9.6)	15
Nicotine inhaler	10.5 vs. 22.8	12.3 (5.9, 18.7)	8
Nicotine spray	13.9 vs. 30.5	16.6 (7.9, 25.3)	6
Nicotine patch	10.0 vs. 17.7	7.7 (6.0, 9.5)	13
Over-the-counter patch*	6.7 vs. 11.8	5.1 (0.8, 4.2)	20
One NRT vs. two NRTs	17.4 vs. 28.6	11.2 (4.3, 18.0)	9
Bupropion SR	17.3 vs. 30.5	13.2 (5.9, 20.5)	8
Second-line treatment options			
Clonidine	13.9 vs. 25.6	11.7 (3.8, 19.7)	9
Noritriptyline	11.7 vs. 30.1	18.4 (6.4, 29.9)	5

*This data is from one study only [61]

NRT Cardiovascular Risks and Drug Dependency

The nicotine patch does not increase the rate of acute cardiovascular events,[62-64] even in patients who smoke on the patch.[65] The Lung Health Study on chronic obstructive pulmonary disease, however, found that 38% of women and 30% of men were still using nicotine gum at 12 months.[66] With free access to nicotine gum, 15-20% of successful abstainers will continue to come for a year or longer.[67] NRT is much less harmful than tobacco use.[68]

Pharmacological Treatment of Tobacco Use in Pregnancy

Pregnant smokers should be encouraged to quit first without pharmacological treatment. Drug treatments may be used in pregnancy and during lactation, if the benefits of tobacco abstinence outweigh the risk of treatment and continued tobacco use. The FDA classification for using these drugs in pregnancy are listed below: Class A (controlled studies demonstrate remote risk) through Class D (some human fetal risk, but the benefits must outweigh the risks), and Class X (drugs are contraindicated in pregnancy).

Class A	None identified yet
Class B	Bupropion SR
Class C	Nicotine patch, clonidine
Class D	Nicotine gum/inhaler/spray, noritriptyline*

*Noritriptyline has been associated with a few case reports of possible limb reduction anomalies.

Nicotine Gum

Nicotine gum improves the smoking cessation rate by approximately 40-60%, compared to control groups at a year follow-up. The dose of the nicotine gum is 2 or 4 mg, of which 50% is absorbed through the mouth. The higher dose gum is more effective with highly dependent smokers. Patients slowly chew the gum until they notice a tingling sensation or peppery taste in their mouth, and then they place the gum between their cheek and gums. After this sensation resolves, patients can start chewing again and go through the same cycle. Chewing too fast can release nicotine rapidly and cause side effects: mouth soreness, hiccups, dyspepsia and jaw ache. The gum can be used up to 12 weeks, with no more than 24 pieces per day. As a guideline, patients can chew a piece of gum every one to two hours for the first six weeks, every two to four hours for the next three weeks and then every four to eight hours for the next three weeks. Adherence to appropriate gum usage is associated with higher smoking cessation rates.[26]

Nicotine Inhaler

Patients can take 6-16 inhalations per day for up to six months, with the goal of gradually decreasing the number of inhalations per day over several weeks.[69;70] Each inhalation delivers 4 mg of nicotine. Side effects include mouth and throat irritation (40%), coughing (32%) and rhinitis (32%); these symptoms decline with continued use.

Patients should avoid drinking and eating 15 minutes before and after each inhalation. The inhaler has the advantage of giving quitters a substitute for the hand-to-mouth behavior of smoking. This method is most similar to the gum, as the inhaler delivers nicotine into the mouth whether or not the patient inhales deeply. In cold weather (below 40^B F), patients need to know that the inhaler does not work well.

Nicotine Patch

These patches come in different dose regimens according to the manufacturer's specifications. The duration of treatment is usually eight weeks, with gradual decrements in the dose regimen every two to six weeks. Treatment of longer than eight weeks does not improve the quit rate; 16- and 24-hour patches work equally as well. Patients may experience mild irritation at the application site of the patch and dizziness as side effects. The patches at least doubled the success rate of other behavioral therapies.[71;72] Half of all users developed local skin reactions. Rotating patch sites and use of topical steroids (1% hydrocortisone cream) may reduce these reactions, but 5% of patients discontinue the patch due to the skin reaction.

Nicotine Spray

With their head tilted slightly back, patients can spray 0.5 mg of nicotine into each nostril, but without inhaling it. They can use 1 to 2 doses per hour (a minimum of 8 and a maximum of 40 doses per day) for three to six months. Users (94%) report moderate to severe nasal irritation in the first two days, which reduces in severity, but 84% still report some irritation after three weeks. The nasal spray method delivers nicotine more quickly than the gum, patch or inhaler but less rapidly than cigarettes. This may explain why 15-20% of patients use the spray for more than six months and 5% use the spray at higher doses than recommended.

Bupropion SR

Bupropion decreases a person's urge to smoke and is effective in helping nondepressed smokers to quit.[73] In a double-blind controlled trial, the rates of smoking cessation at seven weeks were 19.0% in the placebo group, 28.8% in the 100-mg group, 38.6% in the 150-mg group, and 44.2% in the 300-mg group (p < 0.001). At one year, the respective rates were 12.4%, 19.6%, 22.9% and 23.1%. The rates for the 150-mg group (p = 0.02) and the 300-mg group (p = 0.01)—but not the 100-mg group (p = 0.09)—were significantly better than those for the placebo group.[74]

Clonidine

The FDA has not yet approved clonidine for smoking cessation, but it appears an effective treatment. A clear dose-response has not been established. The dose range used in trial is 0.15-0.75 mg per day, or 0.1-0.2 mg/day transdermally (TTS). This initial dose is 0.1 mg twice a day, or 0.1 mg TTS, increasing by 0.1 mg per week, if needed. Treatment may be continued for 3 to 10 weeks. Side effects include dry mouth (40%), drowsiness (33%), constipation (10%), sedation (10%; caution is needed while driving and using machinery) and reduced blood pressure that needs monitoring. Rebound hypertension, agitation, confusion and tremor may occur if this drug is not stopped after two to four days.

Noritriptyline

The FDA has not yet approved noritriptyline for smoking cessation, but it appears an effective treatment. The initial dose is 25 mg per day, increasing gradually to 75-100 mg for up to 12 weeks. This treatment should be started 10-28 days before the quit date. Side effects include sedation (caution is needed while driving and using machinery), dry mouth (64-78%), light-headedness (49%), shaky hands (23%), blurred vision (16%) and urinary retention. Noritriptyline should be used with caution in cardiovascular disease and in patients at risk for suicide because of its toxicity and overdose effects in causing arrhythmias.

Pharmacological and Behavioral Interventions

A question exists whether brief advice improves the outcome of NRT.[26;27] Better outcomes are achieved when nicotine gum is combined with intensive behavioral treatment.[59] Patients, however, use less gum in primary care than in clinic-based programs.[75] The difference in success rates between primary care and clinic-based programs may relate to the improved adherence to NRT rather than the independent effect of behavioral interventions.[26] Such an interpretation of this data only heightens the need to develop more effective behavioral interventions that have an additive or synergistic effect on the beneficial impact of NRT.

THE NEED FOR INNOVATION, IMPROVISATION AND INTEGRATION

As previously noted, the analysis of the smoking cessation data provides a spectrum of different commentaries that span the pessimistic-optimistic continuum. Meta-analyses provide information on aggregate performance about smoking interventions but do not inform you about best practices. Published articles and guidelines do not provide enough information to understand what makes up the different categories of behavioral interventions. Furthermore, these different behavioral methods contain multiple interventions, so it becomes increasingly difficult to identify which aspects of these interventions work best for a particular patient. Thus, guidelines cannot inform you about which are the best practices for particular situations or which specific interventions are best for individual patients.

The AHRQ guideline presents the results of these meta-analyses in isolation from one another, consonant with the reductionistic, scientific method. In contrast, tobacco cessation programs must be integrated into complex systems of health care delivery. Furthermore, these programs must use multimodal, multimethod and interdisciplinary approaches in ways that have additive and synergistic effects on organizations, practitioners and patients. Health care settings must implement and improve complex interventions over time and monitor their impact on helping patients change over time.

These interventions need to address both the organizational processes of implementing tobacco cessation programs but also enhance the potency of behavioral interventions that work in additive or synergistic ways with the drug treatment of nicotine dependence.

In other words, health care systems and settings must innovate, improvise and monitor the impact of using both organizational and behavioral interventions well beyond the duration of randomized controlled trials. No guideline can provide hard evidence on how to do this.

The AHRQ smoking guideline predominantly emphasizes the use of the five A's model: a brief health education and advice approach. The guideline also describes a motivational approach to smoking cessation in terms of risks, relevance, rewards and repetition, but without giving sufficient details about how to implement this approach into practice.[7] The Smokescreen program is another example of such a motivational approach that attempts to enhance patients' readiness to quit smoking.[76] Such an approach to smoking cessation is appropriate when advice-giving approaches do not work.[77] But these approaches are not well developed in terms of helping patients move from not thinking about quitting to thinking about it. Part 16B addresses this issue, and the Web site www.MotivateHealthyHabits.com has a videostreamed demonstration in how to do this.

YOUR SUMMARY

Reflect: write a summary about what you have learned that was new for you.

_____

_____

_____

_____

_____

_____

_____

_____

_____

_____

_____

_____

_____

_____

_____

_____

_____

_____
_____
_____
_____
_____
_____

Enhance: *write down your ideas about how your new learning could improve your interactions with patients. Add your notes to your learning portfolio.*

_____
_____
_____
_____
_____
_____
_____
_____
_____
_____
_____
_____
_____

REFERENCES

1. American Academy of Family Physicians. AAFP Stop Smoking Program: Patient stop smoking guide. American Academy of Family Physicians; 1987

2. National Heart Lung and Blood Institute, American Association for Respiratory Care. How you can help patients stop smoking: Opportunities for respiratory care practitioners. U.S. Department of Health and Human Services; 1989

3. National Heart Lung and Blood Institute, The American Lung Association, and The American Thoracic Society. Clinical opportunities for smoking intervention: A guide for the busy physician [NIH Publication No. 92-2178]. 1992. Bethesda, MD: U.S. Department of Health and Human Services.

4. National Cancer Institute. How to help your patients stop smoking: A National Cancer Institute manual for physicians [NIH Publication No. 89-3064]. 1989. Bethesda, MD: National Institutes of Health.

5. Orleans CT, Glynn TJ, Manley MW, et al. Minimal-contact quit smoking strategies for medical settings. In: Orleans CT, Slade J, eds. Nicotine addiction: Principles and management. New York: Oxford University Press; 1993: 181-220

6. Glynn TJ, Manley MW. How to help your patients stop smoking: A National Cancer Institute Manual for Physicians [NIH Publication No. 89-3064]. Bethesda, MD: U.S. Department of Health and Human Services; 1989

7. The Smoking Cessation Clinical Practice Guideline Panel and Staff. The Agency for Health Care Policy and Research Smoking Cessation Clinical Practice Guideline. Journal of the American Medical Association 1996;275: 1270-1280

8. World Health Organization. Investing in health research and development. Geneva: World Health Organization; 1996

9. Tobacco Advisory Group, Royal College of Physicians. Nicotine addiction in Britain. 2000. London, Royal College of Physicians.

10. Peto R, Lopez A. Future worldwide health effects of current smoking patterns. In: Koop CE, Pearson CE, Schwarz MR, eds. Critical issues in global health. San Francisco: Jossey-Bass; 2000:

11. World Health Organization, Europe. Partnership to reduce tobacco dependence. 2000. Copenhagen, World Health Organization.
   12. West R, McNeill A, Raw M. Smoking cessation guidelines for health professionals: An update. Health Education Authority. Thorax 2000;55: 987-999

13. World Health Organization. Conclusions of conference on the regulation of tobacco dependence treatment products. 1999. Copenhagen, World Health Organization.
   14. Lancaster T, Stead L, Silagy C, et al. Effectiveness of interventions to help people stop smoking: Findings from the Cochrane Library [see comments]. British Medical Journal 2000;321: 355-358

15. Agence National d'Accreditation et d'Evaluation en Sante. Consensus Conference on Smoking Cessation (English summary by Jacques Le Houezec). 1999. Paris, ANAES.
   16. The Cochrane Collaboration. Cochrane Database of Systematic Reviews. 1999. The Cochrane Library.
   17. British Thoracic Society. Smoking cessation guidelines and their cost-effectiveness. Thorax 1998;53: S1-S38

18. Department of Health and Human Services. The health consequences of smoking: Nicotine addiction: A report of the Surgeon General. 88-8406. 1988. Atlanta: US Department of Health and Human Services. Public Health Service, Centers for Disease Control, Center for Chronic Disease Prevention and Health Promotion. Office of Smoking and Health. DHHS Publication No. (PHS) (CDC) 88-8406

19. American Medical Association. American Medical Association guidelines for the diagnosis and treatment of nicotine dependence: how to help patients stop smoking. 1994. Washington, DC: American Medical Association

20. Fiore MC, Bailey WC, Cohen SJ, et al. Treating tobacco use and dependence. Clinical Practice Guideline 2000;343: 1772-1777

21. World Bank. Curbing the epidemic. Governments and the economics of tobacco control. 1999. Washington, DC: World Bank

22. Manning WG, Keeler EB, Newhouse JP, et al. The costs of poor health habits. Cambridge, MA: Harvard University Press; 1991

23. Parrott S, Godfrey C, Raw M, et al. Guidance for commissioners on the cost effectiveness of smoking cessation interventions. Health Educational Authority. Thorax 1998;53 Suppl 5 Pt 2: S1-38

24. Cromwell J, Bartosch WJ, Fiore MC, et al. Cost-effectiveness of the clinical practice recommendations in the AHCPR guideline for smoking cessation. Journal of the American Medical Association 1997;278: 1759-1766

25. Wong JB, Sonnenberg FA, Salem DN, et al. Myocardial revascularization for chronic stable angina: Analysis of the role of percutaneous transluminal coronary angioplasty based on data available in 1989. Annals of Internal Medicine 1990;113: 852-871

26. Lichtenstein E, Glasgow RE. Smoking cessation: What have we learned over the past decade? Journal of Consulting and Clinical Psychology 1992;60: 518-527

27. Hajek P. Current issues in behavioral and pharmacological approaches to smoking cessation. Addictive Behaviors 1996;21: 699-707

28. Raw M. The treatment of cigarette dependence. In: Israel Y, Glaser FB, Kalant H, et al., eds. Research advances in alcohol and drug problems, vol. 4. New York: Plenum Press; 1978: 441-485

29. Lichtenstein E. The smoking problem: A behavioral perspective. Journal of Consulting and Clinical Psychology 1982;50: 804-819

30. Jarvis M. Helping smokers give up. In: Pearce S, Wardle J, eds. The practice of behavioral medicine. London: BPS Books; 1989: 284-305

31. Law M, Tang JL. An analysis of the effectiveness of interventions intended to help people stop smoking. Archives of Internal Medicine 1995;155: 1933-1941

32. Shiffman S. Smoking cessation treatment: Any progress? Journal of Consulting and Clinical Psychology 1993;61: 718-722

33. Glynn TJ. Relative effectiveness of physician-initiated smoking cessation programs. Cancer Bulletin 1988;40: 359-364

34. Orleans CT. Treating nicotine dependence in medical settings: A stepped-care model. In: Orleans CT, Slade J, eds. Nicotine addiction: Principles and management. New York: Oxford University Press; 1993: 145-161

35. Richmond RL, Webster IW. A smoking cessation programme for use in general practice. Medical Journal of Australia 1985;142: 190-194

36. Windsor RA, Cutter G, Morris J, et al. The effectiveness of smoking cessation methods for smokers in public health maternity clinics: A randomized trial. American Journal of Public Health 1985;75: 1389-1392

37. Risser NL, Belcher DW. Adding spirometry, carbon monoxide, and pulmonary symptom results to smoking cessation counseling: A randomized trial. Journal of General Internal Medicine 1990;5: 16-22

38. Fisher EB, Jr., Haire-Joshu D, Morgan GD, et al. Smoking and smoking cessation. American Review of Respiratory Disease 1990;142: 702-720

39. Ockene J, Kristeller JL, Goldberg R, et al. Smoking cessation and severity of disease: The Coronary Artery Smoking Intervention Study. Health Psychology 1992;11: 119-126

40. Gritz ER, Kristeller J, Burns DM. Treating nicotine addiction in high-risk groups and patients with medical co-morbidity. In: Orleans CT, Slade J, eds. Nicotine addiction: Principles and management. New York: Oxford University Press; 1993:279-309

41. Marcus BH, Albrecht AE, King TK, et al. The efficacy of exercise as an aid for smoking cessation in women: A randomized controlled trial [see comments]. Archives of Internal Medicine 1999;159: 1229-1234

42. Shiffman S. Tobacco "chippers": Individual differences in tobacco dependence. Psychopharmacology 1989;97: 539-547

43. Pinto RP, Abrams DB, Monti PM, et al. Nicotine dependence and likelihood of quitting smoking. Addictive Behaviors 1987;12: 371-374

44. Pomerleau CS, Pomerleau OF, Majchrzak MJ, et al. Relationship between nicotine tolerance questionnaire scores and plasma cotinine. Addictive Behaviors 1990;15: 73-80

45. Brandon TH, Tiffany ST, Obremski KM, et al. Postcessation cigarette use: The process of relapse. Addictive Behaviors 1990;15: 105-114

46. Heatherton TF, Kozlowski LT, Frecker RC, et al. The Fagerström Test for Nicotine Dependence: A revision of the Fagerström Tolerance Questionnaire. British Journal of Addiction 1991;86(9): 1119-1127

47. Hughes JR, Hatsukami DK, Pickens RW, et al. Consistency of the tobacco withdrawal syndrome. Addictive Behaviors 1984;9: 409-412

48. Fagerström KO. Effects of nicotine chewing gum and follow-up appointments in physician-based smoking cessation. Preventive Medicine 1984;13: 517-527

49. Killen JD, Fortmann SP, Telch MJ. Are heavy smokers different from light smokers? A comparison after 48 hours without cigarettes. Journal of the American Medical Association 1988;260: 1581-1585

50. Killen JD, Fortmann SP. Role of nicotine dependence in smoking relapse: Results from a prospective study using population-based recruitment methodology. International Journal of Behavioral Medicine 1994;1: 320-334

51. Hughes JR. Combined psychological and nicotine gum treatment for smoking: A critical review. Journal of Substance Abuse 1991;3: 337-350

52. Fagerström KO, Schneider NG. Measuring nicotine dependence: A review of the Fagerström Tolerance Questionnaire. Journal of Behavioral Medicine 1989;12: 159-182

53. Abrams DB, Follick MJ, Biener L, et al. Saliva cotinine as a measure of smoking status in field settings. American Journal of Public Health 1987;77: 846-848

54. Niaura R, Goldstein M, Abrams D. A bioinformational systems perspective on tobacco dependence. British Journal of Addiction 1991;86: 593-597

55. Pomerleau OF, Collins AC, Shiffman S, et al. Why some people smoke and others do not: New perspectives. Journal of Consulting and Clinical Psychology 1993;61: 723-731

56. Killen JD, Fortmann SP, Kraemer HC, et al. Who will relapse? Symptoms of nicotine dependence predict long-term relapse after smoking cessation. Journal of Consulting and Clinical Psychology 1992;60: 797-801

57. Pomerleau OF, Rosecrans J. Neuroregulatory effects of nicotine. Psychoneuroendocrinology 1989;14: 407-423

58. Tang JL, Law M, Wald N. How effective is nicotine replacement therapy in helping people to stop smoking? British Medical Journal 1994;308: 21-26

59. Lam W, Sze PC, Sacks HS, et al. Meta-analysis of randomised controlled trials of nicotine chewing gum. Lancet 1987;2: 27-30

60. Fiore MC, Jorenby DE, Baker TB, et al. Tobacco dependence and the nicotine patch: Clinical guidelines for effective care. Journal of the American Medical Association 1992;268: 2687-2694

61. Leischow SJ, Muramoto ML, Cook G, et al. OTC nicotine patches: Effectiveness alone and with brief physician intervention. American Journal of Health Behavior 1999;23: 61-69

62. Benowitz NL, Gourlay SG. Cardiovascular toxicity of nicotine: Implications for nicotine replacement therapy. Journal of American College Cardiology 1997;29: 1422-1431

63. Joseph AM, Norman SM, Ferry LH, et al. The safety of transdermal nicotine as an aid to smoking cessation in patients with cardiac disease. New England Journal of Medicine 1996;335: 1792-1798

64. Mahmarian JJ, Moye LA, Nasser GA, et al. Nicotine patch therapy in smoking cessation reduces the extent of exercise-induced myocardial ischemia. Journal of American College Cardiology 1997;30: 125-130

65. Working Group for the Study of Transdermal Nicotine in Patients with Coronary Artery Disease. Nicotine replacement therapy for patients with coronary artery disease. Archives of Internal Medicine 1994;154: 989-995

66. Nides MA, Rakos RF, Gonzales D, et al. Predictors of initial smoking cessation and relapse through the first 2 years of the Lung Health Study. Journal of Consulting and Clinical Psychology 1995;63: 60-69

67. Hajek P, Jackson P, Belcher M. Long-term use of nicotine chewing gum. Occurrence, determinants, and effect on weight gain. Journal of the American Medical Association 1988;260: 1593-1596

68. Henningfield JE. Nicotine medications for smoking cessation. New England Journal of Medicine 1995;333: 1196-1203

69. Hjalmarson A, Franzon M, Westin A, et al. Effect of nicotine nasal spray on smoking cessation. Archives of Internal Medicine 1994;154: 2567-2572

70. Sutherland G, Stapleton JA, Russell MAH, et al. Randomised controlled trial of nasal nicotine spray in smoking cessation. Lancet 1992;340: 324-329

71. Fiore MC, Smith SS, Jorenby DE, et al. The effectiveness of the nicotine patch for smoking cessation: A meta-analysis. Journal of the American Medical Association 1994;271: 1940-1947

72. Silagy C, Mant D, Fowler G, et al. Meta-analysis on efficacy of nicotine replacement therapies in smoking cessation. Lancet 1994;343: 139-142

73. Benowitz NL. Treating tobacco addiction—nicotine or no nicotine? New England Journal of Medicine 1997;337: 1230-1231

74. Hurt RD, Sachs DP, Glover ED, et al. A comparison of sustained-release bupropion and placebo for smoking cessation [see comments]. New England Journal of Medicine 1997;337: 1195-1202

75. Jackson PH, Stapleton JA, Russell MA, et al. Nicotine gum use and outcome in a general practitioner intervention against smoking. ddictive Behaviors 1989;14: 335-341

76. Richmond R. Educating medical students about tobacco: Teachers' manual and students' handouts. In: Richmond R, ed. Educating medical students about tobacco: Planning and implementation. Paris, France: Tobacco Prevention Section, Int. Union Against Tuberculosis and Lung Diseases; 1996: 15-59

77. Botelho RJ. When "quit smoking" advice doesn't work: Use motivational approaches. In: Richmond R, ed. Educating medical students about tobacco: Planning and implementation. Paris, France: Tobacco Prevention Section, Int. Union Against Tuberculosis and Lung Disease; 1996: 61-84

CHAPTER 16 Part B

HELPING RESISTANT SMOKERS QUIT

FOR REFLECTION

How can you deal with a patient who does not respond to quit-smoking advice?

OVERVIEW

Health education and advice approaches prepare you to help 10-20% of smokers who are ready to quit. Most smoking cessation programs, however, do not adequately address how to deal with resistant, ambivalent or indifferent smokers. This chapter helps you learn how to motivate such patients to change over time. It discusses how the six-step approach can be used to motivate patients in different stages of the change process, and provides examples of specific questions you can use with your patients to help them quit smoking

In developing new skills, it helps to start with less severe problems: in this case, smokers who are in the contemplation or preparation stage. After developing some basic skills, you can then begin to work with smokers who are in the precontemplation stage. Although these patients are more challenging to work with, they provide the best opportunities for understanding the change process, even though your chances of short-term success is less than with smokers who are in the contemplation or preparation stage.

STEP 1: BUILDING PARTNERSHIPS

The three component parts of this step are crucial for establishing effective partnerships with patients. This process provides the foundation for helping patients to change.

DEVELOP EMPATHY

Communication Skills for Developing Empathy	
Use open-ended questions	*"How does smoking help you?"*
Use reflective listening	*"So, smoking helps you relax and deal with stressful situations."*
Paraphrase	*"And smoking helps soothe your stress and anger away?"*
Validate feelings	*"I can understand why you would feel angry in those situations."*
Normalize behaviors	*"It's normal to want those angry feelings to go away."*
Affirm strengths	*"It takes courage to keep your angry feelings under control."*
Use probing questions	*"How could you control your angry feelings without smoking?"*

USE RELATIONAL SKILLS EFFECTIVELY

Put the Patient in the One-up Position: *"Tell me what convinces you that you will not become addicted to smoking." "What makes you think that you could give up any time you wanted?" "What might convince you to quit now?"*
Take the One-Down Position with a Patient: *"I am not sure (a) what it would take to convince you about the risk of heart disease, (b) what it would take to convince you about the need to quit."*

CLARIFY ROLES AND RESPONSIBILITIES

Clarifying Your Roles
Clarify your prevention role: *"Smoking can damage your health without causing any symptoms. Can I help you protect your health from further damage?"* Clarify the difference between a motivational role (helping patients consider change) and an action-oriented role (treating nicotine addiction): *"I can work with you to help you think more about quitting and increase your chance of setting a quit date [motivational role]."* Or *"Nicotine replacement treatments increase your chance of quitting for good, and I advise you to use one when you set your quit date [fix-it role]."*

Clarifying Your Responsibility
"I'll tell you what I know about the risks and harmful effects related to nicotine addiction and smoking, but we may still see the benefits, risks and harm of smoking differently. If you are willing to work with me on how we see things differently, I may be able to help you increase your motivation to quit. Is that okay?"

STEP 2: NEGOTIATING AN AGENDA

Agenda-setting skills are particularly important because some patients are reluctant or ambivalent about discussing their smoking habit. It is important for you to be sensitive when approaching these patients to avoid evoking undue defensiveness, negative emotions (e.g., anger, irritation), and resistance. The questions and comments in the following tables (prevention- and problem-focused approaches) can help you prevent such reactions from patients.

PREVENTION-FOCUSED APPROACH

This approach is used when patients who do not have any medical problems caused by their tobacco use present with complaints.

Consent-gaining Direct Questions
About smoking: *"I would like to see if there is anything you can do to improve your health. Is it all right to talk about your smoking?"* (Let patient respond. You can then ask,) *"Is there anything that you want to discuss about your smoking, or anything else?"*
About quitting: *"I'd like to talk about whether you are interested in quitting. Is that all right?"* (Let patient respond. You can then ask,) *"Is there anything that you want to discuss about your smoking, or anything else?"*

Leading Questions
"Do you want to continue smoking, at least for the time being?"   *"Would you consider yourself a die-hard smoker?"*   *"Do you think that you will continue smoking for the rest of your life?"*

Prefacing Statements Followed by Challenging Questions
"I would like to talk to you about your smoking in ways that may help you think about it differently. Is that okay?" (Choose any of the following.)   *"Tobacco companies are trying to control your behavior by selling you images about smoking. What are those images? Which of them are important to you? (Let patient respond.) In what way is that image more important to you than your health?"*   *"Tobacco companies benefit if you let yourself become addicted to nicotine. What do you think about what the tobacco industry is trying to do to you?"*

Prefacing Statements Focusing on Lack of Concern about Consequences
"Most young people feel that they can give up smoking any time they want to, and certainly before they damage their health. What do you think?"
"Research shows that most young people think that they can give up smoking, but five years later they have become addicted to nicotine and regret that they ever started smoking. What do you think about this research?"
"Some people are not concerned about how smoking affects their health. What about you?"
"Many people believe that the complications from smoking won't happen to them. This is a normal response because people don't like to think that they are deliberately harming themselves. What do you think?"
"Some people get fed up with people telling them to quit smoking. What has your experience been?"

PROBLEM-FOCUSED APPROACH

Prefacing Statements Followed by Questions
"Smoking can prevent your ulcers [or any other smoking-related problem] from healing." (Pause, let patient respond, and if necessary ask:) *"Did you know that?"* (Let patient respond.)
"I think we need to talk about both your ulcer and your smoking. Is that okay?"
"Most people have tried to quit smoking and experienced withdrawal symptoms. Have you experienced any withdrawal symptoms?"

Exploratory Questions
Open-ended, linear questions: *"How has your bronchitis affected your smoking?"* Or *"How has your smoking affected your bronchitis?"*
Closed-ended, linear questions: *"Has your chest infection affected how much you smoke?"* *"Is smoking affecting your chest infection?"* *"Does your smoking make your cough worse?"* *"Has your cough made you feel like cutting down on your smoking?"*
Circular questions: *"What concerns do your spouse and children have about how smoking affects your health?"*

STEP 3: ASSESSING RESISTANCE AND MOTIVATION

Consider developing your skills to assess patients' readiness to change and how to use a decision balance, in addition to other options listed. In addition to conducting a motivational assessment, you may also have to address the medical complications caused by tobacco use.

MOTIVATIONAL ASSESSMENT

Readiness to Change—Direct Questions
"Where are you in terms of your smoking? Let me explain." (Select any of the following questions, or use them in any sequence that seems compatible with your impression of your patient.) *"Are you interested at all in quitting?"* Or *"Are you not interested in quitting?"* Or *"Are you thinking about quitting smoking?"* Or *"Are you ready to quit anytime soon?"* (Depending on the patient's response, you may proceed with A negative response:) *"I hear that you are not interested in giving up smoking at the moment. Would you mind sharing with me why you don't want to quit?"* (Let patient respond. If patient gives nonverbal indications that he or she does mind, then proceed.) *"Would you rather leave it for a later time?"* (An unsure response:) *"When will you be ready to think more about a quit date?"* (An affirmative response) *"Are you ready to set a quit date?"*
Readiness to Change—Indirect Questions
(Select any one or more of the following:) *"Do you have any regrets about starting smoking?"* *"What do you think might convince you to quit?"* *"Do you think that you will ever stop smoking?"* *"When might you give up smoking?"* *"What, if anything, would help you to decide to quit smoking?"*

Use a Decision Balance with the Patient

The decision balance is considered an essential component of the motivational assessment. Depending on patients' readiness to change, you can provide a stage-specific rationale to them about why you are using it. This process can increase patient cooperativeness in completing a decision balance, particularly for those patients in precontemplation.

Specific Rationale and Gaining Consent to Use the Decision Balance
Precontemplation: *"You just told me that you were not interested in quitting. Would you mind if we did a decision balance together? It can help me better understand why you don't want to quit."* *"You just told me that this is not a good time for you to think about quitting. Would you mind if we did a decision balance together? This may help you think about when it might be a good time to think about quitting."*
Contemplation: *"You told me that you're thinking about quitting. Would you mind if we did a decision balance together? It may help you think more about whether to quit or not."*
Preparation: *"You're thinking about quitting soon. If we did a decision balance together, it could help you set a quit date. Is that okay?"*
Action: *"You are ready to set a date to change. If we did a decision balance together, it could help you prevent a relapse after you quit smoking."*

After providing a rationale for using a decision balance, you can then show the patient what it looks like. You can use a decision balance form or draw one out for the patient.

Sharing the Decision Balance with the Patient
"Let me show you what a decision balance looks like. As we use the decision balance, it can help you better understand your reasons to smoke and your reasons to quit. But first [pointing to the top of the left column]*, what do you like about smoking cigarettes? I would like to make a note of what you say. Is that okay? You can keep this decision balance to use when you go home if you like."*

After gaining the patient's cooperation in doing this task, you can ask one or more questions from each quadrant in the sequence suggested below.

To Quit or Not to Quit: That Is the Question	
1. Benefits of smoking *"What do you like about smoking? And what else?"*	2. Concerns about smoking *"What concerns you about your smoking?"* *"What concerns do others have about your smoking?"*
3. Concerns about quitting *"What concerns do you have if you were to quit?"* *"What effects would quitting have on you?"*	4. Benefits of quitting *"How do you think your health would improve if you were to quit?"* *"In what ways would you benefit from quitting?"*

The primary intent of the assessment is not to help patients decide whether to quit, but to identify benefits and concerns about smoking and quitting without implying they should quit smoking. This approach can give you an insight into the reasons patients smoke in spite of the associated risks and harm. The table below is an example of a patient's response to a practitioner using the decision balance. These responses can help you individualize how to use motivational interventions with a patient; examples of these interventions are provided in subsequent tables.

Reasons to smoke (Cons)	Reasons to change (Pros)
1. Benefits of smoking	2. Concerns about smoking
Pleasurable	Delays healing of ulcer
Enjoy smoking after meals	Feel short of breath on exercise
Makes me feel relaxed	Children don't like my smoking
Enjoy smoking when drinking beer	Smoking too much makes me feel bad
3. Concerns about quitting	4. Benefits of quitting
Difficulty in dealing with stress	Stops my breathing problem from getting worse
Weight gain	Family will be pleased
Withdrawal symptoms	
Resistance	Motivation

Once your patients have completed the decision balance, you can then go on to ask them to provide scores for their motivation and resistance.

Explaining and Obtaining Resistance and Motivation Scores
"The left-hand column represents your reasons to smoke [resistance to change]. The right-hand column represents your reasons to change [motivation to quit]. On a scale of 0–10, 0 meaning none and 10 meaning very high, what score would you give for your reasons to stay the same? [Pointing to the left column] And what score would you give for your reasons to change? Are your resistance and motivation scores based on what you think or feel about change? How would you score your resistance and motivation based on what you feel or think?"

Use a Decision Balance with Family Members

If family members accompany the patient, you can ask them to do a decision balance separately. Afterward, they can compare their perspectives. A family member's decision balance can help you understand how the patient and family members differ in their views about the benefits and concerns of smoking and why they are at different stages of change. When family members are in the action stage (with regard to the patient's smoking habit) and the patient is still in the contemplation stage, family members may nag the patient to change (or be perceived as nagging) and evoke patient resistance toward change.

Negative family influence, such as nagging behavior, is associated with lower smoking cessation rates.[1] The decision balance can help family members understand the patient's resistance and ambivalence about change but, more important, can help them to stop nagging the patient. Such behavior may cause the patient to regress to the stage of precontemplation; in other words, to stop thinking about quitting or even increase the number of cigarettes smoked per day to relieve this family-caused stress.

At the end of the encounter, you can give the decision balance back to the patient and family members. The patient can then add more to his or her decision balance, perhaps in discussion with another family member, as part of an assignment for the next appointment. This task is intended to help patients think more about their smoking and to clarify their ambivalence about change. This activity can provide additional information that can help you summarize the patient's ambivalence and/or highlight discrepancies between the patient's behavior and some aspect of the patient's self-interest.

Assess Motives, Competing Priorities, Energy and Self-efficacy

All these factors can influence a patient's motivation level.

Assess Motives
"Tell me what would make you decide to quit" (Let patient respond, and choose any of the following): *"Would you quit because family and friends want you to?"* *"Would you quit because you felt that you ought to change for your health or any other reason?"* *"Would you quit because it's important to you, or perhaps for a combination of reasons?"* *"Which is most important?"*

Assess Competing Priorities and Energy
"What competing priorities make it difficult for you to quit?"   *"On a scale of 0–10, how much energy are you willing to devote to quitting?"*   *"What is distracting you from putting more energy into quitting?"*
Assess Confidence and Ability (self-efficacy)
"On a scale of 0–10, how would you rate your confidence to quit smoking?"   *"On a scale of 0–10, how would you rate your ability to quit smoking?"*

Assess Supports and Barriers

If you can foster support, you can help maintain the patient's motivation.[2] Social influence can also enhance maintenance or reduce the prospects of relapse.[3] Another predictor of relapse following cessation among adults is the smoking habits of friends and family.[4]

Assess Supports
"What kind of help, if any, would help you quit?"   *"Who or what could help you quit?"*   *"Do you know of any community programs you can attend to help you quit?"*

You can also help patients identify external factors (barriers) that contribute to smoking relapse; for example, drinking alcohol, enjoying a cigarette at the end of the meal, participating in leisure activities with friends who smoke[5] and nagging family members. Sometimes the absence of negative interactions related to smoking may be more important than the presence of positive social support.[1]

Assess Barriers
"Are there smokers around you who would make it more difficult for you to quit?"   *"Do family members and friends nag you about your smoking?"*   *"What is hindering you from quitting?"*   *"What is making it difficult for you to quit?"*

DISEASE-CENTERED ASSESSMENT

The smoking history of the patient is an important, information-gathering component of the disease-focused assessment, in addition to identifying and assessing specific problems caused by smoking.

Smoking History
"How many cigarettes do you smoke a day?"   *"How long have you been smoking?"*   *"At what age did you start smoking?"*   *"Would you be prepared to keep a diary of your smoking to learn more about your habit?"*

Nicotine Addiction and Withdrawal Symptoms
"How soon after getting up do you have your first cigarette?" (Smoking within 30 minutes of waking is indicative of addiction.) *"What is the longest period of time during which you were able to stop smoking? Did you experience any withdrawal symptoms?"* *"When you stopped smoking, did it affect you in any way?"* *"Would you be prepared to fill out this questionnaire to assess whether you might benefit from nicotine replacement therapy?"*
Quit Attempts
"How many times have you been able to quit smoking? What did you learn from trying to give up smoking? What caused you to start smoking again?"

STEP 4: ENHANCING MUTUAL UNDERSTANDING

EDUCATE PATIENTS ABOUT TOBACCO USE

Practitioner-centered and patient-centered ways of providing health education about smoking risks and harm are described to highlight how you can deliver information to patients differently. The use of scare tactics to educate patients about the risks and harm of smoking has the potential to be counterproductive by evoking powerful defense mechanisms or resistance behaviors that avoid or minimize health concerns.[6;7] Self-confidence, not fear, has been linked to success in smoking cessation.[8]

Practitioner-centered Education

Traditionally, the practitioner-centered approach involves educating and advising patients about the consequences of smoking, and telling them to quit. These behavior change messages can be delivered in either a threatening or a nonthreatening manner, without really knowing whether the patient already knows the content of the message or even wants to hear more about it. High-threat communications may elicit statements of agreement from the patients but no change in their behavior. This controlling style of educating patients is a form of practitioner-centered education. When you convey such an informative message in a calm voice, that is autonomy-supportive education.

Practitioner-centered Education
"Most smokers—80%—know many of the harmful effects of smoking, but because they don't know all the harmful effects, they tend to underestimate the hazards of smoking.[9] Most people know that smoking causes lung cancer, but they may not know that smoking kills more patients through heart disease than do all cancers, including lung cancer, and that it is responsible for 89% of chronic bronchitis and emphysema."[10;11] Risks of smoking: *"Smoking is damaging your lungs without causing you any symptoms. It takes many years before you develop symptoms of lung disease."* (Let patient respond.) Harmful effects of smoking: *"Not only has smoking caused your breathing problem, but it will eventually make it much worse. It's just a question of time before you won't be able to walk one hundred yards before having to catch your breath."* (Let patient respond.)

Practitioner-centered Education
Provide educational booklets if patient would like them: *"Here are some pamphlets about quitting and using nicotine replacement treatments."*   Educate patients about nicotine withdrawal symptoms: *"When you stop smoking, it may cause a number of symptoms during the first couple of weeks. (Use all or select any of the following as examples): anxiety, inadequate sleep, irritability, impatience, difficulty concentrating, restlessness, craving for tobacco, hunger, gastrointestinal problems, headaches and/or drowsiness."*   Educate patients about nicotine replacement therapy: *"Nicotine treatment, such as gum, the patch or a nasal inhaler, reduces the withdrawal symptoms and the urge to smoke. This treatment prevents relapses, particularly during the first few weeks after quitting, but it alone will not cure you of your smoking habit. You will still crave cigarettes after you stop using this treatment. Successful quitting still depends on your willpower. Would you like more information about using this treatment to help you over the first four to eight weeks?"*

Patient-centered Education

Health education using the messages (described above) can become patient-centered if your patients seek specific information, and you tailor health information to meet their needs and deliver your message in a personally meaningful way.

Patient-centered Education about Risk and Harm
Risks of smoking: *"At the moment you are not noticing any problems caused by your smoking, but are you aware of the health problems caused by smoking?"* (Let patient respond, and then provide additional information that you think patient is most interested in hearing.) *"Unfortunately, smoking damages people's lungs long before they develop lung cancer and also puts them at an increased risk of developing heart disease, but again, without causing any symptoms. If you are concerned about any breathing problems, would you like me to do some simple tests [peak flow meter] to check up on this?"* (Let patient respond. With a negative answer, ask the patient why he or she is not interested in this suggestion; with a positive answer, proceed.)   Harmful effects of smoking: *"I'm concerned that your smoking has not only caused your breathing problem, but that it's making it much worse, as you know. What concerns do you have about how your shortness of breath will interfere with what it is important for you to do?"* (Let patient respond.)

Alternatively, you can initially focus on the beneficial aspects of smoking and then provide information that helps patients see the benefits less favorably. For example, smoking cigarettes has beneficial effects (pleasure, relaxation and stress reduction) that are not entirely due to the drug effects of nicotine.

Patient-centered Education about Nicotine
Educating patients about nicotine addiction: *"You said that you find smoking pleasurable. However, it's quite complicated to understand how nicotine affects you. Nicotine is a stimulant. When you first smoke a cigarette, it gives you a sense of alertness and also increases your heart rate. After this effect wears off, you get a relaxed feeling. But it's*

Patient-centered Education about Nicotine
important for you to realize that this relaxed feeling is not all due to nicotine. The tobacco companies advertise cigarette smoking as a relaxing activity. In fact, your belief that smoking is relaxing may be just as important as the effect of nicotine. In other words, you have a greater ability to relax than you realize, but the advertisers deceive you into thinking that it's all due to nicotine."
Smoking cigarettes deceives patients about its beneficial effects (relaxation and stress reduction): *"If you're physically addicted to nicotine, you will experience mild withdrawal symptoms, such as feeling stressed or tense, a few hours after not having a cigarette. Cigarette smoking is incredibly deceptive because it makes you think that smoking helps you feel relaxed and relieves your stress, but you're just treating your withdrawal symptoms without knowing it. Does this make sense to you?"* (For patients who need further explanation:) *"Let me see if I can explain it another way. Smoking cigarettes is like a vicious circle. Nicotine makes you first feel alert, but as this effect wears off, you feel relaxed. After a while, you get withdrawal symptoms and start to feel tense or stressed. So you smoke a cigarette to relieve those feelings. It can be difficult to know whether those tense feelings are due to the withdrawal symptoms or due to the stresses you are under. Nicotine teaches you that you need to smoke to cope with tension and stress, but these feelings may just be due to nicotine withdrawal."*
Nicotine addiction convinces some patients to believe that they have no willpower to quit: *"You say that you have no willpower to quit, but you may not understand your nicotine addiction. Nicotine addiction may be stronger than your willpower to quit, but that doesn't mean that you have no willpower. There are a number of ways to treat nicotine addiction—the gum and patch are available over the counter from drugstores. These treatments help you overcome your withdrawal syndrome, but the real test is whether you are willing to use these treatments and put your willpower to the test. I can also work with you to help you build up your willpower to quit for life, but it may take many attempts to do it. People who succeed don't quit trying to quit."*

USE NONDIRECT INTERVENTIONS TO LOWER RESISTANCE

You can use nondirect interventions to understand why patients do not want to quit and to help patients lower their resistance to quitting.

Nondirect Interventions to Lower Resistance
Use simple reflection: *"So, you're getting more shortness of breath when exercising."* Or *"So, your family is concerned about the effects of smoking on your breathing."*
Probe priorities to explore ambivalence: *"So, what do you like most about smoking? And what concerns you most about your smoking?" "What concerns you most about quitting?" "What do you think would be the most important benefit of quitting?"*
Use double-sided reflection to summarize ambivalence: *"On the one hand, you said that smoking helps you relax, but on the other hand, it's making you feel short of breath when you go for walks."*
Acknowledge ambivalence: *"You seem to have mixed feelings about your smoking; you smoke to relax, but your kids are concerned about your smoking."*
Emphasize personal responsibility and choice (useful when patients are being resistant): *"What you decide to do about smoking is entirely up to you, but I'll help you if you like."*

> **Explore the future**: *"So, what was your breathing like five years ago when you were smoking, compared to now? What do you think your breathing will be like in five years?"*

USE DIRECT INTERVENTIONS TO MOTIVATE CHANGE

Direct interventions help patients confront themselves, such that they change their perceptions and values about their smoking and their health. This process helps patients enhance their motivation to change.

Back-to-the-Future Questions

"How short of breath would you have to get before you would decide to quit smoking?" (Provided the patient shows some interest in prevention, continue.) *"Do you want to wait and see if this happens before you decide to quit?"* (If patient remains interested in prevention, continue:) *"What would really convince you to quit?"* (If patient is ambivalent, or not interested in prevention, ask:) *"Would you mind sharing with me why you don't want to quit?"*

Benefit Substitution

"What other ways do you use to help you relax, other than smoking?"
"Can you reward yourself in other ways rather than smoking a cigarette?"

Clarifying Values

Questions that probe values: *"So, what is more important in your life than smoking [or your health]?"*
Questions that contrast values: *"Smoking to relax is more important to you than your lungs and avoiding breathing problems."*
"The pleasure of smoking is worth more than the risk to your health."
Questions that contrast values and behavior: *"If you say that your lungs are more important than smoking to relax, you're saying one thing and doing another. What would convince you to do what you say?"*

Challenging Rationalizations

"Do you mind if I say a few things that might help you think about your smoking in different ways?" (With an affirmative response from the patient:) *"It may even feel a little uncomfortable, but I'm just trying to help you to improve your health and quality of life. If you want me to quit talking about it, just tell me."*
(Choose any of the following approaches.)
"Most young people don't think that they will become addicted to nicotine, but five years later, most of them regret that they ever started smoking. What do you think?" *"Many people believe that they won't die from smoking complications, and that protects them from really thinking about how they are damaging their own health."* (Be silent; if necessary, prompt with a follow-up comment or question.)
"Many people say that they have to die from something and don't want to think about it." (Be silent; if necessary, prompt with a follow-up comment or question.) *"You may or may not agree with that, but what about the quality of your life before you die?"*

Challenging Rationalizations
"Smoking helps you deal with your stress, but you're dealing with that stress much better than you think you are. Nicotine first acts as a stimulant, but as it wears off, it makes you feel relaxed and able to cope with stress better. What may be more important than this effect is your belief that smoking helps relieve your stress. Your mind may be more powerful than nicotine to help you cope with stress. When smokers stop and have a cigarette, they do a number of other things at the same time to cope with stress. They may take a time-out, sit down and maybe say to themselves, 'I deserve a cigarette to relax.' Everything you do at the same time as having a cigarette may be more powerful in relieving your stress than nicotine. What do you think about that?" (Pause, and let the patient respond.) *You're doing a much better job of coping with your stress than you think you are. The problem is that you're kidding yourself that only smoking is helping you relax (or cope with stress). What would it take for you to relax (or deal with this stress), but without kidding yourself that smoking is doing it?"*

Discrepancies
Identify discrepancies: *"You say that smoking helps you relax."* (Let the patient acknowledge your comments nonverbally.) *"But it makes your family worry about your health."* (Let the patient respond. Help the patient develop his or her own discrepancies:) *"You say that you exercise and smoke to relax. Do you see any inconsistency with how you're trying to relax?"*

Reframing Items, Issues or Events
Change a reason to smoke into a reason not to smoke: *"You enjoy smoking, but how does your cough feel in the morning?"* Enhance a reason to quit smoking: *"Your kids are concerned about your smoking. If you quit, they won't worry about your health. What's more, you'll be in a better position to help your kids when they become teenagers and are at risk of developing a smoking habit."* Diminish a reason to smoke: *"You enjoy smoking after meals, but that delays the healing of your ulcer."*

Challenging Claims or Positions
Use amplified reflection: *"So, you're not worried at all about the complications of smoking or dying? And you're not worried at all about how smoking affects the quality of your life before you die?" "So, you're not concerned at all that your children are worried about your smoking and health?"*

Differences in Motivational Reasons
"You take your tablets on a regular basis to control your hypertension [integrated motivation]. *You feel that you ought to lose weight* [introjected motivation] *but you only exercise when your wife goes with you* [extrinsic motivation]. *Nor do you seem interested in quitting* [indifferent motivation]. *What would it take for you to lose weight, exercise and quit smoking in the same way that you take care of yourself by taking your tablets regularly?"* (Let the patient respond.) *"In fact, you would do your health more good by quitting cigarettes than by taking your tablets regularly."*

Monitoring Changes in Resistance and Motivation Scores
"What scores would you now give for your resistance and motivation, using the scale of 0–10? "What *did you change your resistance score? And why did you change your motivation score?"* *"You can learn a lot about yourself even if your scores got worse and went in the wrong direction. Sometimes it helps if your resistance score goes up and your motivation score goes down, as it can teach you what it would take to change for good."*

CLARIFY DIFFERENCES IN PERCEPTION ABOUT PATIENT SELF-EFFICACY

Once you have reached this stage in assessing patient motivation, it is a good idea to assess your and your patient's perception of this motivation before moving on to implement a plan for change. This enables both you and your patient to be at the same stage of change.

Asking about Confidence and Ability (Self-efficacy)
"We've been working together, and I would like you to think about your score on a scale of 0– 10. How would you now rate your ability (and/or confidence) to quit smoking?" (Let patient respond. Address whether you agree with your patient's self-assessment or not.)

Clarifying Persistent Differences in Perceptions
"I think it's important for us to be clear about how we see the benefits, risks and harm of smoking—the same or differently—because that will affect how we work together. I think I understand what you like about smoking, but I seem more concerned about the risks and harms caused by your smoking than you are. What do you think?"

STEP 5: IMPLEMENTING A PLAN FOR CHANGE

This step requires working with your patients toward a plan for change, establishing realistic goals and working toward their implementation.

EVALUATE PATIENT COMMITMENT TOWARD A PLAN OF CHANGE

A number of factors can influence a patient's commitment to the change process.

Evaluating Commitment from the Perspective of Competing Priorities
"What is going on in your life that makes it difficult for you to quit now? Anything else? What would it take for you to put 'quit smoking' at the top of your list of things to do?"
Evaluating Commitment from the Perspective of Patient's Energy
"What is going on that makes it difficult for you to devote your energy to quitting?" *"What would it take for you to put your energy into quitting?"* *"If you don't have any energy to quit, what would it take for you to get your energy back?"*
Evaluating Commitment from the Perspective of Motivational Reasons
"What makes you commit yourself to quit. And what else?" "You say that you are here because your girlfriend wanted you to come. What would it take for you to come for your own reasons?"

DECIDE ON GOALS

The table below lists a range of goals for change that you can give your patients.

Range of Goals
• Think more about quitting. Use a decision balance to consider quitting.
• Prepare for change. Plan how to quit, learn about nicotine addiction and withdrawal, inform family and friends about plans to quit and use the decision balance to build willpower to change.
• Set a quit date.
• Additional options: Nicotine replacement therapy, referral to smoking cessation programs, referral to a counselor for associated problems such as relational conflicts.

Practitioners can selectively use nicotine replacement therapy to treat patients' withdrawal syndromes and thereby increase the smoking cessation rates. While nicotine replacement therapy is invaluable for treating patients' short-term physical addiction (one to two weeks), however, the one-year recidivism rate is high without the concurrent use of behavioral methods.[12-16]

Goal-setting

You can set up goals for change in one of three ways:

1. Practitioner-selected goals

In this scenario, the practitioner takes control of goal-setting, using one of the two following approaches:

An authoritarian, advice-giving monologue: *"You should quit smoking now before you further damage your lungs."*
An authoritative, advice-giving monologue: *"Smoking is damaging your lungs and making you more short of breath when you run. I recommend that you quit smoking, but that's up to you."*

2. Patient-selected goals

Most patients quit smoking without seeking professional help. They decide whether or not they are going to think about quitting and how long they are willing to stay in the different stages of change. You can act as a catalyst, however, to accelerate the pace of change.

An engaging monologue: *"You seemed concerned when we talked about your father developing emphysema that was made worse by his smoking. You're now concerned that you are repeating family history because you're getting more shortness of breath when you run. But you can change the course of family history if you choose to learn from your father. He was told too late to quit smoking because the tobacco companies didn't put warning labels on cigarette packages. What do you want to do about your smoking? Prefer not to think about it? Think about it some more? Prepare yourself to quit, or set a quit date?"*

3. Negotiated approach to goal setting

An engaging dialogue:

MP: *"I'm concerned because your father developed emphysema, and he quit smoking only one year before he died. And now, you're getting short of breath when you run. What do you think about your family history?"*

Patient: *"Well, my grandfather never gave up smoking, and he died from lung disease."*

MP, half-jokingly: *"I suppose you've thought about whether it was worth it for your father to quiting, since he died a year later. He could have enjoyed smoking for another year."*

Patient: *"That was what my brother said to my dad a week before he died. My dad had one cigarette just before he died. He was so exhausted that he inhaled it only once."*

MP: *"Even though it didn't benefit your father, perhaps he gave you a gift by quitting to help future generations. What can you learn from your father about changing family history?"*

Patient: *"I need to quit, but I'm not ready to now. I haven't recovered from my dad's death."*

MP in a low-key tone of voice: *"So, smoking will help you recover from this stress?"*

Patient: *"Yes . . . no, not really."*

MP: *"Are you willing to think more about quitting, or even to prepare for a quit date?"*

Patient: *"I think that I'll try to quit in six weeks, on my fiftieth birthday."*

WORK TOWARD SOLUTIONS[17]

You can use the MED-STAT acronym to help your patients implement a plan.

Interventions	Solution-based Approaches to Implementing a Plan
Miracle question (explore change)	*"Suppose a miracle happened and you quit smoking tomorrow. What would your life be like? How would your family and friends respond?"*
Exceptions (identify strengths)	*"What goes on when you smoke less compared to times when you smoke more than usual?"* Or, *"What's going on when you are stressed, but you don't smoke a cigarette?"*
Difference (use strengths)	*"What makes a difference when you smoke less rather than more? How can you apply your experiences when you don't smoke and you're stressed to those situations when you do smoke when you're stressed?"*
Scaling (assess motivation, self-efficacy and outcome expectancy)	*"On a scale of 0–10, how would you rate your [motivation, competence or confidence] to quit? How would you rate whether you can achieve your goal for change [outcome expectancy]? What would increase or decrease your scores? Can you make a list of those things? Was there a time when your scores were higher than now? What would it take to tip the balance in favor of higher scores?"*
Time-outs (consider alternatives)	*"What ideas do you have about how you could handle your stress differently other than smoking?"* (Check out silences.) *"A moment ago, I asked you a question and you were silent. What was going on?"*
Accolades (enhance efficacy)	*"You clearly have the skills to quit, but what would it take for you to keep using your skills?"*
Task appraisals (encourage action)	*"What would it take for you to think more about quitting, or to quit smoking sooner rather than later? When would be a good time to quit?"*

STEP 6: FOLLOWING

Once the patient has decided to think about quittii
continue to motivate him or her by following up
lapses or a relapse.

RATIONALE, PURPOSE AND REASONS FOR FOLL

You can encourage the patient to make fo
change.

Providing Rationale for Follow-up
"I think it's important for you to come back and discuss [choose one or more of the following:] *how your smoking is affecting your health, how to overcome nicotine addiction or how to deal with the complications from your smoking."* (And then decide whether to set up a follow-up appointment.)
Clarifying Patients' Reasons to Attend Follow-up
"Why is it important for you to attend a follow-up appointment? What do you think is the most important reason for you to attend a follow-up appointment? What health concerns do you want to address at your next appointment?"

ARRANGE FOLLOW-UP

Arranging Follow-up
"Would you like to come back for a follow-up appointment?"   *"How soon do you want to come back and check up on your health concern?"*   *"I think it's important for you to decide when to come back for a follow-up appointment. I will certainly share what I think about this, but I'm more interested in what you think."*

USE METHODS TO ENSURE CHANGE

Behavior modification may involve one of two divergent approaches: negative and positive reinforcement.[18] An aversive approach that is relatively effective involves the patient increasing the number of cigarettes smoked and the rate at which they are smoked.[19] Positive reinforcement that includes self-management procedures (monitoring urges, developing strategies for dealing with temptations and contracting) has limited success.[1;20-25] You can use a diary, relapse prevention strategies and motivational reevaluation approaches to ensure that patients maintain change.

A Diary to Track Thoughts, Feelings and Behavior over Time

A Diary for Tracking Change
"Are you interested in keeping a diary to understand your smoking habit better so that you can anticipate when you're likely to relapse after quitting? It would also help if you were to record your thoughts and feelings during situations when you feel tempted to smoke."

...n Approach

...ation of the relapse prevention approach is that patients who maintain ...pared with those who relapse have similar skills for coping with stresses; ...o relapse, however, do not use their coping skills at times of heightened ...ility.[3] In essence, patients relapse not because of a lack of skills but from a ...e to use their skills. Consequently, approaches to help patients develop relapse ...vention skills may be unwarranted if patients lack sustained motivation to use the skills they have. Studies that have examined relapse prevention strategies are, at best, only moderately encouraging.[1;26] Some strategies are listed below.

Relapse Prevention Approach
Management of risk situations: *"The physical urges to smoke are worse during the first two weeks of the withdrawal syndrome, but the psychological cravings for cigarettes can persist for months or years after smoking. In what situations are you likely to start smoking again? How about making a list of how to deal with those urges and cravings?"*
Pharmacological management: *"How do you think you will benefit from nicotine replacement therapy? Do you have any concerns about using nicotine replacement therapy?"*
Emotional management: *"When you feel stressed [or any other negative emotions], how do you think you can deal with those feelings other than by lighting up a cigarette?"*
Reevaluation of supports: *"Would it help to have someone help you quit?"*
Reevaluation of barriers: *"What do you think is making it difficult for you to quit? How do you think you're going to handle those difficulties?"*
Use of positive reinforcement: *"Would it be helpful you to set up a reward for quitting? What would that be?"*

Motivational Reevaluation

When patients have lapsed, relapsed or are struggling to maintain change, you can revisit their decision balance to reassess their think and feeling scores for their resistance and motivation.

Motivational Reevaluation
"Let's look again at your decision balance so you can tell me how your think and feeling scores for your resistance and motivation are changing. (Let patient respond.) What's making your resistance score go up and your motivation score go down? (Let patient respond.) What could help to make your scores better?"

YOUR SUMMARY

Reflect*: write a summary about what you have learned that was new for you.*

_____
_____
_____
_____
_____
_____
_____
_____
_____
_____
_____
_____
_____
_____
_____
_____
_____
_____
_____
_____
_____
_____
_____
_____

Enhance*: write down your ideas about how your new learning could improve your interactions with patients. Add your notes to your learning portfolio.*

_____
_____
_____
_____
_____
_____
_____
_____
_____
_____
_____
_____

REFERENCES

1. Antonuccio DO, Boutilier LR, Ward CH, et al. The behavioral treatment of cigarette smoking. Progress in Behavior Modification 1992;28: 119-181

2. Fisher EB, Jr., Haire-Joshu D, Morgan GD, et al. Smoking and smoking cessation. American Review of Respiratory Disease 1990;142: 702-720

3. Fisher EB, Jr., Rost K. Smoking cessation: A practical guide for the physician. Clinics in Chest Medicine 1986;7: 551-565

4. Fisher EB, Jr., Fondren DP. Undirected smoking cessation: A survey of successful quitters. Washington University; 1986

5. Shiffman S. A cluster-analytic classification of smoking relapse episodes. Addictive Behaviors 1986;11: 295-307

6. Job RFS. Effective and ineffective use of fear in health promotion campaigns. American Journal of Public Health 1988;78: 163-167

7. Orleans CT. Understanding and promoting smoking cessation: Overview and guidelines for physician intervention. Annual Review of Medicine 1985;36: 51-61

8. Condiotte MM, Lichtenstein E. Self-efficacy and relapse in smoking cessation programs. Journal of Consulting and Clinical Psychology 1981;49: 648-658

9. U.S. Department of Health & Human Services. Reducing the Health Consequences of Smoking: 25 Years of Progress: A Report of the Surgeon General (DHHS publication No. [CDC] 89-8411). Rockville, MD: U.S. Government Printing Office; 1989

10. U.S. Department of Health & Human Services. The health consequences of smoking: Chronic obstructive lung disease: A report of the Surgeon General (DHHS publication No. [PHS] 84-50205). Rockville, MD: U.S. Government Printing Office; 1984

11. U.S. Department of Health & Human Services. The health consequences of smoking: Cardiovascular disease: A report of the Surgeon General (DHHS Publication No. [PHS] 84-50204). Washington, DC: Office on Smoking and Health; 1984

12. Tonnesen P, Norregaard J, Simonsen K, et al. A double-blind trial of a 16-hour transdermal nicotine patch in smoking cessation. New England Journal of Medicine 1991;325: 311-315

13. Wong JG. How to help your patients quit smoking: Strategies that work. Postgraduate Medicine 1993;94: 197-201

14. Miller GH, Golish JA, Cox CE. A physician's guide to smoking cessation. Journal of Family Practice 1992;34: 759-760, 762-766

15. Benowitz NL, Jacob P, Savanapridi C. Determinants of nicotine intake while chewing nicotine polacrilex gum. Clinical Pharmacology & Therapeutics 1987;41: 467-473

16. Blum A. Nicotine chewing gum and the medicalization of smoking. Annals of Internal Medicine 1984;101: 121-123

17. Giorlando ME, Schilling RJ. On becoming a solution-focused physician: The MED-STAT acronym. Families, Systems & Health 1997;15: 361-373

18. Schwartz JL. Methods of smoking cessation. Medical Clinics of North America 1992;76: 451-476

19. Danaher BG. Research on rapid smoking: Interim summary and recommendations. Addictive Behaviors 1977;2

20. Glasgow RE. Smoking. In: Holroyd K, Creer T, eds. Self-management of chronic disease and handbook of clinical interventions and research. Orlando, FL: Academic Press; 1986: 99

21. Lichtenstein E, Brown RA. Current trends in the modification of cigarette dependence. In: Bellak AS, Hersen M, Kazdin AE, eds. International Handbook of Behavior Modification and Therapy. New York: Plenum Press; 1983: 575
22. Pechacek TF. Modification of smoking behavior. In: Krasnegor NA, ed. The behavioral aspects of smoking (NIDA Res Monogr 26) (DHEW publication No. 79-882). Bethesda, MD: U.S. Department of Health, Education and Welfare; 1979: 127
23. Schwartz JL. Smoking cures: Ways to kick an unhealthy habit. In: Jarvik ME, Cullen JW, Gritz ER, et al., eds. Research in smoking behavior (NIDA Research Monogr 17) (DHEW publication No. [ADM] 78-581). Bethesda, MD: U.S. Department of Health, Education and Welfare; 1977: 308-335
24. Schwartz JL. Review and evaluation of smoking cessation methods: The United States and Canada. [DHHS publication no. 87-2940]. Rockville, MD: National Cancer Institute, Department of Health and Human Services; 1987
25. Schwartz JL, Dubitzky M. Requisites for success in smoking withdrawal. In: Borgatta EF, Evans RR, eds. Smoking, health, & behavior. Chicago, IL: Aldine Publishing; 1968: 231-247
26. Curry SJ, McBride CM. Relapse prevention for smoking cessation: Review and evaluation of concepts and interventions. Annual Review of Public Health 1994;15: 345-366

CHAPTER 17

FACILITATING SELF-CARE OF DIABETES

FOR REFLECTION

How can you help patients adhere to multiple recommendations in order to
- *Lower hemoglobin A1c as much as possible?*
- *Reduce the rate of diabetic complications?*
- *Slow the deterioration rate of diabetic complications?*
- *Lessen the impact of complications when they occur?*

OVERVIEW

This chapter describes how you can develop individualized interventions to help patients take better care of their diabetes. You can negotiate with patients about whether and how to adhere to the diabetic guidelines and thereby work toward reducing Hb A1c levels, the complication rates and the impact of those complications.

Diabetes is used as a self-care example of a chronic disease because it involves multiple behavioral tasks: for example, exercising more, losing weight, keeping to a diabetic diet, and taking medications as prescribed. This chapter will not address current key facts and specific issues about the medical recommendation for this chronic disease because practitioners can access updated evidence-based guidelines online and adapt them for their purposes.

Diabetes is a good example of a chronic disease because the lifestyle ramifications (such as diet) has an impact beyond the individual and affects family members directly or indirectly. During the course of chronic diabetes, practitioners, patients and families have different perceptions and priorities about the need to address adherence and the goal of achieving normoglycemia. They often have different levels of investment in addressing these issues and are therefore at different stages in terms of their readiness to address any aspect of adherence to self-care of diabetes. When this occurs, practitioners, patients and families usually experience resistance in working together. To avoid this, they can collaborate in ways that help them begin to work through the stages of change together.

To work toward this goal, practitioners can use their agenda-setting skills to help patients and family members become more willing to discuss, think about and address the multiple issues related to self-care of diabetes. Practitioners also can conduct the agenda-setting phase in ways that help patients and families change their priorities so that patients become more activate in their self-care of diabetes.

In addition to practitioners, patients and families having different agendas and priorities in dealing with multiple issues, they often perceive the benefits of and concerns about nonadherence or adherence to a diabetic regimen differently. Patients often change their perceptions over time about preventive issues. For example, some patients are least motivated to adhere to their self-care regimen during the phase of primary prevention because they feel relatively well and rarely suffer any ill consequences from complications; they may become more motivated to change when early complications occur.

STEP 1: BUILDING PARTNERSHIPS

Communication Skills for Developing Empathy	
Use open-ended questions	*"Tell me how diabetes interferes with enjoying life."*
Use reflective listening	*"So, you enjoy eating doughnuts and . . ."*
Paraphrase	*"You know how to control your diabetes, but other things seem to have a higher priority than your diabetes."*
Validate feelings	*"So, sometimes you do feel a little guilty about eating doughnuts."*
Normalize behaviors	*"It's quite common for people not to keep to their diet all the time."*
Affirm strengths	*"But you take your medication regularly and watch your diet most of the time."*
Use probing questions	*"What would it take for you to keep more on top of your diabetes?"*

Relational Skills
Put the patient in the one-up position: *"What might convince you that you're at risk of developing diabetic complications?" "What might convince you to take better control of your diabetes?"*   *"You know what to do, but what do you think is stopping you from doing it?"*
Take the one-down position with a patient: *"I'm not sure what it would take to convince you about your risk of developing complications." "I'm not sure what would convince you to take better control of your diabetes."*

Clarifying Roles
Clarify your prevention role: *"Diabetes can damage your health even when you feel well and before you get any symptoms. Can I help to keep you from letting diabetes damage your health?"*
Clarify your motivational role: *"There's a lot you can do to stop diabetes from damaging your health, particularly when you're feeling so well. Can I help you so you can take better care of your diabetes?"*

Clarifying Responsibility
"I'll tell you what I know about the risk of developing diabetic complications (practitioner's responsibility), but we may still see the benefits and risks of good diabetic control differently. We can work together to understand our differences (a shared responsibility). I can help you increase your motivation to change [practitioner's responsibility], but it's up to you whether you can keep your hemoglobin A1c in the normal range [patient's responsibility]."

STEP 2: NEGOTIATING AN AGENDA

PREVENTION-FOCUSED APPROACH[a]

Consent-gaining, Direct Questions
"I'd like to check on whether there is anything you can do to improve your diabetes. Is that all right?" (Let patient respond. You can then ask some direct questions.) **Opened-ended questions:** *"There are several things we could discuss about diabetes. What would you like to talk about?"* (Ask one or more of the following questions.) *"How are you doing with the diet?"* *"What's it like for you to live with diabetes?"* *"What are you doing to control your blood glucose levels?"* *"How does your living with diabetes affect your family?"* **Or** *"I would like to talk about whether you're interested in doing anything more to deal with your diabetes. Is that all right?"* (Let patient respond. You can then ask,) *"Is there anything that you want to discuss?"*
Focused, open-ended questions: *"In what ways does your busy life cause difficulties in caring for your diabetes?"* *"How does your family help you deal with the care of your diabetes?"*
Closed-ended questions: *"Do you take your tablets?"* *"Do you keep to your diet?"* *"Do you check your blood glucose regularly?"*
Leading Questions
"I'd like to ask about the kinds of food you like to eat. Do you have a favorite food that you know you shouldn't eat?" *"What do you like to eat when you go out with friends?"* *"How often do you forget to take your tablets?"*
Prefacing Statements
"It is difficult to deal with all the diabetic recommendations. What do you find most difficult to deal with?"

PROBLEM-FOCUSED APPROACH

Prefacing Statements Followed by Leading Questions
"Your hemoglobin A1c is 11.8. What you do understand about that result?" *"Most patients find it difficult to remember to take their tablets every day, particularly when they feel well. How often do you forget to take your tablets?"* *"Most patients find it difficult to keep to the diabetic diet. What do you find most difficult or inconvenient about this diet?"* *"Many patients get fed up with checking their blood glucose levels. What do you find is most inconvenient about checking your sugar levels?"* **Normalizing and validating comments:** *"Patients find it difficult to keep to the diabetic diet and to lose weight. What do you find difficult about keeping to a diet and losing weight?"* **Preparing patients for nonpharmacological interventions (type 2 diabetes):** *"We need to talk about either adding another drug, using insulin injections or losing weight. Let me*

303

explain. If you lose weight, you might be able to lower your blood glucose to a point where you won't need to take another tablet or use insulin injections. Perhaps we can talk about your diet and weight reduction as a way to avoid adding another tablet or using insulin injections. " (Let patient respond.)

Comments that explore patients' concerns about consequences: *"Have you any concerns about having hypoglycemic episodes if we try to keep your blood glucose at normal levels?"*

Exploratory Questions

Open-ended, linear questions: *"How has your infection affected your blood glucose levels?"* *"How have your concerns about angina affected what you do in dealing with your diabetes?"*

Closed-ended, linear questions: *"Has the infection affected your appetite?"* *"Has your illness affected how often you check your blood sugar?"* *"Have your symptoms made you feel less inclined to keep on top of your diabetes?"* (Let patient respond.)

Circular questions: *"What concerns does your spouse have about how diabetes affects your health? What does your spouse think about how you're dealing with your diabetes?"*

STEP 3: ASSESSING RESISTANCE AND MOTIVATION

Readiness to Change
"Where are you in terms of dealing with [diabetic diet, weight reduction goals glucose monitoring, exercise]?" (You can select one of the following three questions, or sequence them according to your impression of the patient.) *"Are you not really thinking about changing?"* *"Are you thinking about it?"* *"Are you willing to make a change?"*

Providing Stage-specific Rationale and Gaining Consent to Use the Decision Balance
Precontemplation: *"You just told me that you're not thinking about changing your diet or losing weight. We could do a decision balance together because it could help both of us better understand why you want to continue as you are. Is that okay?"*
Contemplation: *"You told me how much you struggle with trying to keep to your diet and lose weight. We could do a decision balance together because it could help you think more seriously about change."*
Preparation: *"You're seriously thinking about keeping to your diet better and losing weight. We could do a decision balance together because it could help motivate you to set a date to change."*
Action: *"You seem ready to set a date to change. We could do a decision balance together because it could help prevent you relapsing to your old ways."*

Showing the Decision Balance to the Patient
"Let me show you what a decision balance looks like. As we use the decision balance, it can help you better understand your reasons to stay the same and your reasons to lose weight and go on a diet. But first [pointing to the top middle column], *I would like you to list as many benefits as possible from eating what you like. I would like to make a note of what you say. Is that okay? You can keep this decision balance to use when you go home if you like."* (You can ask one or more of the following questions from each quadrant.)

Reasons to Stay the Same	Reasons to Change
1. Benefits of eating anything *"What are the benefits of eating what you want, as opposed to sticking to the diabetic diet? Does eating food benefit you in other ways; for example, to relax or relieve stress?"* (Let patient respond.) *"And what else?"*	**2. Concerns about eating anything** *"What concerns you about eating what you want?"* (Pause and let patient respond.) *"How might diabetic complications interfere with any other parts of your life?"* (Pause and let patient respond.) *"What, if anything, concerns you about not having a normal Hb A1c?"*
3. Concerns about dieting and weight loss *"What concerns you about keeping to the diabetic diet?"* *"What, if anything, concerns you about losing weight?"* *"Do you have any concerns about achieving good diabetic control or about hypoglycemic episodes?"*	**4. Benefits about dieting and weight loss** *"Tell me what you understand about the benefits of achieving good diabetic control."* *"How would your family respond if you were to lower your Hb A1c?"*

Reasons to Stay the Same (Cons)	Reasons to Change (Pros)
1. Benefits of nonadherence[b] Less work for spouse preparing family meals Less work in checking glucose levels Relieve stress by eating candy	2. Concerns about nonadherence Family nags me to look after myself better Risk of hospitalizations Eye, kidney and feet complications
3. Concerns about adherence Extra costs Hypoglycemic episodes Interferes with work	4. Benefits of adherence Improve health Live longer Keep my heart in good shape
Resistance	**Motivation**

Explaining and Obtaining Resistance and Motivation Scores
"The left-hand column represents your reasons to stay the same [resistance to change]. The right-hand column represents your reasons to change [motivation to change]. On a scale of 0–10, 0 meaning none and 10 meaning very high, what score would you give for your reasons to stay the same? [Pointing to the left column.] And what score would you give for your reasons to change? Are your resistance and motivation scores based on what you think or feel about change? Now, how would you score your resistance and motivation based on what you feel or think?
Assessing Motives
"What would persuade you to take better care of your diabetes [or try to lower your Hb A1c, or any other specific aspect of self-care of diabetes]?" (Let patient respond; if necessary, prompt the patient.) *"Would you do it because family and friends wanted you to? Would you do it because you felt that you ought to take better care of your diabetes for your health or any other reason? Would you do it because it is important to you? Or perhaps for a combination of reasons? Which is most important?"*
Assessing Competing Priorities and Energy
"What competing priorities do you face in taking care of your diabetes?" *"On a scale of 0–10, how much energy can you put into taking better care of your diabetes?"*
Assessing Confidence and Ability (self-efficacy)
"On a scale of 0–10, how would you rate your confidence to keep your hemoglobin A1c within normal range [or deal with any other aspect of diabetic self-care]?" *"On a scale of 0–10, how would you rate your ability to keep your hemoglobin A1c within normal range [or deal with any other aspect of diabetic self-care]?"*
Assessing Supports
"Would you like others to help you with your diabetes? Who or what could help your diabetes? Do you know of any community programs you can attend to help your diabetes?"
Assessing Barriers
"Do you have difficulties in getting the care that you need?" *"Do you have money problems that make it difficult for you look after your diabetes?"* *"Are there people around you who make it more difficult for you to deal with your diabetes?"*

STEP 4: ENHANCING MUTUAL UNDERSTANDING

EDUCATE PATIENTS ABOUT HEALTH BEHAVIOR CHANGE

Practitioner-centered Education

Authoritarian advice-giving (limited applications): State in a firm tone of voice: *"I think you should lose weight, keep to the diabetic diet, check your blood glucose regularly and keep your blood glucose levels normal with your insulin regimen so that you can reduce your risk of going blind and developing kidney failure."*
 Authoritative advice-giving: *"Checking your blood sugar at home helps you know if your levels are normal, but the Hb A1c is the best way to know whether you're keeping good control of your diabetes. If you keep your Hb A1c at normal levels, you can reduce your chance of*
 • *Eye damage [retinopathy] by 76%*
 • *Progression of eye damage [retinopathy] by 54%*
   [proliferative or severe nonproliferative retinopathy by 47%];
 • *Protein in your urine*
   [microalbuminuria: > 40 mg per 24 hours by 39% and > 300 micrograms per 24 hours by 54%]
 • *Nerve damage [neuropathy[by 60%*
 But tight control of your blood glucose [intensive insulin therapy] may cause a two- to threefold increase in severe hypoglycemia."

Patient-centered Education about Risk and Harm
Risk of diabetic complications: *"At the moment, you are not noticing any problems with your diabetes, but are you aware of the problems?"* (Let patient respond, and then provide additional information that you think the patient is most interested in hearing.) *"Unfortunately, it can damage your [eyes, kidneys, feet, nerves and heart] without your being aware of it until it causes symptoms years later. The way to reduce your risk of complications is to check your Hb A1c on a regular basis. Are you willing to have this blood test every three months or so?"*   Complications of diabetes: *"What concerns do you have about your health?"* (Let patient respond.) *"I'm concerned that your diabetes is causing eye damage [or any other complication needing specialist care] and that it will progress unless you see the eye doctor."*

Family-centered Education
Family-centered advice-giving: *"You and your family both know that high sugar levels put you at risk for complications and increase your risk of dying. You seem to be willing to accept the fact you may die from diabetic complications."* (Pause and let patient respond. Assuming an affirmative response, continue.) *"But your family doesn't seem ready for you to die, and they want to help reduce your risk of complications. How about you and your family working together to avoid diabetic complications so that you can maintain your quality of life before you die?"*

USE NONDIRECT INTERVENTIONS TO LOWER PATIENT RESISTANCE

Use simple reflection to elicit ambivalence: *"Keeping to the diet [losing weight or checking your blood glucose] regularly is difficult. You feel well even when your blood glucose is high."*
Probe priorities to explore ambivalence: *"In what ways is your life easier by not keeping your diabetes under tight control?"* *"This may seem an unusual request, but take a moment to think about the most important benefit of not sticking strictly to the diabetic recommendations."* (Pause for silence; if necessary, ask) *"What is it?"* *"What concerns you most about not keeping your hemoglobin A1c within normal range?"* *"What would concern you most if you tried harder to control your weight, blood glucose and/or diabetes? What are the most important benefits of controlling your diabetes?"*
Use double-sided reflection to summarize ambivalence: *"On the one hand, if you achieve normal glucose levels, you will reduce your risk of complications, but on the other hand, you are more likely to have hypoglycemic attacks."*
Acknowledge ambivalence: *"People often have mixed feelings about not keeping strictly to the diabetic diet." "People often have mixed feelings about not following the recommendations."*
Emphasize personal responsibility and choice (useful when patients are being resistant): *"Whether you decide to try and keep your hemoglobin A1c within the normal range is up to you, but I'm willing to help you prevent diabetic complications."*
Explore the future questioning: *"What was your diabetes like a few years ago, what is it like now and what do you think it will be like in five to ten years?"*

USE DIRECT INTERVENTIONS TO MOTIVATE PATIENT CHANGE

Back-to-the-future Questioning
"If you developed a diabetic complication now, would you try to keep your diabetes in better control in the future?" (Provided that the patient shows some interest in prevention, continue.) *"Do you want to wait and see if you develop a complication before deciding to change?"* (If the patient remains interested in prevention, continue.) *"What would it take for you to decide to take better control of your diabetes?"* (If the patient is ambivalent or not interested in prevention, ask:) *"Can you share with me what is difficult about changing?"*
Benefit Substitution
"Are there ways for you to enjoy your food but at the same time stay within the dietary recommendations or simply reduce the amount that you eat? For example, when you overeat on some occasions, can you check your glucose levels before such an occasion and give yourself some extra regular insulin?"

Clarifying Values
Questions that probe values: *"What is more important in your life than trying to prevent the complications of diabetes?"*   **Questions that contrast values:** *"Is eating regular meals with your family more important to you than trying to avoid the long-term complications of diabetes?"*   *"Is being a parent and spouse more important to you than trying to avoid the long-term complications of diabetes?"*   **Questions that contrast values and behavior:** *"If you say that your health is more important than eating regular meals with your family, you're saying one thing and doing another. What would convince you to do what you say?"*
Challenging Rationalizations
"May I propose a few things that might help you think about your diabetes differently?" (With an affirmative response from the patient, continue.) *"It may make you pause and think about how much effort you want to put into preventing complications. You don't have to say anything if you don't feel like it, and if you want me to stop talking about diabetes, just tell me."*   (Choose any of the following questions and, if necessary, prompt with a follow-up comment.) *"Some diabetics don't think that they will ever get any complications, but later regret that they didn't take better care of themselves."*   *"Diabetes is deceptive. It makes you think that you don't have a disease because you can feel so well. But, by the time you develop symptoms, the damage is often done and difficult to reverse."*   *"Many people say that they have to die sometime from something, so they live as they please for now and don't have any concerns about dying or the quality of their life before they die."*   *"Your blood glucose levels are good when you check them at home, but your Hb A1c is still high."*   (These statements help patients to reexamine their rationalizations for not changing.)
Discrepancies
Identify discrepancies between a behavior and self-interest: *"You say that you want to stay well, but your increased level of Hb A1c is putting you at risk of diabetic complications."*   **Identify differences in motivational reasons:** *"What would it take for you to care for yourself in terms of taking the tablets and sticking to the diet in the same way that you look after your feet?"*
Reframing Items, Issues or Events
Change a reason not to adhere into a reason to adhere: *"Although you can have high blood glucose levels and feel well, it still puts you at high risk for developing complications."*   **Enhance a reason to adhere to diabetic recommendations:** *"Your spouse nags you about not sticking to your diet, but could this show how much he or she is really concerned about your health?"*   **Diminish a reason not to adhere:** *"You say that you enjoy eating out with your friends, but can you enjoy your friends and also stick to your diet?"*

Amplified Reflection
"So, you're not worried at all about diabetic complications?" *"So, you believe that you are in some way specially protected from the complications of diabetes."*
Differences in Motivational Reasons
"You put so much effort into taking great care of your family, but what would it take for you to put more effort into taking care of your diabetes?" *"You regularly check your feet because you don't want to have any more ulcers* [integrated motivation]. *You feel that you ought to take medication* [introjected motivation]. *You check your blood glucose levels when your spouse prompts you to* [extrinsic motivation], *but you don't seem at all concerned about sticking to your diet* [indifferent motivation]. *What would it take for you to lower your Hb A1c as much as possible in the same way that you look after your feet?"*
Monitoring Changes in Resistance and Motivation Scores
"What scores would you now give for your resistance and motivation, using the scale of 0–10?" "Why did you change your resistance score? And why did you change your motivation score?" "You can learn a lot about yourself even if your scores got worse and went in the wrong direction. Sometimes it helps if your resistance score goes up and your motivation score goes down, because this can teach you what it would take to change for good."

CLARIFY DIFFERENCES IN PERCEPTION ABOUT PATIENT SELF-EFFICACY

Confidence and Ability (self-efficacy)
"On a scale of 0–10, how would you now rate your ability to lower your Hb A1c [or any other self-care task for diabetes]? And how would your rate your confidence to lower your Hb A1c to below 7?" (Let patient respond; address whether you agree with your patient's self-assessment.)

STEP 5: IMPLEMENTING A PLAN FOR CHANGE

Clarifying Persistent Differences in Perceptions
"I think it's important for us to be clear about whether we see the benefits, risks and harm the same way or differently, because that will affect how we work together. I understand what you like about eating whatever you want, but I seem to be more concerned about the risks and harm caused by your poor diabetic control than you are. What do you think?"

EVALUATE PATIENT COMMITMENT TOWARD A PLAN OF CHANGE

Competing Priorities
"What is going on in your life that makes it difficult for you to take better care of your diabetes? And anything else?"
"What would it take for you to put good diabetic care at the top of your list of things to do?"
Or *"What is stopping you from putting good diabetic care at the top of your list of things to do?"*

Energy
"What is going on that makes it difficult for you to devote your energy to taking better care of your diabetes?"
"What would it take for you to put your energy into taking better care of your diabetes?"
"If you don't have any energy to change, what would it take for you to get your energy back?"

Motives
"What makes you commit yourself to this change? And what else?"
"You say that you're here because your spouse wanted you to come, but what would it take for you to come for your own reasons?"

DECIDE ABOUT GOALS FOR CHANGE

Range of Goals for Improving Self-care of Diabetes

Think about change
    Think more about what it would take to achieve normal Hb A1c
    Use a decision balance to address any behavior change issues
Prepare for change
    Plan how to take better care of diabetes
    Learn about managing diabetic complications
    Involve family and friends in plans to change
Take action
    Set a change date to change behavior or address any diabetic issues
Additional goals
    Referral to specialists
    Referral to community resources

WORK TOWARD SOLUTIONS (INCORPORATING MED-STAT)[1]

Interventions	Solution-based Language for Behavior Change[1]
Miracle question (explore change)	*"Suppose a miracle happened, and you lost 15-20 pounds in a year so that you could stop taking diabetic tablets. What would your life be like then? How would you and your family respond?"*
Exceptions (identify strengths)	*"How did you stop yourself from overeating on an occasion when you felt depressed?"*
Differences (use strengths)	*"How does this occasion compare to other situations when you felt depressed and overate?"*
Scaling (assess motivation, self-efficacy and outcome expectancy)	*"On a scale of 0–10, how would you score your [motivation, competence and confidence] to keep to a diabetic recommendation [lose weight, keep to a diet, maintain weight loss and/or normalize your Hb A1c]?"* *"How would you rate whether you can achieve your goal for change [outcome expectancy]?"* *"Was there a time when your scores were higher than now? What would increase your scores? Can you make a list of that? What would it take to tip the balance in favor of higher scores?"*
Time-outs (consider alternatives)	*"What other ideas do you have about how you could handle depression and diabetes better? What would it take for you to put those ideas into practice?"*
Accolades (enhance efficacy)	*"You managed to keep your Hb A1c below 9 most of the time, but how could you build on what you are doing right to do better still?"*
Task appraisals (encourage action)	*"What would it take for you to keep your Hb A1c as low as possible?"*

STEP 6: FOLLOWING THROUGH

ARRANGING FOLLOW-UP

Providing Rationale and Purpose for Follow-up
"I think a follow-up would be important in order for us to [choose one or more of the following]: 　　*Check up on your Hb A1c* 　　*Monitor for complications* 　　*Provide care for the complications."* (and then make a follow-up appointment.)
Clarifying Patients' Reasons to Attend Follow-up
"What do you understand as your reasons for your attending a follow-up appointment? What is important for you to address at the next appointment?"
Timing, Duration and Frequency of Follow-up Appointments
"How often do you think you should come back to see me?" *"I think it's important for you to decide when to come back for a follow-up appointment. I will certainly share what I think about this, but I'm more interested in what* you *think."*

USE METHODS TO ENSURE CHANGE AND PREVENT RELAPSE

A diary to track change:
"Are you interested in keeping a diary to understand your diabetes better so that you can anticipate when you are likely to relapse from good diabetic control? It would also help if you were to record your thoughts and feelings during situations when you feel tempted to relapse."
Relapse prevention
Management of risk situations: *"Which kind of situations will make it difficult for you to keep to your goals for good diabetic control? What ways can you deal with those difficulties?"* Pharmacological management: *"What difficulties do you have in taking your tablets on a regular basis? Do you feel that you know how to alter your insulin dose according to blood glucose readings and meal sizes?"*
Emotional management: *"When you feel upset [or any other negative emotions], how do you deal with those feelings instead of eating?"* Reevaluation of supports: *"Would it help to have someone help you work toward your goal of change?"*
Reevaluation of barriers: *"What do you think is making it difficult for you to maintain your goal for change? How do you think you're going to handle those situations?"*
Use of positive reinforcement: *"Would rewards help you keep to your goals for change? What would those be?"*
Motivational reevaluation: *"Let's look again at your motivational balance and talk about whether you still think your reasons to change are really more important than your reasons to stay the same. This may help you stick to the diabetic recommendations when you have difficulties in keeping to them."*

313

YOUR SUMMARY

Reflect: *write a summary about what you have learned that was new for you.*

_____
_____
_____
_____
_____
_____
_____
_____
_____
_____
_____
_____
_____
_____
_____
_____
_____
_____
_____
_____
_____
_____
_____
_____
_____
_____

Enhance*: write down your ideas about how your new learning could improve your interactions with patients. Add your notes to your learning portfolio.*

_____
_____
_____
_____
_____
_____
_____
_____
_____
_____
_____
_____
_____

REFERENCES

1. Giorlando ME, Schilling RJ. On becoming a solution-focused physician: The MED-STAT acronym. Families, Systems & Health 1997;15: 361-373

AFTERWORD

Patients with unhealthy habits often feel like that they are trapped in a locked room without a key to the door. Your dialogue with patients can help them cut a key to open the door. Yet, many patients may still get stuck at the door's threshold. Your ongoing dialogue can also help them cross the threshold to escape from their unhealthy habits. This art of dialogue is a lifelong learning process, a journey of professional enrichment without end.

The six-step approach provides you with ways of initiating dialogues with patients in new ways. The motivational principles (listed in Chapter 1) provide you with guidance with your ongoing dialogues with patients. As you develop new skills, you will encounter awkward moments and impasses in working with your patients. To help you handle such situations, you can use any of the following bail-out strategies.

BAIL-OUT STRATEGIES

The bail-out strategies (described below) can help you learn how to overcome impasses and awkward moments that are bound to happen when developing new skills. You take a risk whenever you use a new skill with a patient. If you feel particularly uncomfortable about using a technique, try to understand why you feel reluctant about using it, and identify a specific bail-out strategy that you can use in the event that the technique does not work for you.

1. Check whether an intervention is working.

When using new interventions, you may have difficulty knowing what effect they have on a patient. Sometimes, you will be surprised. Check it out with your patients, because you may find you are doing a better job than you thought.

> *Suggested language: "I just tried a new approach for helping people think about change. I'd like to know whether or not you found it helpful. What do you think?"*

2. Clarify the source of awkwardness.

When practicing using any new skill, you may initially feel awkward because it does not fit in with your normal pattern of interacting with patients. Patients may sense your awkwardness but still feel that the interaction itself was effective. Sometimes awkwardness arises from the practitioner-patient interaction itself; at other times, you yourself may not feel awkward using a new skill but may still make the patient feel awkward. You may even find it difficult to know where the sense or feeling of awkwardness is coming from. Addressing and clarifying the source of your awkward or uncomfortable feelings can help you better understand the challenge of change for the patient as well as for yourself.

> *Suggested language: "I felt awkward when I said_____. Did it affect you in any way?"*
> *"When I said_____, it felt awkward between us. How did it feel to you?"*
> *"When I said_____, I felt that it made you feel awkward.* [Let patient respond and, if prompting is necessary, proceed further.] *Can you help me understand that?"*

Remember that these options are to create opportunities for you and your patients to learn from your interactions in ways that will facilitate change.

3. Comment on the process.

You can comment on the process of what is happening or not happening in the interaction, rather than pushing to work on what you think the patient needs to address.

> *Suggested language: "I sense that we're not working on the same wavelength."*
> *"I sense that we're working at cross purposes."*
> *"I get the sense that you don't think that I'm trying to work on your side."*
> *"A moment ago, I tried to help you increase your motivation to change, but it isn't clear to me whether or not you want me to help you."*

4. Take a timeout.

On rare occasions when none of these bail-out strategies seem to work for you, you can tell patients that you need to take a timeout.

> *Suggested language: "I get a sense that what we're trying to do is just not working. I'm wondering whether we should drop this for now so that we can think more about it and come back to it later. What do you think?"*

5. Consult others.

When you get stuck, reach an impasse, or are uncertain about what to do about a health care issue, you can consult your colleagues or encourage patients to consult family members and friends. This strategy sends your patient the message that more time and attenton is needed to address the issue.

> *Suggested language: "I'm not quite sure how to proceed from this point. I think it's very important that we address this issue more, but I would like to speak to a colleague first to think through how you and I can work together more effectively."*
> *"I think this issue is particularly important for you, but I think it might be worthwhile for you to talk to your family members and friends to find out what they think about this issue. Afterward, we can get back together and talk about it more."*

APPENDIX 1
Worksheet for Enhancing Your Partnership-Building Skills

After reading Chapter 9 (Parts A-C) and/or the relevant sections in Chapters 15-17, use the 0-10 scale to rate your level of competence (C-score).

0	1	2	3	4	5	6	7	8	9	10
None					Moderate					Very High

How would you rate your C-score?	After reading the chapter	After a practice session
Develop empathic skills		
a. Use open-ended questions		
b. Use reflective listening		
c. Paraphrase		
d. Validate feelings		
e. Normalize behaviors		
f. Affirm strengths		
g. Use probing questions		
Use relational skills		
a. Put patient in the one-up position		
b. Take the one-down position		
Clarify roles and responsibilities		

After doing the practice session, write down your reasons for the change in your scores.

APPENDIX 2
Worksheet for Enhancing Your Agenda-Setting Skills

After reading Chapter 10 and/or the relevant sections in Chapters 15-17, use the 0-10 scale to rate your level of competence (C-score).

0	1	2	3	4	5	6	7	8	9	10
None					Moderate					Very High

How would you rate your C-score?	After reading the chapter	After a practice session
Prevention-focused approach a. Consent-gaining, direct questions		
b. Leading questions		
c. Prefacing statements		
Problem-focused approach a. Prefacing statements		
b. Exploratory questions		
c. Leading questions		

After doing the practice session, write down your reasons for the change in your scores.

APPENDIX 3
Worksheet for Enhancing Your Skills at Assessing Resistance And Motivation

After reading Chapter 11 and/or the relevant sections in Chapters 15-17, use the 0-10 scale to rate your level of competence (C-score).

0	1	2	3	4	5	6	7	8	9	10
None					*Moderate*					*Very High*

How would you rate your C-score?	After reading the chapter	After a practice session
Ask about readiness to change		
Provide a stage-specific rationale for using the decision balance		
Use a decision balance with a patient		
Explain "think" and "feeling" score for resistance and motivation		
Assess motives for change		
Assess competing priorities and energy		
Assess confidence and ability to change		
Assess supports and barriers		

After doing the practice session, write down your reasons for the change in your scores.

APPENDIX 4
Worksheet for Enhancing Your Skills in Developing Mutual Understanding
After reading Chapter 12 and/or the relevant sections in Chapters 15-17, use the 0-10 scale to rate your level of competence (C-score).

0	1	2	3	4	5	6	7	8	9	10
None					Moderate					Very High

How would you rate your C-score?	After reading the chapter	After a practice session
Educate about the need for behavior change in patient-centered way		
Use nondirect interventions		
a. Probe priorities		
b. Use double-sided reflection		
c. Explore the future		
d. Acknowledge ambivalence		
e. Emphasize personal responsibility/choice		
f. Use simple reflection		
Use direct interventions		
a. Use back-to-the future questioning		
b. Use benefit substitution		
c. Clarify values		
d. Challenge rationalizations		
e. Use discrepancies		
f. Reframe items, issues or events		
g. Challenge claims or positions		
h. Use differences in motivational reasons		
Clarify differences in perceptions about confidence and ability		

After doing the practice session, write down your reasons for the change in your scores

APPENDIX 5
Worksheet for Enhancing Your Skills at Implementing a Plan
After reading Chapter 13 and/or the relevant sections in Chapters 15-17,
use the 0-10 scale to rate your level of competence (C-score).

0	1	2	3	4	5	6	7	8	9	10
None					Moderate					Very High

How would you rate your C-score?	After reading the chapter	After a practice session
Evaluate patient commitment (competing priorities, energy and motives)		
Decide about goals		
b. Patient-selected goals		
c. Negotiated approach to goal setting		
Set a goal for change		
b. Prepare for a change		
c. Set a quit date		
d. Additional options		
Clarify persistent differences in perceptions		
Use solution-based approaches		

After doing the practice session, write down your reasons for the change in your scores.

APPENDIX 6
Worksheet for Enhancing Your Skills at Following Through

After reading Chapter 14 and/or the relevant sections in Chapters 15-17, use the 0-10 scale to rate your level of competence (C-score).

0	1	2	3	4	5	6	7	8	9	10
None					*Moderate*					*Very High*

How would you rate your C-score?	After reading the chapter	After a practice session
Provide rationale for follow-up		
Clarify patient's reason for follow-up		
Arrange follow-up		
Use methods to ensure change		
a. A diary to track change		
b. Relapse prevention approach		
Management of risk situations		
Pharmacological management		
Emotional management		
Reevaluation of supports		
Reevaluation of barriers		
Use of positive reinforcement		
c. Motivational reevaluation		

After doing the practice session, write down your reasons for the change in your scores.

Printed in the United Kingdom
 by Lightning Source UK Ltd.
112999UKS00001B/3